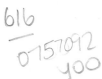

616
0757092
400
2010

Chest Radiographic Interpretation in Pediatric Cardiac Patients

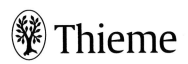

Chest Radiographic Interpretation in Pediatric Cardiac Patients

Shi-Joon Yoo, MD, PhD, FRCPC
Section Head of Cardiac Imaging
Department of Diagnostic Imaging
Hospital for Sick Children
Professor
Departments of Medical Imaging and Paediatrics
University of Toronto
Toronto, Canada

Cathy MacDonald, MD, FRCPC
Radiologist
Department of Diagnostic Imaging
Hospital for Sick Children
Assistant Professor
Department of Medical Imaging
University of Toronto
Toronto, Canada

Paul Babyn, MD, FRCPC
Radiologist-in-Chief
Department of Diagnostic Imaging
Hospital for Sick Children
Associate Professor
Department of Medical Imaging
University of Toronto
Toronto, Canada

Thieme
New York • Stuttgart

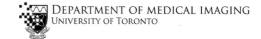
DEPARTMENT OF MEDICAL IMAGING
UNIVERSITY OF TORONTO

Thieme Medical Publishers, Inc.
333 Seventh Ave.
New York, NY 10001
Editorial Director: Michael Wachinger
Managing Editor: Timothy Y. Hiscock
Editorial Assistant: Jacquelyn DeSanti
International Production Director: Andreas Schabert
Production Editor: Kenneth L. Chumbley, Publication Services
Vice President, International Marketing and Sales: Cornelia Schulze
Chief Financial Officer: James W. Mitos
President: Brian D. Scanlan
Compositor: Thomson Digital
Printer: Sheridan Books, Inc.

Library of Congress Cataloging-in-Publication Data

Chest radiographic interpretation in pediatric cardiac patients / [edited by] Shi-Joon Yoo, Cathy MacDonald, Paul Babyn.
    p. ; cm.
  Includes bibliographical references.
  ISBN 978-1-60406-036-2 (alk. paper)
  1. Pediatric cardiology—Diagnosis. 2. Pediatric radiography. I. Yoo, Shi-Joon. II. MacDonald, Cathy, MD. III. Babyn, Paul S.
  [DNLM: 1. Heart Diseases—radiography. 2. Child. 3. Infant. 4. Radiography, Thoracic. WS 290 C525 2010]
  RJ423.C44 2010
  618.92′1207572—dc22
                                            2009043190

Important note: Medical knowledge is ever-changing. As new research and clinical experience broaden our knowledge, changes in treatment and drug therapy may be required. The authors and editors of the material herein have consulted sources believed to be reliable in their efforts to provide information that is complete and in accord with the standards accepted at the time of publication. However, in view of the possibility of human error by the authors, editors, or publisher of the work herein or changes in medical knowledge, neither the authors, editors, nor publisher, nor any other party who has been involved in the preparation of this work, warrants that the information contained herein is in every respect accurate or complete, and they are not responsible for any errors or omissions or for the results obtained from use of such information. Readers are encouraged to confirm the information contained herein with other sources. For example, readers are advised to check the product information sheet included in the package of each drug they plan to administer to be certain that the information contained in this publication is accurate and that changes have not been made in the recommended dose or in the contraindications for administration. This recommendation is of particular importance in connection with new or infrequently used drugs.

Some of the product names, patents, and registered designs referred to in this book are in fact registered trademarks or proprietary names even though specific reference to this fact is not always made in the text. Therefore, the appearance of a name without designation as proprietary is not to be construed as a representation by the publisher that it is in the public domain.

Printed in the United States of America

5 4 3 2 1

ISBN 978-1-60406-036-2

Contents

Foreword

Appropriate management of children with cardiovascular disease in the 21st century relies heavily on an armamentarium of sophisticated imaging techniques, such as echocardiography, computed tomography, magnetic resonance imaging (including functional techniques), angiography, and interventional procedures guided by angiography. No modern hospital can provide appropriate care for the child with cardiovascular disease without the availability of this full range of modalities.

Plain radiographs of the chest are still used in these children at the time of their initial presentation and during follow-up of medical management and after corrective surgical or interventional procedures. Although the plain radiograph does not provide the definitive anatomic and functional information depicted by the more sophisticated modalities, it serves as an initial part of the evaluation at the time of the diagnosis and is essential (usually repeatedly) following surgical correction. Accurate interpretation of the plain radiograph of the chest therefore remains vitally important. However, in recent decades there has been tremendous interest in the newer, more exciting, sophisticated modalities, and more time has been spent learning how to derive maximum information from these modalities. In this era, learning to optimize the interpretation of plain radiographic findings often assumes a less important role.

This book, authored by Drs. Yoo, MacDonald, and Babyn, highlights the plain radiographic interpretation in cardiovascular abnormalities manifesting in neonates, infants, and children. The information is presented in an organized and interesting manner. The quality of the illustrations is outstanding, and they are accompanied by extremely clear and straightforward explanations of the findings. The text also describes the common cardiovascular surgical procedures (past and present) in detail to facilitate the understanding of what can be expected to be found on the chest radiograph in these conditions postoperatively.

At the Hospital for Sick Children, Toronto, Canada, there has long been a close relationship between the pediatric radiologists, whose prime interest has been in cardiovascular disease, and the pediatric cardiologists and cardiac surgeons. This close relationship began decades ago, when the cardiac radiologist Dr. Fred Moes forged a close collaboration with Drs. Rowe, Mustard, and Freedom in cardiology and cardiovascular surgery. Over the years, other outstanding cardiac radiologists have joined the staff, such as Gordon Culham and Pat Burrows and more recently Shi-Joon Yoo and Cathy MacDonald.

This collaboration has led to the publication of many outstanding papers and books on the subject of pediatric cardiovascular disease. The present book on interpretation of the plain radiograph in these patients finds its niche by filling a specific area of interest among the other books on pediatric cardiovascular diseases published from this institution.

The information in this book is important not only to pediatric cardiovascular radiologists but also to pediatric cardiologists and cardiac surgeons. The book will become standard reading for all those training in these specialties. The manner in which it has been written and illustrated will reignite interest in the interpretation of the plain chest radiograph even for those whose main interest is in the more sophisticated modalities.

Dr. Alan Daneman
Professor of Medical Imaging
University of Toronto
Head of Body Imaging
Department of Diagnostic Imaging
Hospital for Sick Children
Toronto, Canada

Foreword

It is with great pleasure that I write this foreword to Drs. Yoo, MacDonald, and Babyn's tour de force, *Chest Radiographic Interpretation in Pediatric Cardiac Patients.*

With the ever-increasing technology available to image cardiovascular disease, it is sometimes easy to forget the value of basic clinical assessment and investigations. If ever there was an illustration that such an evolution was mistaken, it exists in this text. The extraordinary wealth of diagnostic and therapeutic information that may exist within the chest radiograph shouts out from almost every page of this extraordinary contribution. Replete with up-to-the-minute examples of virtually every abnormality imaginable, I am convinced that this book will rapidly establish itself as a seminal work in the field.

On behalf of all of the potential readers of this text, I would like to commend the extraordinary efforts of the authors for their painstaking collection and analysis on our behalf. Accrued over the course of five years, and representing many thousands of hours of analysis, illustration, writing, and production, this book is a credit not only to Drs. Yoo, MacDonald, and Babyn, but also to the combined Divisions of Cardiology and Radiology at the Hospital for Sick Children. I am proud to be associated with the authors and, in this small way, with the book itself.

Andrew Redington, MD
Head, Division of Cardiology
Department of Paediatrics
Hospital for Sick Children
University of Toronto
Toronto, Canada

Preface

Don't be intimidated by the size of this book!
This book contains more images and drawings than words. By voyaging through many examples, the readers will become very familiar with the important radiographic features in a very short time.

Why a new book for an old topic?
Despite the enormous recent strides in medical imaging with the introduction of a variety of cross-sectional imaging techniques, chest radiography remains the gateway for initial evaluation of the child who presents with cardiovascular symptoms and/or signs. Chest radiographs are still routinely obtained when the patients present with cardiovascular symptoms and signs, after the medical, surgical, or image-guided treatments, and at regular clinic visits. There are many books and book chapters available on this topic, most of which are structured according to disease entities or findings. A few suggest a systematic approach to chest radiographs but with only a few case examples. In addition, the discussions on basic cardiac anatomy, pathology, terminology, and surgical procedures are essential but not properly tailored for those who do cardiac imaging or interpret the chest radiographs. We decided to write this book to provide the essential background knowledge needed for cardiac imaging interpretation and systematic approach to chest radiographs with an ample number of case examples. Our previous and current trainees motivated us to teach them in a logical and easy-to-understand manner. Most importantly we found ourselves in a great position to write this book, as we are engaged in reading numerous chest radiographs of excellent radiographic quality at the Hospital for Sick Children, which is one of the largest pediatric cardiac centers worldwide.

How is this book structured?
This book provides an up-to-date and tailored approach to the interpretation of chest radiography in pediatric cardiac patients providing an important foundation for today's sophisticated medical and surgical management.

The text consists of three main sections. Section I, "Getting Started," includes chapters on normal cardiovascular anatomy, a sequential segmental approach to congenital heart disease and relevant terminology, and cardiac function and hemodynamics. A listing of current and important surgical procedures and appropriate radiographic techniques are also provided. The detailed information in this section provides a better understanding of basics of pediatric cardiology and cardiac imaging and facilitates communication among imagers, clinicians, and surgeons. Section II, representing the central part of the book, details how chest radiographs should be evaluated systematically. Each chapter includes an ample number of example cases allowing the reader to build perceptual skills and improve accuracy in interpretation of normal and abnormal radiographic findings across the spectrum of pediatric ages. Section III summarizes the pathology, clinical manifestation, and radiographic findings of a variety of individual cardiovascular lesions. Although chest radiography may not play a major role in the exact diagnosis of cardiac disease, knowledge of the usual expected radiographic findings in individual cardiac lesions will help in recognition of problems that may not already have been diagnosed or suspected, or in detection of the unusual presentation or complication of the known disease. This section utilizes a bullet form approach for quick review and reference during day-to-day practice.

Who are the target readers?
We hope that this text is useful to radiology and cardiology residents and fellows as well as pediatric and general radiologists, pediatric cardiologists and cardiac surgeons, neonatologists, and chest intensivists who are involved in the daily interpretation in reporting of the chest radiographs or direct care for pediatric cardiac patients.

Shi-Joon Yoo
Cathy MacDonald
Paul Babyn

Acknowledgments

First and above all, I should thank all patients and their families who trusted the Hospital for Sick Children in Toronto and provided us with such tremendous opportunities to improve our knowledge and skills in managing the children with cardiac problems.

I would like to thank the past and current residents and fellows of our department and the Division of Cardiology, Department of Paediatrics, who motivated and stimulated us to write a book from our teaching materials.

This book could not have become what it is now without the dedication of the radiology technologists at the Hospital for Sick Children who always take the best quality radiographs with the least amounts of radiation dose.

I would like to express my gratitude to the following people for their contributions in writing this book:

- Eul Kyung Kim, for preparing illustrations
- Dorris Kellenberger for retrieving and managing the radiographs
- Katherine McLaren, Jennifer Russell, and Vicki Corris for their administrative work and reference management
- Drs. Michael Seed, Brian Grant, Kelly Wong, Perry Choi, Christian Drolet, and Mary Louise Greer for proofreading the draft manuscripts and for their valuable comments
- All contributors for their time and effort in retrieving the materials and writing the chapters

I would like to thank my wife, Eul Kyung Kim, for her understanding, support, and patience. She made a special effort in working on the illustrations despite her carpal tunnel syndrome and trigger fingers.

Finally, I would like to dedicate this book to late Dr. Robert M. Freedom, who was my teacher, mentor, and great friend.

Shi-Joon Yoo

First, I would like to thank Dr. Shi-Joon Yoo for letting me share in his passion for pediatric cardiac imaging and his zeal for new ways of learning.

To my wife Elizabeth and my children, Andre, Laura, Michael, and Jonathan, for their spirit and encouragement.

To all our trainees who continue to challenge and teach us.

Paul Babyn

First, I would like to thank Dr. Shi-Joon Yoo, who put forth the idea of writing this book, for inviting me to participate in this project.

To my husband Rick and my children, Brandon, Kyle, and Jamie, for their patient endurance and encouragement.

To Linda Halpert and Danny Aguilar, for the production of the text and figures.

Finally, to all the fellows, residents, and students, whose enthusiastic quest for learning was the nidus for this book.

Cathy MacDonald

Contributors

Paul Babyn, MD, FRCPC
Radiologist-in-Chief
Department of Diagnostic Imaging
Hospital for Sick Children
Associate Professor
Department of Medical Imaging
University of Toronto
Toronto, Canada

Christopher Caldarone, MD
Staff Cardiac Surgeon
Department of Surgery
Hospital for Sick Children
Professor of Surgery, Chief of Cardiac Surgery
University of Toronto
Toronto, Canada

Ellen Charkot, MRT(R)
Management Director
Department of Diagnostic Imaging
Hospital for Sick Children
Toronto, Canada

Monica Epelman, MD
Director of Neonatal Imaging
Department of Radiology
The Children's Hospital of Philadelphia,
University of Pennsylvania
Philadelphia, Pennsylvania

Anne Geoffray, MD
Chief of Pediatric Imaging
Fondation Lenval
Nice, France

Christian J. Kellenberger, MD
Radiologist-in-Chief
Department of Diagnostic Imaging
University Children's Hospital
Zurich, Switzerland

Cathy MacDonald, MD, FRCPC
Radiologist
Department of Diagnostic Imaging
Hospital for Sick Children
Assistant Professor
Department of Medical Imaging
University of Toronto
Toronto, Canada

Donald G. Perrin, PhD
Pathologists' Assistant
Department of Pathology and Laboratory Medicine
Hospital for Sick Children
Departments of Paediatrics and Pathology
University of Toronto
Toronto, Canada

Kevin S. Roman, MD
Consultant in Congenital Heart Disease
Congenital Cardiac Centre
Southampton University Hospital Trust
Southhampton, England

Derek Wong, MD
Senior Fellow
Division of Cardiology
Department of Paediatrics
Hospital for Sick Children
Toronto, Canada

Shi-Joon Yoo, MD, PhD, FRCPC
Section Head of Cardiac Imaging
Department of Diagnostic Imaging
Hospital for Sick Children
Professor
Departments of Medical Imaging and Paediatrics
University of Toronto
Toronto, Canada

Abbreviations

Aa	aortic arch
ALCAPA	anomalous origin of the left coronary artery from the pulmonary artery
Ao	ascending aorta
ao	descending aorta
AP	anteroposterior
AV	aortic valve; atrioventricular
CS	coronary sinus
CSV	crista supraventricularis
CT	computed tomography; computed tomogram; cardiothoracic
FO	fossa ovalis
GB	gallbladder
IS	infundibular septum
IVC	inferior vena cava
LA	left atrium
LAA	left atrial appendage
LAD	left anterior descending coronary artery
LAO	left anterior oblique
LB	left main bronchus
LCA	left coronary artery
LCX	left circumflex coronary artery
LIV	left innominate vein
LPA	left pulmonary artery
LUL	left upper lobe
LV	left ventricle
lv	rudimentary left ventricle
LVOT	left ventricular outflow tract
MAPCA	major aortopulmonary collateral arteries
MB	moderator band
MPA	main pulmonary artery
MR	magnetic resonance
MV	mitral valve
os	outlet septum
PA	pulmonary artery; posteroanterior
PCWP	pulmonary capillary wedge pressure
PD	posterior descending coronary artery
PV	pulmonary valve; pulmonary vein
PVOD	pulmonary veno-occlusive disease
RA	right atrium
RB	right main bronchus
RAA	right atrial appendage
RAO	right anterior oblique
RCA	right coronary artery
RPA	right pulmonary artery
RPO	right posterior oblique
RPV	right pulmonary vein
RUL	right upper lobe
RUPV	right upper pulmonary vein

RV	right ventricle
rv	rudimentary right ventricle
RVOT	right ventricular outflow tract
SVC	superior vena cava
TSM	trabecula septomarginalis
TV	tricuspid valve
VA	ventriculoarterial
VACTERL	vertebral abnormalities, anal atresia, cardiac abnormalities, tracheoesophageal fistula, esophageal atresia, renal agenesis, and limb defects
VIF	ventriculoinfundibular fold

Getting Started

1 Normal Cardiovascular Anatomy for Imaging

Shi-Joon Yoo and Donald G. Perrin

■ General Consideration

The heart lies within the pericardial sac in the mediastinum with two thirds placed to the left of the midline and one third to the right (**Fig. 1.1**). This asymmetric position of the heart within the thorax is called levocardia. The heart is shaped like an ice-cream cone that is tilted to the right and backward with its apex directed downward, to the left, and forward.

The heart consists of three segments: the atria, the ventricles, and the arterial trunks (**Fig. 1.2**).[1] The three segments are joined together at the atrioventricular and ventriculoarterial junctions that are guarded by valves. The four cardiac valves that demarcate these two junctions are arranged in a single plane. This plane is called the base of the heart or more precisely the base of the ventricles.

The apex of the heart refers to the most pointed part of the ventricular mass. In the normal heart, it is composed of the tip of the left ventricle. The long axis of the heart is a line that connects the apex and the center of the base (**Fig. 1.3A**). The planes that are parallel to the long axis are called the long axis planes (**Fig. 1.3B**). The long axis planes that are oriented in a vertical plane to the body are

called vertical long axis planes. The two-chamber views of the right and left ventricles are typical vertical long axis planes. The long axis planes that are oriented in a transverse plane to the body are called horizontal long axis planes. The four-chamber view is a typical horizontal long axis plane. The left ventricular long axis view is a plane midway between the vertical and horizontal planes. The planes that are perpendicular to the long axis are called the short axis planes. Examples are the atrial, basal ventricular, midventricular, and apical ventricular short axis planes (**Fig. 1.3C**).

The ventricular part of the cardiac cone is not entirely circular. Its anterior surface is slightly convex, the posterior surface more rounded, and the inferior surface flat. The anteroinferior margin of the cardiac cone, which is composed of the right ventricle, forms an acute angle as it molds itself into the recess of the thoracic cage between the anterior chest wall and the diaphragm (**Fig. 1.4**). This part of the cardiac cone is therefore called the acute margin of the ventricular mass. In contrast, the posterior margin of the heart that is composed of the left ventricular free wall is called the obtuse margin as this part of the heart is more rounded.

Externally, the four cardiac chambers are demarcated by grooves: the interatrial, interventricular, and atrioventricular

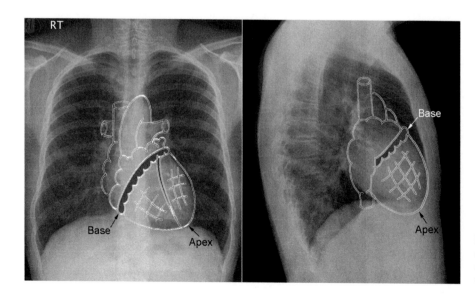

Fig. 1.1 The heart is shaped like an ice-cream cone. The base of the cone is the atrioventricular junction and the apex is composed of the tip of the left ventricle.

3

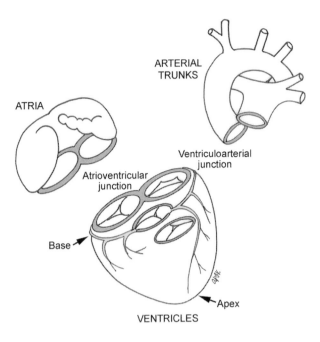

ARTERIAL TRUNKS

ATRIA

Ventriculoarterial junction

Atrioventricular junction

Base

Apex

VENTRICLES

Fig. 1.2 Cardiac segments and junctions. (Modified from Anderson RH, Ho SY. Sequential segmental analysis—description and categorization for the millennium. Cardiol Young 1997;77:98–116).

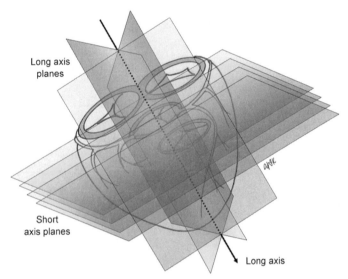

Long axis planes

Short axis planes

Long axis

A

Fig. 1.3 Long and short axis planes of the heart. **(A)** Diagrammatic representation of the cardiac axis and planes. **(B,C)** Examples of magnetic resonance images obtained along the long and short axis planes. LV, left ventricle; RV, right ventricle.

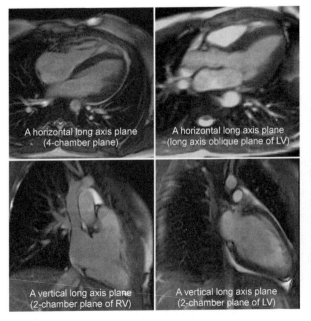

A horizontal long axis plane (4-chamber plane)

A horizontal long axis plane (long axis oblique plane of LV)

A vertical long axis plane (2-chamber plane of RV)

A vertical long axis plane (2-chamber plane of LV)

B

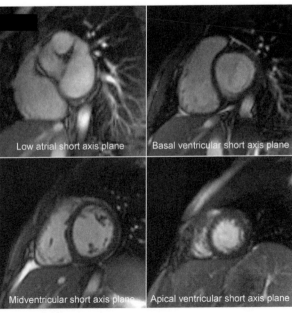

Low atrial short axis plane

Basal ventricular short axis plane

Midventricular short axis plane

Apical ventricular short axis plane

C

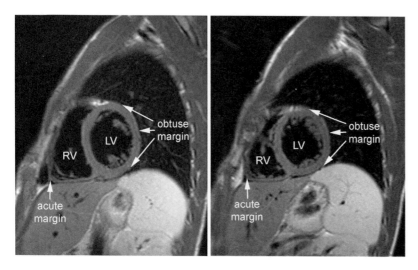

Fig. 1.4 Acute and obtuse margins of the ventricles shown on short axis magnetic resonance images. RV, right ventricle; LV, left ventricle.

grooves (**Fig. 1.5**). The atrioventricular and interventricular grooves are distinct as they contain a large amount of epicardial fat on which the major epicardial coronary arteries and veins are located. The interatrial groove is less distinct. Posteriorly, the interatrial and interventricular grooves are continuous with one another and are crossed by the atrioventricular groove. This point of intersection is called the crux cordis.

■ Base of the Ventricles

The base of the ventricles can be exposed by removing the atria and arterial trunks from the ventricles (**Fig. 1.6**). When the base of the heart is seen from above, the four cardiac valves are closely related to each other in a slanted plane. Familiarity with the arrangement of the cardiac valves in this plane facilitates the understanding of many important aspects of the cardiac anatomy.

The atrioventricular valves, that is, the tricuspid and mitral valves, are located more posteriorly and inferiorly relative to the semilunar valves, that is, the aortic and pulmonary valves. The tricuspid valve is the most rightward and inferior valve and the mitral valve is the most posterior. The aortic valve has a deeply wedged position between the tricuspid and mitral valves. The pulmonary valve lies anterior and leftward of the aortic valve. The aortic valve is tilted slightly rightward and forward; the pulmonary valve is tilted slightly leftward and backward.

The tricuspid, mitral, and aortic valves are firmly attached together through a dense fibrous tissue core called the central fibrous body. As will be discussed later in this chapter, the interventricular and atrioventricular membranous septum is the septal extension of the central fibrous body. The aortic and pulmonary valves, on the other hand, are loosely attached to each other.

The aortic and mitral valves are in direct contact with one another in the left ventricle. In the right ventricle, the pulmonary and tricuspid valves are apart from one

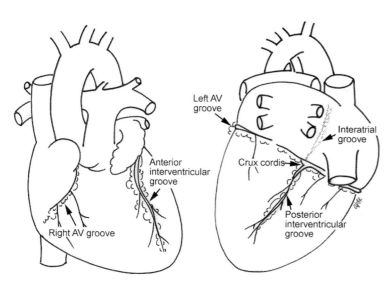

Fig. 1.5 Interatrial, interventricular, and atrioventricular (AV) grooves. The point where the atrioventricular groove is crossed by the interatrial and interventricular groove is called the crux cordis.

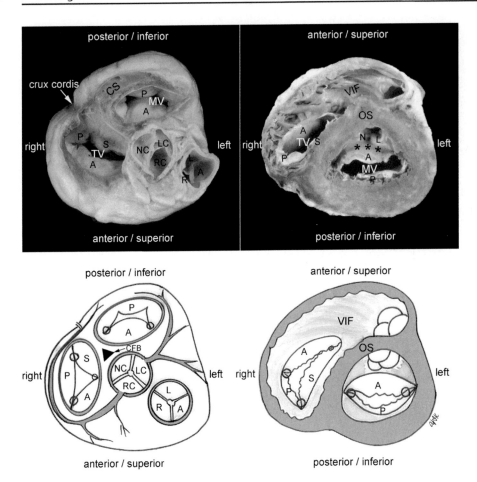

Fig. 1.6 Photographs and drawings showing the base of the ventricles seen from above (left panel) and below (right panel). The arterial trunks and atria are removed above the valve and the apical parts of the ventricles are removed. The tricuspid, mitral, and aortic valves are firmly attached to a dense fibrous tissue core called the central fibrous body (CFB). The mitral and aortic valves are in direct contact (*asterisks*) in the left ventricle. The tricuspid and pulmonary valves are separated by the intervening crista supraventricularis. The crista supraventricularis consists of the ventriculoinfundibular fold (VIF) and outlet septum (OS). The tricuspid valve (TV) consists of the septal (S), anterior (A), and posterior (P) leaflets. The mitral valve (MV) consists of the anterior (A) and posterior (P) leaflets. The aortic valve consists of the right coronary (RC), left coronary (LC), and noncoronary (NC) cusps. The pulmonary valve consists of the right (R), left (L), and anterior (A) cusps. The coronary sinus (CS) is seen along the posterior margin of the mitral valve.

another with an intervening fold of right ventricular myocardium called the crista supraventricularis.[2,3] Because of the wedged position of the aortic valve between the tricuspid and mitral valves, the aortic and tricuspid valves, despite belonging to different ventricles, are in close proximity with only the membranous septum separating them. Therefore, a pathologic defect in the membranous septum brings the aortic and tricuspid valves in direct contact with each other.

■ Atria

The right atrium is located rightward, anterior, and inferior to the left atrium (**Fig. 1.7**). The right atrium receives blood flow from the body through the superior and inferior venae cavae. The right atrium also receives blood flow from the myocardium through the coronary sinus and small direct coronary venous channels. The right atrium communicates with the right ventricle, which is anterior and leftward. The left atrium is a midline posterosuperior chamber in front of the vertebral column. Interposed between the left atrium and the vertebral column are the esophagus on the right and the descending aorta on the left. The carina of the trachea and the left main bronchus are located immediately above the left atrium. The left atrium receives the pulmonary veins, usually two from each lung. The left atrium communicates with the left ventricle, which is anterior and leftward.

Each atrium consists of a smooth-walled main body and a trabeculated appendage or auricle. The main bodies of the right and left atria are opposed to each other

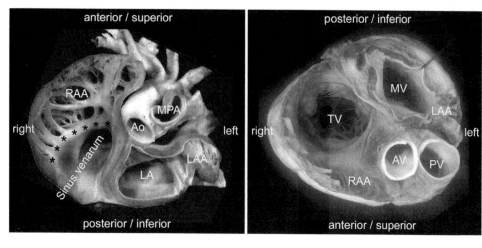

A

B

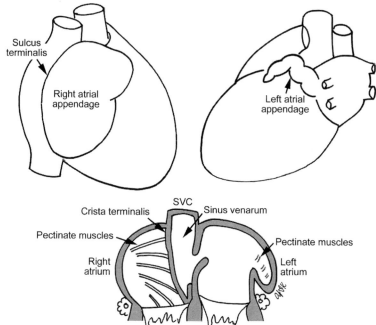

C

Sulcus
terminalis

Right atrial
appendage

Left atrial
appendage

Crista terminalis   SVC   Sinus venarum

Pectinate muscles

Right
atrium

Pectinate muscles

Left
atrium

Fig. 1.7 Morphologic characteristics of the right and left atria. **(A)** The atria and arterial trunks are seen from below after the ventricles together with the atrioventricular and semilunar valves are removed (asterisks indicate crista terminalis). **(B)** The base of the heart is seen from above after removal of the cranial parts of the atria. Note that the pectinate muscles extend to the atrioventricular junction in the right atrium, but not in the left atrium. **(C)** Drawings showing the morphologic characteristics of the right and left atria. Ao, ascending aorta; RAA, right atrial appendage; MPA, main pulmonary artery; LA, left atrium; LAA, left atrial appendage; TV, tricuspid valve; MV, mitral valve; AV, aortic valve; PV, pulmonary valve; SVC, superior vena cava. (**[A]** Reproduced with permission of Professor Robert H. Anderson.)

centrally with the atrial septum in an oblique plane behind the ascending aortic root. The atrial appendages project laterally from the main bodies to embrace the arterial trunks from behind. The right atrial appendage is shaped like a blunt triangle and has a broad base at its junction with the main body of the right atrium. The left atrial appendage is a finger-like, crenellated tube and has a narrow orifice at its junction with the main body of the left atrium.

In the right atrium, the superior and inferior venae cavae form a furrow-like confluence called the sinus venarum. Medially, the sinus venarum is bounded by the atrial septum with an indistinct demarcation. Laterally, the sinus venarum is bounded by the appendage. The C-shaped muscular ridge that demarcates the sinus venarum and appendage is the crista terminalis. Externally, this

junction is demarcated by a shallow depression called the sulcus terminalis. In the left atrium, the pulmonary venous confluence does not form a furrow; therefore, there is neither a crista nor a sulcus terminalis.

Superiorly, the crista terminalis extends to the atrial septum in front of the superior vena caval orifice (**Fig. 1.8A**). Inferiorly, the crista is transformed to a thin membranous flap that extends to the atrial septum in front of the inferior caval orifice. This membranous flap is the Eustachian valve of the inferior vena cava (**Fig. 1.8B**). The Eustachian valve varies in size and is often perforated. Infrequently, it reaches the superior vena caval orifice and appears as a septum with multiple perforations, which is called Chiari's network. Immediately medial and posterior to the inferior vena caval orifice is the orifice of the coronary sinus. The coronary sinus is the terminal drainage root of

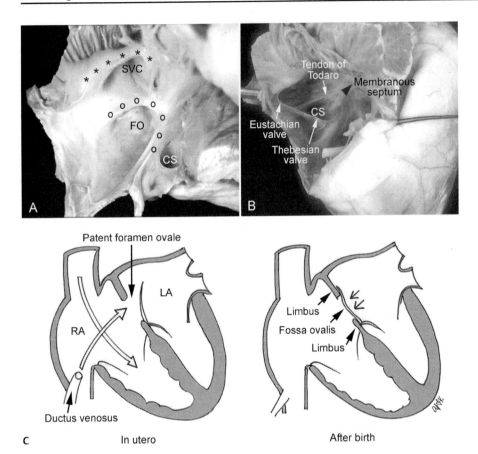

Fig. 1.8 Anatomy of the atrial septum. **(A)** The atrial septum is seen from the right atrium. There is an oval depression called the fossa ovalis (FO) which is demarcated by a muscular limb (marked by "o's") called the limbus of the fossa ovalis. The superior vena cava (SVC) is demarcated anteriorly by the crista terminalis (*asterisks*). **(B)** The anterior wall of the right atrium is removed to show the Eustachian valve of the inferior vena cava (probed) and the Thebesian valve of the coronary sinus. The tendon of Todaro is the fibrous ridge extending from the commissure between these two valves to the atrioventricular membranous septum. The triangle of Koch is demarcated by the tendon of Todaro, coronary sinus opening, and the base of the septal leaflet of the tricuspid valve. The atrioventricular node is located in the triangle of Koch. **(C)** Drawings show how the foramen ovale conveys the oxygenated blood from the placenta to the left side of the heart and how the fossa ovalis is formed after birth. The tissue forming the fossa ovalis is the embryologic septum primum and the surrounding limbus is the embryologic septum secundum. SVC, superior vena cava; CS, coronary sinus; LA, left atrium; RA, right atrium.

most of the coronary venous blood and courses along the posterior aspect of the left atrioventricular groove to open into the right atrium immediately near the crux cordis (**Fig. 1.6A**). The coronary sinus orifice is either unguarded or partially concealed by a membranous flap, which is called the Thebesian valve (**Fig. 1.8B**). In contrast to the right atrium, the main body of the left atrium is smooth-walled without any recognizable muscular ridges or membranous valves. Usually two, infrequently one and rarely three, pulmonary veins from each lung are connected to each side of the posterior wall.[4]

The internal walls of the atrial appendages are roughly trabeculated (**Fig. 1.7**). These trabeculations are called the pectinate muscles. The pectinate muscles of the right atrial appendage extend inferiorly to the posterior and lateral parts of the atrioventricular junction (**Figs. 1.7B, 1.7C**).[5] In the left atrium, the pectinate muscles are confined

to the tubular appendage and only rarely do a few tiny strands reach the atrioventricular junction. In other words, the right atrial appendageal orifice reaches the atrioventricular junction, whereas the orifice of the left atrial appendage is located at some distance from the atrioventricular junction.

The atrial septum seen from the right atrium is rather complex (**Fig. 1.8A**). The atrial septum appears quite large when it is observed in an opened specimen. However, only a small part that appears to be interatrial is truly between the atrial chambers. The rest of the dividing wall between the atria is the infolding of tissue from the superior and posterior parietal wall of the atrium.[6] The right atrial side of the atrial septum has a central depression with a surrounding muscular rim, called the fossa ovalis and limbus of the fossa ovalis, respectively. Anteroinferiorly, the limbus merges with the supratricuspid part of the septum in front of the coronary sinus orifice. The upper posterior region of the supratricuspid part of the septum is between the atria as is the floor of the fossa ovalis; the lower anterior region is between the right atrium and the left ventricle. This is because the tricuspid valve is attached to the septum more apically than the mitral valve.

In the supratricuspid part of the septum, a fibrous fascicle arises from the commissure between the Eustachian and Thebesian valves and inserts into the central fibrous body (**Fig. 1.8B**). This is designated the tendon of Todaro,[7] which is an important landmark forming the posterosuperior boundary of the triangle of Koch that contains the atrioventricular node (**Fig. 1.8B**). The other boundaries of the triangle of Koch are the attachment of the septal leaflet of the tricuspid valve and the orifice of the coronary sinus. The anterior apical part of the triangle is the membranous septum. The atrioventricular node is located immediately behind the membranous septum and gives rise to the atrioventricular conduction axis of His.

Unlike the right atrial side, the left atrial side of the atrial septum is smooth. The only recognizable structure is a fibrous strand of tissue in its anterosuperior part. This strand represents the ventral edge of the floor of the fossa ovalis, which has fused to the limbus of the fossa ovalis after birth.

The fossa ovalis is of vital importance during fetal life. In the fetus, it is a one-way valve or door-like structure with its hinge along the posteroinferior part of the limbus and its free edge against the door-frame of the limbus on the left side (**Fig. 1.8C**). Embryologically, the valve is the septum primum, and the limbus the septum secundum. The inferior vena caval blood flow hits the floor of the fossa ovalis and opens the valve, allowing the oxygenated blood from the placenta via the ductus venosus to pass into the left atrium, left ventricle, and aorta to perfuse the myocardium and brain. In contrast, the superior vena caval blood flows directly into the right ventricle through the tricuspid valve and then to the pulmonary arterial trunk, allowing the deoxygenated blood to reach the placenta through the ductus arteriosus, descending aorta, and umbilical arteries. The opening in the atrial septum in fetal life is called the foramen ovale. After birth, with breathing of air and establishment of the pulmonary circulation, the increased left atrial blood flow and pressure result in functional closure of the door of the foramen ovale against the limbus of the fossa ovalis. Subsequently, the foramen ovale closes completely by fibrous adhesions. Not infrequently, the fusion is incomplete, leaving the foramen ovale patent. A patent foramen ovale (PFO) is seen in over 25% of both autopsy and healthy adult studies.[8,9] The presence of a PFO has no adverse consequence in otherwise healthy adults. However, a systemic venous thrombus can migrate into the systemic arterial circulation during a Valsalva maneuver. Patients who suffer a stroke or transient ischemic attack in the presence of a PFO and without any other cause are considered for prophylactic medical therapy and/or surgical or nonsurgical closure of the PFO to reduce the risk of a recurrent embolic event.

■ Ventricles

Mostly, the right ventricle is located anterior and rightward of the left ventricle. The right ventricle is pyramidal in shape, and the left ventricle is a truncated ellipsoid (**Fig. 1.9**). In short axis planes, the left ventricle is circular, whereas the right ventricle is crescentic encircling the left

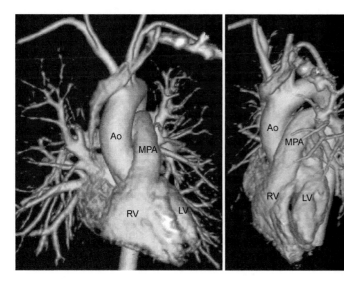

Fig. 1.9 Morphology and spatial relationship of the right and left ventricles. Volume rendered contrast-enhanced magnetic resonance angiograms are reconstructed as seen from front and the left side. The right ventricle (RV) is pyramidal; the left ventricle (LV) is elliptical. Note that the ventricular outflow tracts and arterial trunks spiral around each other. Ao, Ascending aorta; MPA, main pulmonary artery.

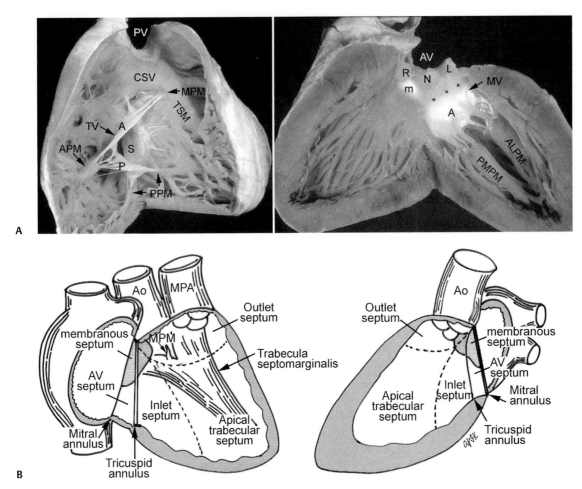

Fig. 1.10 (A) Interior of the right and left ventricles. Note the difference in trabeculation patterns of the ventricles. The trabecular septomarginalis (TSM) is the most-stout trabeculation on the septum. The pulmonary and tricuspid valves are separated by an intervening muscular crest that is called the crista supraventricularis (CSV). The aortic and mitral valves are in direct contact (*asterisks*). The mitral valve is supported by two stout papillary muscles called the anterolateral and posteromedial papillary muscles (ALPM and PMPM, respectively). The tricuspid valve (TV) consists of the septal (S), anterior (A) and posterior (P) leaflets. They are supported by the medial, anterior, and posterior papillary muscles (MPM, APM, and PPM, respectively). The membranous part (m) of the ventricular septum is transilluminated from the right side. The atrioventricular (AV) septum is present because of the offset attachment of the mitral valve (MV) and tricuspid valve leaflets to the septum. The ventricular septum is arbitrarily divided into the inlet, apical, trabecular, and outlet parts. **(B)** Rendered drawing of interior of the right and left ventricles. Ao, ascending aorta; MPA, main pulmonary artery; AV, atrioventricular.

ventricle (**Figs. 1.4, 1.6B**). The left ventricle is approximately three times thicker than the right ventricle.

Each ventricle consists of three anatomic and functional units: the inlet, apical trabecular, and outlet components (**Fig. 1.10**). Although there are no discrete boundaries between the components, the overall arrangement of the three components can readily be appreciated. The inlet and trabecular components of the right ventricle are positioned to the right and anterior to the corresponding components of the left ventricle. The outlet of the right ventricle, however, is to the left and anterior to the outlet of the left ventricle. This rather complicated spatial relationship of the ventricles can easily be understood in the plane at the base of the ventricles (**Fig. 1.6**). There are three important features:

1. In the right ventricle, a prominent muscular crest called the crista supraventricularis separates the atrioventricular and arterial valves. In the left ventricle, there is no crista supraventricularis and the atrioventricular and arterial valves are in fibrous continuity.
2. The inlet–outlet relationship is right-left in the right ventricle, whereas it is left-right in the left ventricle.
3. The left ventricle is oval in its short axis; the right ventricle is crescentic. The right ventricle wraps around the right and anterior aspect of the left ventricle.

The atrioventricular valves of the right and left ventricles are the tricuspid and mitral valves, respectively (**Figs. 1.6, 1.10**). Each valve is supported by a tension apparatus that consists of chordae tendineae and papillary muscles. The three leaflets of the tricuspid valve are the septal, anterior (superior), and posterior (inferior) leaflets. The septal leaflet is related to the septum, the posterior leaflet the posterolateral wall of the right ventricle, and the anterior leaflet the anterior wall toward the outlet part of the right ventricle. The slits between the leaflets are called the commissures, which are called the anteroseptal, the posteroseptal, and anteroposterior commissures. Along each commissure, the chordae tendineae arise from the ventricular surfaces of the adjacent leaflets and converge to the tip of the papillary muscle. The chordae tendineae from the septal and anterior leaflets converge to a small papillary muscle that arises from the ventricular septum at the junction between the inlet and outlet parts. This papillary muscle is called the medial or conal papillary muscle (of Lancisi). The papillary muscle(s) supporting the anteroposterior commissure is called the anterior papillary muscle and arises from the moderator band or from the anterior wall of the right ventricle adjacent to the moderator band. The posteroseptal commissure is usually supported by a few small papillary muscles that arise from the diaphragmatic surface of the right ventricular wall and lower part of the ventricular septum and are called the posterior papillary muscles. There is further support of the tricuspid leaflets by additional chordae tendineae that insert directly into the right ventricular septum or wall.

The mitral valve consists of two leaflets: the anterior or aortic leaflet and the posterior or mural leaflet (**Figs. 1.6, 1.10**). The anterior leaflet makes up one third of the circumference of the valve ring and faces the aortic valve, which justifies its alternative name, the aortic leaflet. The anterior leaflet of the mitral valve has a limited attachment to the posterior part of the septum around the crux cordis because of the deeply wedged position of the aortic valve between the tricuspid and mitral valves. The posterior leaflet makes up two thirds of the valve ring along the free wall and is called the mural leaflet. The anterior leaflet is twice as tall as the posterior leaflet, which results

in the two leaflets of the mitral valve having similar areas. The posterior leaflet is scalloped along its free edge. Most commonly there are three scallops: the medial, central, and lateral. There are two commissures between the two mitral leaflets, which are supported by the anterolateral and posteromedial (posteroseptal) papillary muscles. In contrast to those of the tricuspid valve, the papillary muscles of the left ventricle do not arise from the ventricular septum and there is no direct insertion of chordae tendineae to the left ventricular septum or wall.

The apical trabecular components of the right and left ventricles show characteristic trabeculations (**Fig. 1.10**). The trabeculations of the right ventricle are heavier and more irregular in shape and arrangement than those of the left ventricle. There is a stout trabeculation in the right ventricular aspect of the septum, which is called the trabecula septomarginalis. It is a Y-shaped trabeculation. The body of this Y-shaped trabecula runs from the crista supraventricularis area toward the apex. The anterior limb of the Y supports the pulmonary valve, whereas the posterior limb extends toward the anteroseptal commissure of the tricuspid valve. The medial papillary muscle supporting the anteroseptal commissure of the tricuspid valve arises from the septum above the bifurcation of the trabecula septomarginalis. From the apical part of the body of the trabecula, a muscular bundle arises and crosses the right ventricular cavity to insert to the parietal wall (**Fig. 1.11**) and is designated the moderator band. As mentioned, the anterior papillary muscle(s) usually arises from the moderator band although it can also arise from the adjacent right ventricular free wall.

The outlet components of the ventricles also exhibit important morphologic differences. The right ventricular outlet consists of a completely muscular conus or infundibulum due to a prominent muscular crest, the crista supraventricularis in the roof of the right ventricle between the tricuspid and pulmonary valves (**Figs. 1.6, 1.9, 1.10**). The left ventricular outlet, on the other hand,

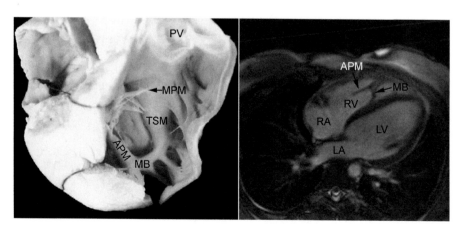

Fig. 1.11 Moderator band and anterior papillary muscle. The anterior free wall of the right ventricle is removed in the specimen photograph. The moderator band (MB) arises from the apical part of the trabecula septomarginalis (TSM) and inserts to the parietal wall. The anterior papillary muscle (APM) arises from the moderator band. MPM, medial papillary muscle; PV, pulmonary valve; RA, right atrium; LA, left atrium; LV, left ventricle; RV, right ventricle.

is less conspicuous and is not completely muscular because of the fibrous continuity between the mitral and aortic valves. Because the left ventricle is devoid of the crista supraventricularis, it does not have a muscular conus or infundibulum. The crista supraventricularis of the right ventricle has two components: the parietal and septal parts (**Fig. 1.6**). The parietal part is the superior wall of the right ventricle that is seen in the plane of the base of the heart, between the tricuspid and pulmonary valves. This part of the crista supraventricularis is called the ventriculoinfundibular fold. The septal part is the small triangular part of the crista that is cradled between the anterior and posterior limbs of the trabecula septomarginalis. This part is the outlet or infundibular component of the ventricular septum. Different names have been introduced for the components of the crista supraventricularis and ventricular septum. The ventriculoinfundibular fold has also been named the parietal band, whereas the outlet septum and trabecular septomarginalis together the septal band.

The ventricular septum consists of the muscular and membranous parts (**Fig. 1.10**). As mentioned, the membranous septum is the septal extension of the central fibrous body. The membranous septum is in direct contact with the anterior leaflet of the mitral valve, the septal leaflet of the tricuspid valve at the anteroseptal commissure, and the non- and right coronary cusps of the aortic valve. Most of the ventricular septum is muscular. The muscular septum is divided into the inlet, apical trabecular, and outlet components. Each component occupies a triangular area with a common apex at the membranous septum. As the left ventricular outlet is less conspicuous than the right ventricular outlet, the outlet septum occupies a much smaller area in the left ventricle than in the right ventricle. It is also important to note that the upper part of the inlet septum seen from the right ventricle is in fact between the right ventricular inlet and left ventricular outlet because of the deeply wedged position of the aortic valve. Only the posterior part of the inlet septum seen from the right ventricle is truly between the two inlets (**Figs. 1.10, 1.11, 1.12**).

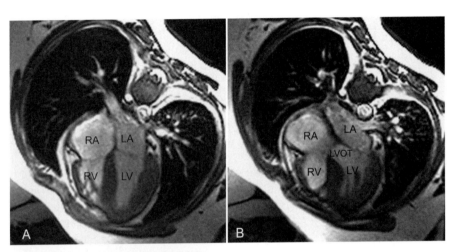

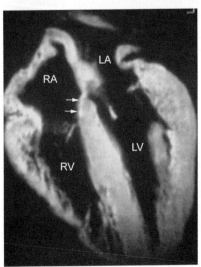

Fig. 1.12 Septal components of the right and left ventricles. **(A,B)** Magnetic resonance (MR) images obtained in four-chamber and five-chamber planes. The septum seen in four-chamber view is truly between the right and left ventricular inlets. The septum seen in a five-chamber view separates the inlet part of the right ventricle from the outlet part of the left ventricle (LVOT). In the four-chamber plane, the tricuspid valve has a more apical attachment to the septum than the mitral valve. The part of the septum between the insertions of the mitral and tricuspid valves is the atrioventricular septum. **(C)** T1-weighted MR image of a heart specimen in a four-chamber plane shows the offset attachments of the tricuspid and mitral valves. Note that a thin white layer of fat tissue (*arrows*) is seen along the right atrial side of the atrioventricular septum. This is a subendocardial extension of the epicardial fat tissue from the crux cordis to the region of the membranous septum. RA, right atrium; LA, left atrium; RV, right ventricle; LV, left ventricle.

As stated, a small area of septum is present between the right atrium and the left ventricle, which is called the atrioventricular septum (**Figs. 1.10, 1.12**). This part of the septum exists because of the more apical attachment of the tricuspid valve to the septum compared with that of the mitral valve and deeply wedged position of the aortic valve. The atrioventricular septum, as well, consists of a muscular part posteriorly and a membranous part anterosuperiorly.[10] The atrioventricular part of the membranous septum is continuous with the interventricular part of the membranous septum. In other words, the membranous septum is divided into the atrioventricular and interventricular parts by the attachment of the tricuspid valve. The right atrial aspect of the muscular part of the atrioventricular septum is covered by fatty tissue underneath the endocardium (**Fig. 1.12B**). As this fatty tissue is continuous with the epicardial fatty tissue in the atrioventricular sulcus, Anderson et al regard this part of the septum as an infolding of the parietal wall rather than a true septum.[11]

■ Great Arteries

The aortic and pulmonary valves are identical in design with three equally sized cusps contained in a short connective tissue sleeve. Unlike the atrioventricular valves, these valves are not supported by tension apparatus. The cusps are semilunar in shape, and the commissures between the cusps are shaped like a Mercedes-Benz sign (**Fig. 1.6**). The valves are arranged so that two of the three cusps of each valve face two cusps of the other valve, and the commissures between the facing cusps of the aortic and pulmonary valves are aligned in most individuals. The right and left facing cusps of the aortic valve are called the right and left coronary cusps because the right and left coronary arteries arise from the aortic sinuses above these cusps. The nonfacing cusp of the aortic valve is called the noncoronary cusp. The three pulmonary cusps are the right, left, and anterior cusps. The sleeves containing the aortic and pulmonary valves show rounded bulges, forming the sinuses above the insertion of the cusps. The aortic and pulmonary sinuses are bounded superiorly by the tubular parts of the aorta and pulmonary artery at the sinotubular junction or ridge (**Fig. 1.13**).

The ascending aorta and the main pulmonary artery have a partially spiral arrangement (**Fig. 1.9**). The ascending aorta courses slightly to the right and forward in its proximal part and forms a gentle curve to subsequently course slightly to the left and backward to continue as the aortic arch after it gives rise to the innominate (or

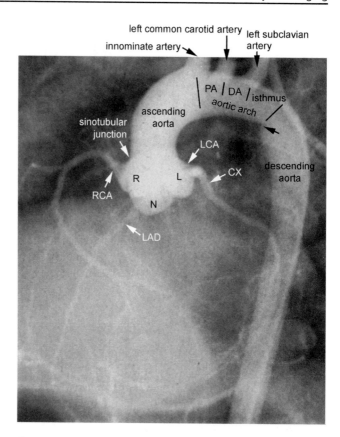

Fig. 1.13 Segments of the aorta seen in an aortogram in left anterior oblique view. The aortic arch is divided into the proximal arch (PA) and distal arch (DA) by the origins of the head and neck branches. The last segment of the aortic arch is the aortic isthmus. The arrow indicates the site of ductal insertion. R, L, and N indicate right, left, and noncoronary sinuses, respectively. RCA, right coronary artery; LCA, left coronary artery; LAD, left anterior descending coronary artery; CX, circumflex coronary artery.

brachiocephalic) artery. The aortic arch is the transverse part of the aorta extending from the origin of the innominate artery to the insertion site of the ductus arteriosus (**Fig. 1.13**). It is subdivided into the proximal and distal arches and the isthmus by the origins of the left common carotid and left subclavian arteries, respectively. The aortic arch courses backward and slightly to the left on the left side of the trachea above the left pulmonary artery and left main bronchus. The aortic arch is described as a left or right aortic arch according to its relative position to the trachea. The aorta distal to the insertion of the ductus is the descending aorta.

The main pulmonary artery courses upward and backward to bifurcate into the right and left pulmonary arteries. The right pulmonary artery has a transverse course in the mediastinum in front of the left and right main bronchi (**Fig. 1.14**) and gives rise to the right upper lobe branch in the mediastinum. As it reaches the right pulmonary hilum, it courses backward and downward below

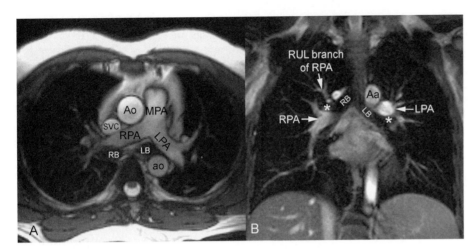

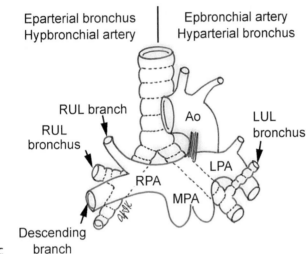

Fig. 1.14 (A–C) Pulmonary arterial and bronchial anatomy seen in magnetic resonance images and drawing. The right pulmonary artery courses rightward in front of the left and right main bronchi (LB and RB, respectively) in the mediastinum. It gives rise to the right upper lobar (RUL) branch before it reaches the lung hilum. Then it courses backward below the right upper lobar bronchus (*asterisk*). The left pulmonary artery courses leftward and backward above the left main bronchus in the mediastinum. It reaches the lung hilum before it gives rise to the branches to the lung. Aa, aortic arch; Ao, ascending aorta; MPA, main pulmonary artery; RPA, right pulmonary artery; LPA, left pulmonary artery; ao, descending aorta; SVC, superior vena cava; LUL, left upper lobar.

the right upper lobar bronchus. Therefore, the right pulmonary artery is called the hypbronchial artery, and the right upper lobar bronchus is called the eparterial bronchus. The left pulmonary artery courses backward and to the left above the left main bronchus. Therefore, the left pulmonary artery is called the epbronchial artery, and the left main bronchus is called the hyparterial bronchus. The left pulmonary artery gives rise to its first branch to the upper lobe at the pulmonary hilum. In association with the asymmetric course and branching of the right and left pulmonary arteries, the bronchial branching is also asymmetric. The left main bronchus is longer than the right main bronchus with the left/right ratio of more than 1.5.[12]

During fetal life, the ductus arteriosus is a large open channel between the roof of the main pulmonary artery near the origin of the left pulmonary artery and proximal part of the descending aorta. Within 24 to 48 hours after birth, the ductus arteriosus closes by vasoconstriction in response to increased oxygen tension.[13] Within the next

2 to 3 weeks, the ductus is completely sealed by fibrosis and remains as the ligamentum ductus.

■ Coronary Arteries

The normal coronary arterial system consists of the right and left coronary arteries and their branches. The major coronary arteries form a circle around the atrioventricular groove and a loop along the interventricular grooves.

The right coronary artery arises from the right coronary sinus and courses to the right and backward along the right atrioventricular groove (**Figs. 1.5, 1.15**). It gives rise to the following branches to the right ventricle in sequence: the conal artery, the right ventricular artery, the acute marginal artery, and posterior descending artery. The posterior descending artery gives rise to septal branches to the interventricular septum. After the right coronary artery gives rise to the posterior descending

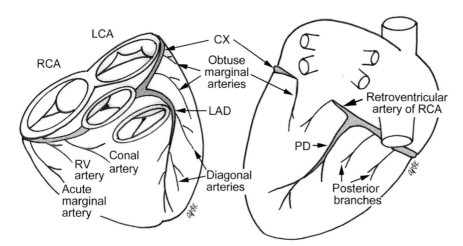

Fig. 1.15 Coronary arterial system. CX, circumflex artery; LAD, left anterior descending artery; LCA, left coronary artery; PD, posterior descending artery; RCA, right coronary artery, RV, right ventricular.

artery at the crux cordis, it continues along the left atrioventricular groove as the retroventricular artery. In 60% of hearts, the right coronary artery gives rise to the sinus nodal artery from the proximal part of the right coronary artery immediately distal to the origin of the conal artery. In the remainder, the sinus nodal artery arises from the circumflex artery. The atrioventricular nodal artery arises from the retroventricular artery.

The left coronary artery arises from the left coronary sinus and immediately bifurcates into the left anterior descending and circumflex arteries (**Figs. 1.13, 1.15**). In 20% of cases, the left coronary artery gives rise to an intermediate branch, the ramus intermedius, to the left ventricular free wall. The left anterior descending artery courses along the anterior interventricular groove and gives rise to multiple branches to the anterior wall of the left ventricle called diagonal arteries. It also gives rise to small branches to the interventricular septum called septal (perforating) branches. The circumflex artery courses along the left atrioventricular groove and gives rise to branches to the posterior wall of the left ventricle called obtuse marginal arteries. It also gives rise to small branches to the left atrium. In 10–15% of cases, the posterior descending artery is a branch of the left coronary artery. This variation is called a dominant left coronary artery. There are many variations in coronary arterial branching.[14]

Although there is tremendous variability in the coronary arterial blood supply to the myocardium, the ventricles can be segmented into areas assigned to specific coronary arterial territories. As a standard segmentation system for all cardiac imaging modalities, the American Heart Association suggested the use of the 17-myocardial segment model of the left ventricle in 2002 (**Fig. 1.16**).[15] Myocardial segments should be named and localized with reference to the long axis of the ventricle and the 360-degree circumferential locations on the short axis views. Using *basal*, *midcavity*, and *apical* as part of the name defines the location along the long axis of the ventricle from the apex to base. With regard to the circumferential location, the basal and midcavity slices should be divided into six segments of 60 degrees each (**Fig. 1.16**). The attachment of the right ventricular wall to the left ventricle should be used to identify and separate the septum from the left ventricular anterior and inferior free walls. The circumferential locations in the basal and midcavity are anterior, anteroseptal, inferoseptal, inferior, inferolateral, and anterolateral. Segments 1, 2, 7, 8, 13, 14, and 17 are assigned to the left anterior descending coronary artery distribution. Segments 3, 4, 9, 10, and 15 are assigned to the right coronary artery when it is dominant. Segments 5, 6, 11, 12, and 16 generally are assigned to the left circumflex artery. The greatest variability in myocardial blood supply occurs at the apical cap (segment 17), which can be supplied by any of the three arteries.

■ Cardiac Veins and Coronary Sinus

The venous drainage of the myocardium is through three different systems. First, the coronary sinus system drains the left ventricle (**Fig. 1.17**). The coronary sinus is a wide venous channel situated in the posterior part of the atrioventricular groove, and covered by muscular fibers from the left atrium. It ends in the right atrium between the opening of the inferior vena cava and the atrioventricular orifice. The coronary sinus orifice is usually guarded by a semilunar valve, the Thebesian valve of the coronary sinus. The coronary sinus receives the great, small, posterior, and middle cardiac veins. The great cardiac vein or left coronary vein originates at the apex of the heart and ascends along the anterior interventricular groove to reach the atrioventricular groove where it merges with the oblique vein of the left atrium (of Marshall) to form the coronary sinus. The great cardiac vein receives tributaries from both ventricles and the left atrium. As the coronary

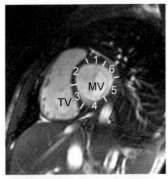
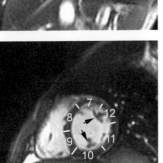
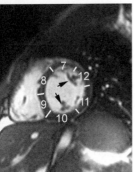
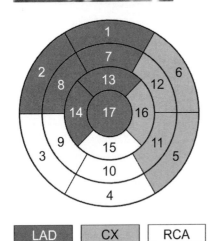

Basal
short axis view

Midcavity
short axis view

Apical
short axis view

A

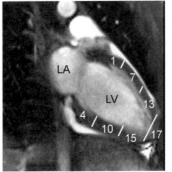
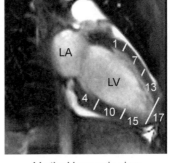

Horizontal long axis view
(4-chamber view)

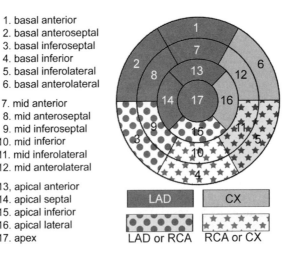

Vertical long axis view
(2-chamber view)

1. basal anterior
2. basal anteroseptal
3. basal inferoseptal
4. basal inferior
5. basal inferolateral
6. basal anterolateral

7. mid anterior
8. mid anteroseptal
9. mid inferoseptal
10. mid inferior
11. mid inferolateral
12. mid anterolateral

13. apical anterior
14. apical septal
15. apical inferior
16. apical lateral
17. apex

B

LAD | CX | RCA

C

LAD | CX
LAD or RCA | RCA or CX

Fig. 1.16 Standard 17-myocardial segmentation and nomenclature proposed by the American Heart Association in 2002.[15] **(A)** Cardiac segments seen on short axis, 4-chamber, and vertical long axis views. **(B)** Circumferential polar plot of 17 myocardial segments with the most common pattern of coronary artery territory. **(C)** Circumferential polar plot with common variations of coronary artery territory. RA, right atrium; LA, left atrium; RV, right ventricle; LV, left ventricle; TV, tricuspid valve; MV, mitral valve; CX, circumflex artery; LAD, left anterior descending artery; RCA, right coronary artery.

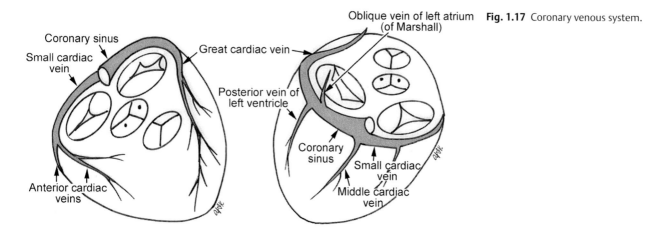

Fig. 1.17 Coronary venous system.

sinus courses along the left atrioventricular groove, it receives the posterior cardiac and middle cardiac veins. The posterior cardiac vein drains the posterior wall of the left ventricle. The middle cardiac vein originates at the apex of the heart and courses along the posterior interventricular groove to connect to the coronary sinus at the crux cordis. It drains the posterior part of the ventricles and interventricular septum. The small cardiac vein courses in the atrioventricular sulcus between the right atrium and right ventricle and opens into the terminal part of the coronary sinus or directly into the right atrium. It drains the posterior wall of the right atrium and right ventricle. The coronary sinus opens into the right atrium as mentioned earlier (**Figs. 1.6A, 1.8B**). Second, three or four anterior cardiac veins drain the anterior wall of the right ventricle. The anterior cardiac veins or their confluence may open directly into the right atrium at the right anterior part of the atrioventricular groove. Third, the Thebesian veins drain the right atrium and the base of the right ventricle. Thebesian veins are several minute veins that open directly into the right atrium or right ventricle. Readers who have a further interest in variations of the cardiac venous system are advised to refer to the references 16 and 17.

■ Systemic Veins

The internal jugular and subclavian veins merge to form the innominate (or brachiocephalic) veins bilaterally (**Fig. 1.18**). The left innominate vein courses rightward in front of the aortic arch and joins the right innominate vein to form the superior vena cava in the right superior mediastinum. The superior vena cava descends along the posterolateral aspect of the ascending aorta and in front of the distal right pulmonary artery. The azygos vein arches forward over the right main bronchus and empties into the superior vena cava.

The thoracic and abdominal wall drains into the azygos–hemiazygos venous system. The azygos–hemiazygos system is an anastomotic route between the superior and inferior vena caval systems. The azygos and hemiazygos veins are continuations of the right and left lumbar veins. Both veins ascend along the sides of the thoracic vertebral column. On the right side, the azygos vein intercepts most of the right intercostal veins and terminates in the superior vena cava. On the left side, the anatomy is more complex and variable. Commonly the eighth to twelfth left

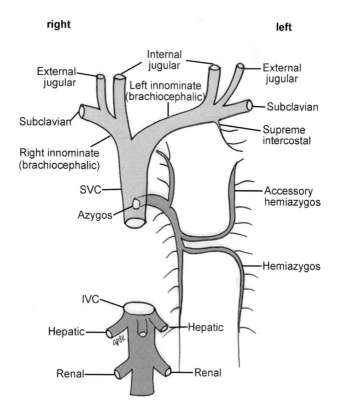

Fig. 1.18 Systemic venous system. IVC, inferior vena cava; SVC, superior vena cava

intercostal veins drain into the hemiazygos vein. In contrast to the azygos vein that directly connects to the superior vena cava, the hemiazygos vein crosses the midline in front of the spine to connect to the azygos vein. The first to third or fourth left intercostal veins make a confluence to the supreme intercostal vein that connects to the inferior surface of the left innominate vein. The rest of the left intercostal veins form a confluence to the accessory hemiazygos vein that connects to the azygos or hemiazygos vein. Pericardial and some bronchial veins also drain to the azygos–hemiazygos venous system.

The inferior vena cava receives both renal veins and hepatic veins. The suprahepatic part of the inferior vena cava traverses the diaphragm and joins the inferior surface of the right atrium.

■ Conduction System

The conduction system of the heart is the pathway for the electrical impulse from the atrial pacemaker in the right atrium to its final destination in the ventricles and the left atrium. The atrioventricular conduction pathway consists of five parts: (1) the sinus node, (2) the internodal pathways, (3) the atrioventricular node, (4) the atrioventricular bundle of His, and (5) the ventricular bundle branches (**Fig. 1.19**). The first three parts are exclusively the structures of the right atrium. The sinus node is the pacemaker. This small cigar-shaped structure is located underneath

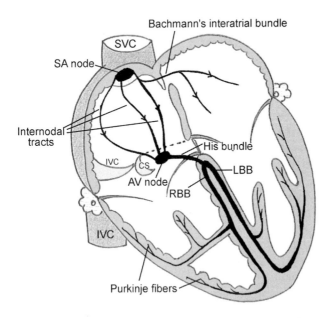

Fig. 1.19 Conduction system. AV node, atrioventricular node; CS, coronary sinus; LBB, left bundle branch; RBB, right bundle branch; SA node, sinuatrial node; SVC, superior vena cava; IVC, inferior vena cava.

the epicardium at the junction between the superior vena cava and the right atrium. The internal landmark is the transverse part of the crista terminalis. It is supplied by the sinus nodal artery that arises from the right coronary artery distal to the origin of the conal artery or less frequently from the circumflex coronary artery. The sinus node is connected to the atrioventricular node through the internodal pathways in the atrial musculature in the atrial septum and crista terminalis. The atrial impulse is gathered in the atrioventricular node located underneath the endocardium in the center of the triangle of Koch. The triangle is composed of the tendon of Todaro posterosuperiorly, the septal attachment of the tricuspid valve anteroinferiorly, and the orifice of the coronary sinus posteroinferiorly (**Fig. 1.8B**). It is supplied by the atrioventricular nodal artery, a branch of the retroventricular branch that arises from the right coronary artery or less frequently the circumflex coronary artery. The atrioventricular node extends anteriorly toward the membranous septum, which is the apex of the triangle of Koch, to become the atrioventricular bundle of His. The bundle of His courses on the muscular ventricular septal crest along the posteroinferior margin of the atrioventricular and interventricular membranous septum, which is the septal extension of the central fibrous body. At this point, the bundle of His branches, becoming the right and left bundle branches. The right bundle branch is a thin cord-like structure, which courses toward the base of the medial or conal papillary muscle in the intramyocardial position, and then descends toward the ventricular apex in the trabecula septomarginalis. It ramifies in the apex and a part of it crosses the ventricular cavity in the moderator band. The left bundle branch spreads out in fan-like fashion toward bases of the two papillary muscles of the mitral valve. As the electrical impulse reaches the ventricular myocardium, it is transmitted to the myocardial cells through the Purkinje fibers that are the specialized myocardial conduction cells. The pacemaking impulses from the sinoatrial node are conducted to the left atrial myocardium through the muscular continuity between the right and left atria, which is called Bachmann's bundle. It is most frequently found as a subendocardial bridge at the anterosuperior margin of the interatrial groove (**Fig. 1.19**).[18]

■ Pericardium

The heart and the roots of the great vessels are contained within a conical sac of pericardium. The pericardium consists of two sacs: the outer fibrous pericardium and inner serous pericardium (**Fig. 1.20**). The serous pericardium is composed of two layers of delicate membrane with a

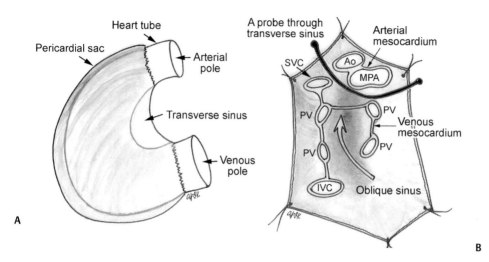

Fig. 1.20 Pericardium. **(A)** The visceral pericardial reflections at the arterial and venous poles of the heart tube are the arterial and venous mesocardium, respectively. The pericardial cavity between the arterial and venous mesocardium along the lesser curvature side of the cardiac tube is the transverse sinus. **(B)** The venous mesocardium is a complex structure that forms an inverted "u"-shaped cul-de-sac that is called the oblique sinus. Ao, ascending aorta; MPA, main pulmonary artery; PV, pulmonary vein; IVC, inferior vena cava; SVC, superior vena cava.

pericardial cavity between them. The outer layer of the serous pericardium is the parietal pericardium that is intimately connected to the fibrous pericardium. The inner layer of the serous pericardium is the visceral pericardium that covers the heart like a layer of skin and is also known as the epicardium. The adipose tissue underneath the epicardium is called epicardial fat. It tends to accumulate in the atrioventricular, interventricular, and interatrial grooves and along the acute margin of the right ventricle and the coronary branches. The pericardial cavity contains a small amount of lubricant fluid. The fibrous pericardium forms a flask-shaped bag. Its neck is closed by its fusion with the external coats of the aorta, the superior vena cava, the right and left pulmonary arteries, and the four pulmonary veins. Its base is attached to the central tendon and to the muscular fibers of the left side of the diaphragm. The inferior vena cava enters the pericardium through the central tendon of the diaphragm; therefore, it is not covered by the fibrous layer. The fibrous pericardial sac is securely anchored within the thoracic cavity by connections to the manubrium and xyphoid process anteriorly, to the deep cervical fascia posteriorly as well as attachments to the diaphragm. The outer surface of the fibrous pericardium contains a variable amount of adipose tissue that is designated pericardial fat. The visceral pericardium is reflected from the heart and the root of the great vessels onto the inner surface of the fibrous pericardium to become continuous with the parietal layer. The visceral pericardial reflection forms two separate exit routes for the vessels entering and leaving the heart (**Fig. 1.20**). The pericardial reflection enclosing the aorta and pulmonary artery is the arterial mesocardium. The reflection enclosing

the superior and inferior venae cavae and the four pulmonary veins is the venous mesocardium. The venous mesocardium is shaped like an inverted "u." The cul-de-sac enclosed between the limbs of the "u" lies behind the left atrium and is known as the oblique pericardial sinus. The portion of the pericardial cavity between the arterial and venous mesocardium is termed the transverse sinus. As the pericardial reflection extends onto the vessels, the pericardial cavity and its sinuses form various recesses including the postcaval recess, right and left pulmonary vein recesses, superior and inferior aortic recesses, and the posterior pericardial recess. Readers having further interests in the pericardial recesses are advised to refer to the reference 19.

■ Cardiovascular Anatomy in Plain Chest Radiographs

The frontal and lateral radiographs are the routine views for chest examinations (**Fig. 1.21**). In frontal radiograms, the cardiothoracic ratio, the ratio between the transverse diameter of the cardiac silhouette and the inner diameter of the thorax, is 60% or less in newborns and 50% or less in children and adults. The right side of the cardiovascular silhouette is divided into two segments. The upper segment is nearly vertical in children and young adults and is usually formed by the right innominate vein and superior vena cava. In older adults, the aorta tends to dilate and elongate so that the right upper border is formed by the ascending aorta and becomes

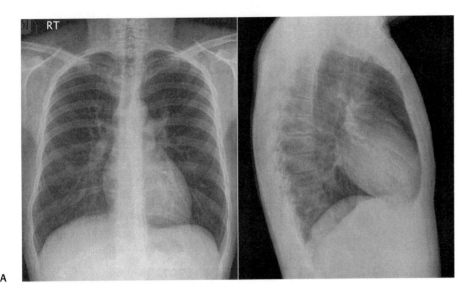

A

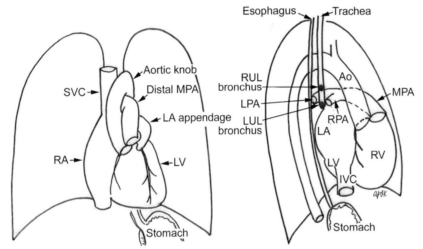

B

Fig. 1.21 (A) Chest radiographic anatomy. **(B)** Rendered drawing of chest radiographic anatomy. Ao, ascending aorta; IVC, inferior vena cava; LA, left atrium; LPA, left pulmonary artery; LUL, left upper lobar bronchus; LV, left ventricle; MPA, main pulmonary artery; RA, right atrium; RPA, right pulmonary artery; RUL, right upper lobar bronchus; RV, right ventricle; SVC, superior vena cava.

convex. The lower segment of the right heart border is usually convex and represents the lateral border of the right atrium. The left side of the cardiovascular silhouette is considered to consist of four segments. The uppermost is the rounded contour of the distal part of the aortic arch, which is continuous with the left lateral wall of the descending aorta behind the heart in the left paraspinal area. The second segment is the contour of the distal main pulmonary arterial trunk. The contour of this segment varies considerably. Usually, it is straight or slightly convex. Less often, especially in young females, this segment shows considerable convexity. The third segment is an indistinct segment of the left atrial appendage, which occupies a short segment below the pulmonary arterial segment. As the left atrial appendage does not project outward, it is not discernable unless it is enlarged or prolapsed through a defect of the adjacent parietal pericardial covering. The lowermost segment is the convex contour of the left lateral free wall of the left

ventricle. The left ventricular contour tends to be less convex and the cardiac axis more vertical with increasing degree of inspiration. The left ventricular contour tends to be more convex and the cardiac axis more horizontal in overweight individuals. The left ventricular contour forms the cardiac apex at or near the diaphragmatic silhouette. Both the right and left sides of the cardiovascular silhouette can be concealed by the overlying thymic shadow in young children.

In lateral radiographs, the cardiovascular silhouette is seen as an American football sitting obliquely on the diaphragmatic shadow. The anterior aspect of the cardiovascular silhouette consists of three segments. The uppermost segment is the slightly convex contour of the anterior wall of the ascending aorta and is usually not a distinct segment. The middle segment is a short segment of forward and upward convexity that represents the proximal part of the main pulmonary arterial trunk. The lowermost segment is formed by the right ventricle that leads to the main pulmonary arterial trunk. Inferiorly, most of this segment is in direct contact with the sternum. Only the subpulmonary part of the right ventricular outflow forms a visible convex contour that is continuous with the main pulmonary arterial trunk. The posterior side of the cardiovascular silhouette consists of two segments. The upper segment is the slightly convex contour of the left atrium. The lower segment is the convex contour of the posterior wall of the left ventricle. As the left ventricular contour intersects the diaphragmatic silhouette, an acute angle is formed between the two silhouettes. In the well-taken lateral radiogram, this acute angle is filled with the web-like shadow of the inferior vena cava.

The hilar anatomy seen in the frontal radiograph is asymmetric with the left pulmonary artery being located slightly higher than the right pulmonary artery. The left pulmonary artery is seen above the angle formed by the left main bronchus and its upper lobar bronchus. The descending branch of the right pulmonary artery is seen below the angle formed by the right main bronchus and its upper lobar bronchus. In well-taken frontal radiograms, the discrepancy in length between the right and left main bronchi can be appreciated. In the lateral radiogram, the structures of the pulmonary hila are seen behind and above the left atrial contour. The right and left upper lobar bronchi are seen as round circles that are arranged superoinferiorly. As the right pulmonary artery has a transverse course in the mediastinum in front of the right main bronchus, it is seen in front of the round lucent circles of the upper lobar bronchi. The left pulmonary artery is seen above and behind the left upper lobar bronchial shadow.

It is important to be familiar with a normal pulmonary vascular pattern. The pulmonary vascularity should be symmetric. One may feel that the pulmonary vascularity is less prominent in the left lung than in the right lung. This faulty impression is due to the fact that the cardiac silhouette overlaps a significant part of the left lower lung. Unfortunately, there are no available normal ranges for the size of the pulmonary vessels for various age groups. As a rule of thumb, the diameter of the descending branch of the right pulmonary artery is approximately equal to the diameter of the trachea within the thorax. It is also important to be familiar with the size of the pulmonary arteries seen on a lateral view.

The right and left posterior or anterior oblique views of the chest are rarely obtained now.

References

1. Anderson RH, Ho SY. Sequential segmental analysis – description and categorization for the millennium. Cardiol Young 1997;7:98–116
2. Anderson RH, Becker AE, Van Mierop LH. What should we call the 'crista'? Br Heart J 1977;39(8):856–859
3. Kosiński A, Nowiński J, Kozłowski D, Piwko G, Kuta W, Grzybiak M. The crista supraventricularis in the human heart and its role in the morphogenesis of the septomarginal trabecula. Ann Anat 2007;189(5):447–456
4. Marom EM, Herndon JE, Kim YH, McAdams HP. Variations in pulmonary venous drainage to the left atrium: implications for radiofrequency ablation. Radiology 2004;230(3):824–829
5. Uemura H, Ho SY, Devine WA, Kilpatrick LL, Anderson RH. Atrial appendages and venoatrial connections in hearts from patients with visceral heterotaxy. Ann Thorac Surg 1995;60(3):561–569
6. Anderson RH, Brown NA, Webb S. Development and structure of the atrial septum. Heart 2002;88(1):104–110
7. Ho SY, Anderson RH. How constant anatomically is the tendon of Todaro as a marker for the triangle of Koch? J Cardiovasc Electrophysiol 2000;11(1):83–89
8. Hagen PT, Scholz DG, Edwards WD. Incidence and size of patent foramen ovale during the first 10 decades of life: an autopsy study of 965 normal hearts. Mayo Clin Proc 1984;59(1):17–20
9. Meissner I, Whisnant JP, Khandheria BK, et al. Prevalence of potential risk factors for stroke assessed by transesophageal echocardiography and carotid ultrasonography: the SPARC study. Stroke Prevention: Assessment of Risk in a Community. Mayo Clin Proc 1999;74(9):862–869
10. Becker AE, Anderson RH. Atrioventricular septal defects: What's in a name? J Thorac Cardiovasc Surg 1982;83(3):461–469
11. Anderson RH, Ho SY, Becker AE. Anatomy of the human atrioventricular junctions revisited. Anat Rec 2000;260(1):81–91
12. Deanfield JE, Leanage R, Stroobant J, Chrispin AR, Taylor JF, Macartney FJ. Use of high kilovoltage filtered beam radiographs for detection of bronchial situs in infants and young children. Br Heart J 1980;44(5):577–583
13. Schneider DJ, Moore JW. Patent ductus arteriosus. Circulation 2006;114(17):1873–1882
14. Cademartiri F, La Grutta L, Malagò R, et al. Prevalence of anatomical variants and coronary anomalies in 543 consecutive patients studied with 64-slice CT coronary angiography. Eur Radiol 2008;18(4):781–791
15. Cerqueira MD, Weissman NJ, Dilsizian V, et al; American Heart Association Writing Group on Myocardial Segmentation and Registration for Cardiac Imaging. Standardized myocardial segmentation and nomenclature for tomographic imaging of the heart: a statement for healthcare professionals from the Cardiac Imaging Committee of the Council on Clinical Cardiology of the American Heart Association. Circulation 2002;105(4):539–542
16. Jongbloed MR, Lamb HJ, Bax JJ, et al. Noninvasive visualization of the cardiac venous system using multislice computed tomography. J Am Coll Cardiol 2005;45(5):749–753
17. Chiribiri A, Kelle S, Götze S, et al. Visualization of the cardiac venous system using cardiac magnetic resonance. Am J Cardiol 2008;101(3):407–412
18. Saremi F, Channual S, Krishnan S, Gurudevan SV, Narula J, Abolhoda A. Bachmann Bundle and its arterial supply: imaging with multidetector CT—implications for interatrial conduction abnormalities and arrhythmias. Radiology 2008;248(2):447–457
19. Broderick LS, Brooks GN, Kuhlman JE. Anatomic pitfalls of the heart and pericardium. Radiographics 2005;25(2):441–453

2 Sequential Segmental Approach to Congenital Heart Disease

Morphologically, malformations affecting the heart can be categorized into two broad categories. The first category is the malformations affecting the heart in which the cardiac chambers and the great arteries are normally related and connected. Typical examples are septal defects and valvular stenosis. The second category includes more complex malformations that are characterized by an abnormal relationship between the components of a segment or segments and abnormal connections between cardiac segments. Examples include various forms of so-called single ventricles or univentricular hearts, complete and corrected transposition of the great arteries, and double-outlet ventricles. These complex malformations require a systematic analysis in a step-by-step fashion that is called the sequential segmental approach.[1–6] The concept of sequential segmental approach was first introduced by Van Praagh et al in 1964.[7] Since then, there have been discussions and debates regarding the system of segmental analysis and its terminology. The most intense and serious debates have been between Richard Van Praagh of Boston, Massachusetts, and Robert H. Anderson of London, UK. Unfortunately, the debates have polarized the pediatric cardiology group into two schools, Van Praaghnians and Andersonians. On reading the published book chapters and articles regarding this important subject, one may be overwhelmed by the semantic controversies and debates. In this chapter, we will introduce the compromised system and terms that we find most useful in day-to-day clinical practice without discussion of the scholastic origins of the terms.

■ Basic Cardiac Segments and Steps of Sequential Segmental Analysis

As discussed in Chapter 1, the heart consists of three morphologically and functionally distinct segments: the atria, the ventricles, and the arterial trunks (**Fig. 2.1**). They are joined together by two connecting units, the atrioventricular junction and the ventriculoarterial junction, both of which are usually guarded by the valves. Each component of each segment of the heart is characterized by its own morphologic characteristics. The components of each segment

can be related in various ways, and the components of a segment can be connected to the components of the next segment in various ways. Therefore, there are three facets in the make-up of the heart: the *morphologies*, the *connections*, and the *relations*.[6] Sequential segmental analysis is the systematic approach to the diagnosis of congenital heart disease in which the three facets of the make-up in the heart are analyzed in a segment-by-segment fashion. The major steps of sequential segmental approach include (**Fig. 2.2**)

1. Determination of the visceral situs and cardiac position
2. Morphologic identification of the cardiac chambers and great arteries
3. Analysis of the connections and the relations
   a. Determination of the atrial situs
   b. Evaluation of the atrioventricular connections and ventricular relationship
   c. Evaluation of the ventriculoarterial connections and great arterial relationship
4. Evaluation of the associated anomalies at each segment

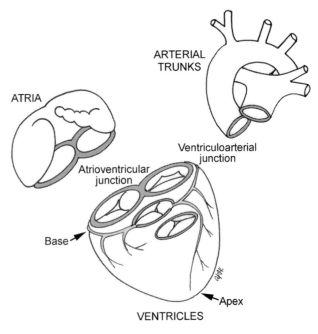

Fig. 2.1 Basic cardiac segments and intervening junctions.

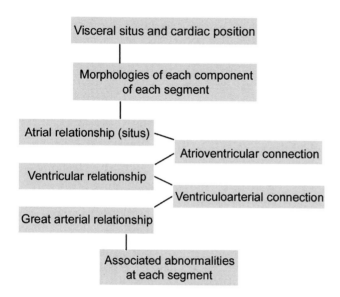

Fig. 2.2 Steps of the sequential segmental approach.

■ Determination of the Visceral Situs and Cardiac Position

Congenital heart disease is common and usually complex when the visceral situs is abnormal or the heart is abnormally positioned. As will be discussed later in this chapter, the visceral situs is highly predictive of the atrial situs, which is called the visceroatrial concordance rule. Therefore, the visceral situs should be determined as the first step of a segmental approach.

The visceral situs is classified into the situs solitus, situs inversus, and heterotaxy. In situs solitus, the larger lobe of the liver is seen on the right, and the stomach and spleen are seen on the left (**Fig. 2.3**). The abdominal aorta is located posteriorly at the left anterior aspect of the spine, and the inferior vena cava is located more anteriorly on the right as it connects to the right atrium. In situs inversus, this right–left relationship is reversed. Rarely, the arrangement of the abdominal organs does not conform to the orderly and lateralized pattern of the situs solitus or the situs inversus. This condition is called visceral heterotaxy.[3,4] Usually visceral heterotaxy is associated with either polysplenia or asplenia. It is important,

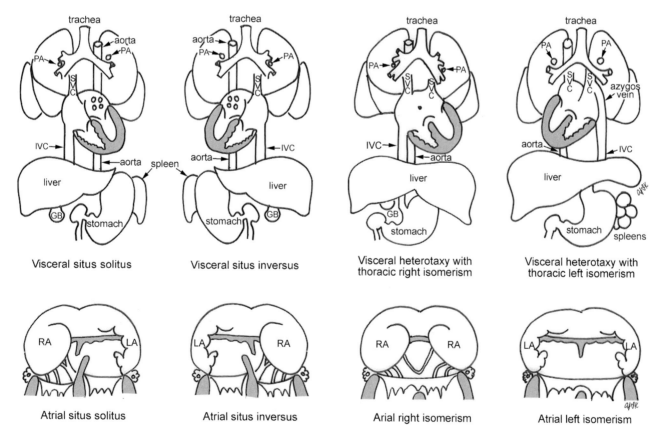

Fig. 2.3 Types of visceral and atrial situs. PA, pulmonary artery; SVC, superior vena cava ; IVC, inferior vena cava; GB, gallbladder; RA, right atrium; LA, left atrium.

therefore, to evaluate the splenic status by scrutinizing the perigastric area when the abdominal situs is neither solitus nor inversus. In polysplenia, multiple spleens of similar size are seen behind the stomach as they are aggregated on both sides of the mesogastrium. Occasionally, multiple spleens may be fused to form a single but multi-lobulated mass. Polysplenia is commonly associated with interruption of the suprarenal segment of the inferior vena cava with continuation through the azygos or hemi-azygos venous system. Although it can also occur with any other body situs, interruption is highly suggestive of polysplenia.[8,9] In most cases of asplenia, the abdominal aorta and inferior vena cava are juxtaposed on the same side of the spine.[8–10] In the thorax, visceral heterotaxy is characterized by a symmetric lobation of the lungs and a symmetric branching pattern of the bronchi and pulmonary arteries. Visceral heterotaxy with asplenia is typically associated with a right isomeric arrangement of the lungs, bronchi, and pulmonary arteries, whereas visceral heterotaxy with polysplenia is usually associated with a left isomeric arrangement.

The cardiac positions are classified into levocardia, dextrocardia, and mesocardia according to where the main part of the heart is located relative to the midline (**Fig. 2.4**). With rare exceptions, the main part of the heart is positioned on the side where the cardiac apex is located. In mesocardia, the cardiac apex may point to the right, left, or midline. These terms should not be used for those conditions where the heart is displaced to either side secondary to a noncardiac pathology such as hypoplasia or hyperinflation of a lung. Complex terms, such as dextroversion, levoversion, and dextroposition should be abandoned.

■ Morphologic Identification of the Cardiac Chambers and Great Arteries

After determination of the visceral situs and cardiac position, the cardiac chambers and great arteries are identified according to the morphologic characteristics. In this regard, one should be aware that the adjectives "right" and "left" for the cardiac chambers are not to describe the sidedness within the body, but to describe the morphology of the atria and ventricles. Therefore, the atrium that is located on the right, but shows the morphologic characters of the normal left atrium should be called "the right-sided (morphologically) left atrium." The morphologic criteria for atrial, ventricular, and great arterial identification are discussed in Chapter 1 and summarized in **Tables 2.1, 2.2, 2.3**.

■ Analysis of the Segmental Connections and Relations

Determination of the Atrial Situs

The atrial situs means how the atria are related to each other relative to the midline. It is categorized into the situs solitus, situs inversus, right isomerism, and left isomerism (**Fig. 2.3**). As discussed, determination of the atrial situs is based on the morphology of the atrial appendages and the extent of the pectinate muscles relative to the atrioventricular junction.[11] Although these criteria are easy to apply at pathologic examination, they are often inapplicable during

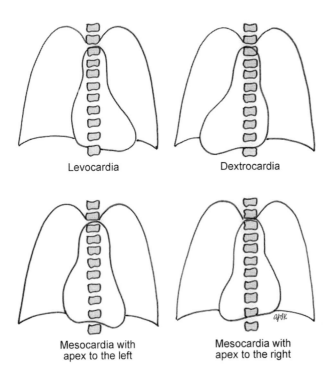

Levocardia

Dextrocardia

Mesocardia with apex to the left

Mesocardia with apex to the right

Fig. 2.4 Cardiac positions.

Table 2.1 Morphologic Criteria for Identification of the Right and Left Atria

	Right Atrium	Left Atrium
Sulcus and crista terminalis	Yes	No
Appendage	Triangular	Finger-like
Appendageal orifice	Wide	Narrow
Extent of pectinate muscles	Extend to the atrioventricular junction	Do not extend to the atrioventricular junction
Fossa ovalis with limbus	Yes	No

Table 2.2 Morphologic Criteria for Identification of the Right and Left Ventricles

	Right Ventricle	Left Ventricle
Trabeculation	Heavy and irregular	Fine and relatively regular
Trabecular septomarginalis	Yes	No
Moderator band	Yes	No
Septal attachment of the atrioventricular valve	More apical	More cranial

Table 2.3 Morphologic Criteria for Identification of the Great Arteries

	Aorta	Main Pulmonary Artery	Common Truncus
Gives rise to	Coronary arteries	Branch pulmonary arteries	Coronary arteries
	Systemic arteries		Systemic arteries
			Branch pulmonary arteries

diagnostic imaging of living individuals. It is well known, however, that the atrial situs is harmonious with the visceral situs in the majority of cases. Therefore, the atrial situs can be accurately predicted by analyzing the bronchial branching pattern and splenic situs. Lastly, it should be emphasized that an atrioventricular block in the presence of structural heart disease is highly suggestive of left atrial isomerism.[12]

Evaluation of the Atrioventricular Connection and Ventricular Relationship

The patterns of how the atria are connected to the underlying ventricles or ventricle are divided into biventricular and univentricular connections (**Fig. 2.5**).[2,5,6] Biventricular atrioventricular connection refers to one-to-one connection between the atria and ventricles; univentricular connection refers to two-to-one connection. Both atria are connected to a ventricle regardless of whether there are only one or two ventricles. When one or both atrioventricular valves override the ventricular septum, this

simple rule does not work. In this rather uncommon situation, a "50% rule" is applied: the atrium is judged to connect to the ventricle that takes more than half of the area of its atrioventricular valve (**Fig. 2.6**).

When there are two ventricles, the ventricular relation is described as either D-loop or L-loop (**Fig. 2.7**). D-loop denotes the ventricular relationship in which the right ventricle is located to the right of the left ventricle, which is considered as the consequence of D-looping of the straight heart tube in early embryogenesis. L-loop denotes the ventricular relationship in which the right ventricle is located to the left of the left ventricle, which is considered as the consequence of L-looping of the embryonic heart. The ventricles of either D- or L-loop can be related side-by-side, anteroposterior or superoinferior fashion.

Biventricular atrioventricular connection is either concordant or discordant when there is atrial situs solitus or

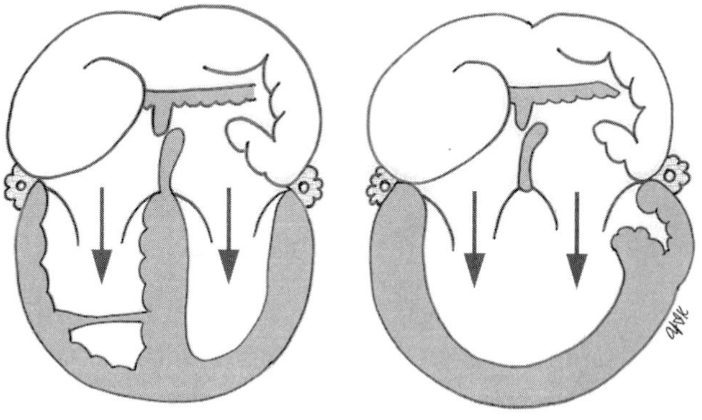

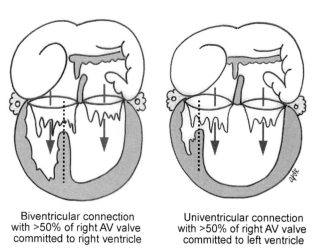

Biventricular connection with >50% of right AV valve committed to right ventricle

Univentricular connection with >50% of right AV valve committed to left ventricle

Fig. 2.6 Biventricular versus univentricular atrioventricular connection. When an atrioventricular (AV) valve overrides the ventricular septum, the "50%" rule is applied.

Biventricular connection   Univentricular connection

Fig. 2.5 Biventricular versus univentricular atrioventricular connection.

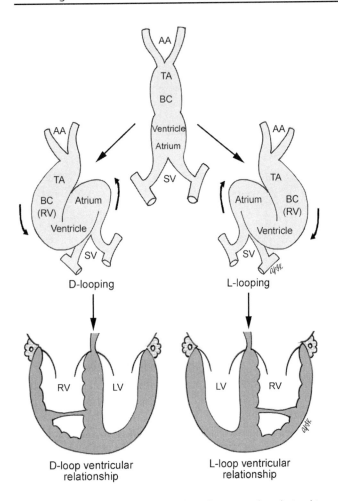

Fig. 2.7 Types of ventricular relationship: The ventricular relationship with the morphologically right ventricle (RV) on the right side of the morphologically left ventricle (LV) is called a D-loop ventricular relationship because it is a consequence of rightward looping of the straight heart tube during embryogenesis. The reversed relationship is called an L-loop relationship as it is a consequence of leftward looping of the heart tube. AA, aortic arches; BC, bulbus cordis; SV, sinus venosus; TA, truncus arteriosus.

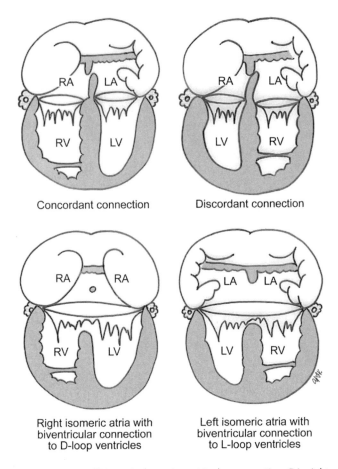

Fig. 2.8 Types of biventricular atrioventricular connection. RA, right atrium; LA, left atrium; RV, right ventricle; LV, left ventricle.

situs inversus (**Fig. 2.8**, upper panels). The biventricular connection in the setting of right or left isomerism is, however, neither concordant nor discordant. Traditionally, these have been described as an "ambiguous connection."[2,5] Nevertheless, the atrioventricular connections in these particular situations are not ambiguous. Instead, they simply need a long, but proper description (**Fig. 2.8**, lower panels).[6]

Univentricular atrioventricular connection includes double inlet ventricles and the absence of one atrioventricular connection (**Fig. 2.9**). A double inlet connection implies that both atria are connected to the same ventricular chamber through separate atrioventricular valves or a common valve. Therefore, this ventricle has two inlets. An absent atrioventricular connection implies that one atrium and the underlying ventricle are separated by the

intervening atrioventricular sulcus tissue. The only outlet of that atrium is the interatrial septal defect or patent foramen ovale. Therefore, there is only one atrioventricular valve that connects to the ventricular mass. The absence of an atrioventricular connection may affect the right or left side. The absence of the right or left atrioventricular connection is different from an imperforate right or left atrioventricular valve, although the hemodynamic consequence is the same. Conceptually, there is a potential biventricular connection in the latter.

The ventricular mass in hearts with a univentricular atrioventricular connection usually consists of two ventricles: one dominant and the other rudimentary. The dominant ventricle may be the morphologically right or left. Uncommonly, only one ventricular chamber of indeterminate morphology is found. Therefore, the univentricular connection may be to a dominant right or left ventricle or to a solitary and indeterminate ventricle (**Fig. 2.10**). When there is a univentricular connection, it is often difficult to identify the morphologic characteristics of the right and left ventricles. In this setting, the morphology of the ventricles

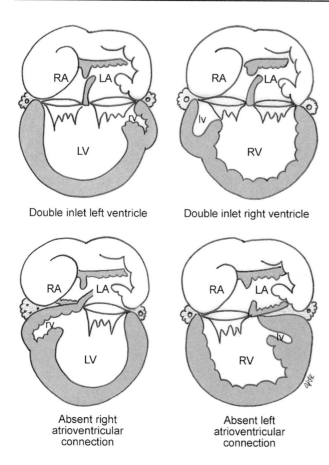

Fig. 2.9 Types of univentricular atrioventricular connection. RA, right atrium; LA, left atrium; RV, right ventricle; LV, left ventricle.

can be defined just by observing where the rudimentary chamber is located. The presence of the rudimentary ventricular chamber at the anterior and superior aspect of the main ventricular chamber indicates that the main ventricular chamber is the morphologically left ventricle (**Fig. 2.10**, upper panel). On the contrary, the presence of the rudimentary ventricular chamber at the posterior and inferior corner of the main chamber indicates that the main ventricular chamber is the morphologically right ventricle (**Fig. 2.10**, two left diagrams in lower panel). In other words, the position of the rudimentary chamber relative to the crux cordis determines whether it is the morphologically right or left ventricle. The rudimentary left ventricle is located at either corner of the crux cordis; the rudimentary right ventricle is not directly related to the crux cordis. When only one ventricle is present, it is hard to determine the morphology of the ventricle.

When there is a biventricular atrioventricular connection, each atrium is connected to the ventricle on the same side and the blood flow axes from the atria to the ventricular apices are parallel to each other. Uncommonly, the cardiac chambers and great arteries show unexpected spatial relationship for the given segmental connections, and the atrioventricular blood flow axes spiral each other. The abnormal spatial relationship and spiral atrioventricular connection in this condition can be understood if the heart is assumed to be twisted around the base-apex cardiac axis by a hand placed on the cardiac apex (**Fig. 2.11**).[13,14] Usually, the twisting occurs in a clockwise

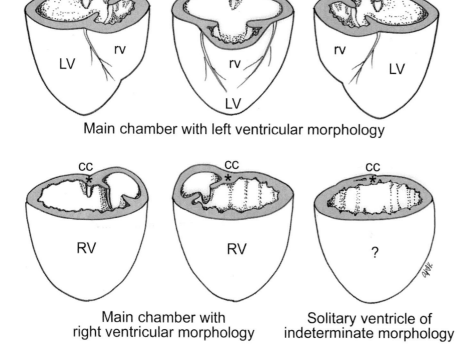

Main chamber with left ventricular morphology

Main chamber with right ventricular morphology

Solitary ventricle of indeterminate morphology

Fig. 2.10 Morphology of the ventricles in hearts with univentricular atrioventricular connection. When the rudimentary chamber is located anterior to the main ventricular chamber and therefore is away from the crux cordis (cc), the rudimentary chamber is the morphologically right ventricle, and the main chamber is the morphologically left ventricle. When the rudimentary chamber of the left ventricular chamber is located posteroinferiorly at either side of the crux cordis, the rudimentary chamber is the morphologically left ventricle, and the main chamber is the morphologically right ventricle. When only one chamber is present, the morphology is hard to define. cc, crux cordis; rv, rudimentary right ventricle; RV, right ventricle; LV, left ventricle.

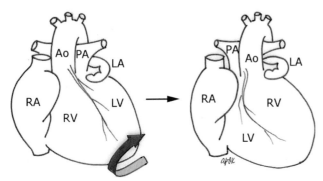

Clockwise twisting in a heart with D-loop ventricles

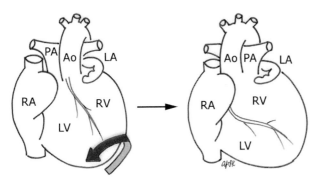

Conterclockwise twisting in a heart with L-loop ventricles

Fig. 2.11 Twisted atrioventricular connections in complete (upper panel) and congenitally corrected (lower panel) transpositions of the great arteries. RA, right atrium; LA, left atrium; RV, right ventricle; LV, left ventricle; Ao, ascending aorta; PA, pulmonary artery.

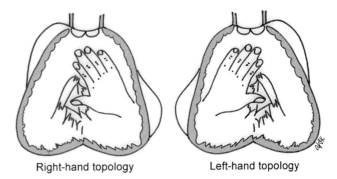

Right-hand topology   Left-hand topology

Fig. 2.12 Ventricular topology. The palmar surface of the hand is placed on the right ventricular septal surface with the wrist on the apex, the thumb in the atrioventricular valve and the fingers in the ventriculoarterial valve. In right-hand topology, the right ventricular septum accepts the palm of the right hand. In left-hand topology, the right ventricular septum accepts the palm of the left hand.

or counterclockwise direction that places the right ventricle superiorly. Therefore, the ventricles are superoinferiorly related in most cases with twisted atrioventricular connection.[15] With further twisting, the atrioventricular connection may appear criss-crossed.[16,17] To determine the ventricular relationship in this condition, one should mentally untwist the twisted connection. One can utilize the concept of so-called chirality or ventricular topology for this purpose instead of mentally reconstructing the untwisted status.[6] This concept works well if one has a pathologic specimen in one's hand, but is very difficult to apply during image interpretation or at surgery. This concept is introduced here not necessarily for improved understanding, but for the sake of completeness of the information. In this concept, the internal organization of the right ventricle is determined by placing the palm of the observer's right or left hand on the ventricular septum with the thumb in the inlet, the fingers in the outlet, and the wrist in the apical part (**Fig. 2.12**). If the septum of the morphologic right ventricle accepts the observer's right hand as in a normal D-loop ventricle, the ventricular

topology is defined as a right-hand pattern. If the septum of the morphologically right ventricle accepts the observer's left hand as in classic corrected transposition, the ventricular topology is defined as a left-hand pattern. The atrioventricular connection is predictive of the ventricular topology in the majority of cases. Very rarely, the atrioventricular connections are not harmonious with the ventricular topology.[18] Also very rarely, a twisted connection may be associated with double inlet ventricles.[19]

Evaluation of the Ventriculoarterial Connections and Great Arterial Relationship

In the presence of two ventricles and two arterial trunks arising from the heart, the ventriculoarterial connection is classified into concordant, discordant, or double outlet from right ventricle and double-outlet left ventricle (**Fig. 2.13**).[1–6] A concordant ventriculoarterial connection indicates that the morphologically right ventricle gives rise to the main pulmonary artery and the morphologically left ventricle gives rise to the aorta. A discordant ventriculoarterial connection indicates that the morphologically right ventricle gives rise to the aorta and the morphologically left ventricle gives rise to the main pulmonary artery. "Discordant ventriculoarterial connection" is synonymous with "transposition of the great arteries." Complete transposition denotes discordant ventriculoarterial connection in the presence of concordant atrioventricular connection. Congenitally corrected transposition denotes discordant ventriculoarterial connection in the presence of a discordant atrioventricular connection in which a wrong connection at one level is congenitally corrected by a wrong connection at another level. A double-outlet ventricle

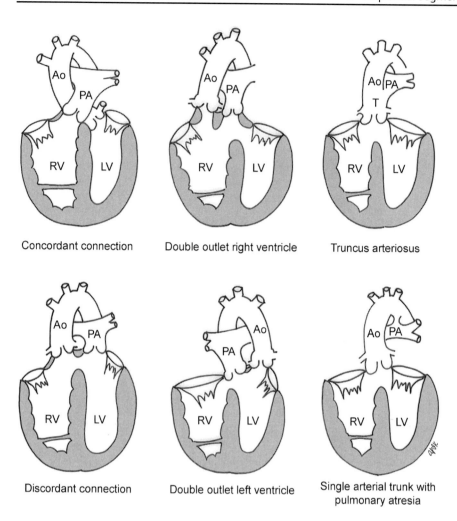

Fig. 2.13 Types of ventriculoarterial connections. RV, right ventricle; LV, left ventricle; Ao, ascending aorta; PA, pulmonary artery; T, truncus arteriosus.

Concordant connection

Double outlet right ventricle

Truncus arteriosus

Discordant connection

Double outlet left ventricle

Single arterial trunk with pulmonary atresia

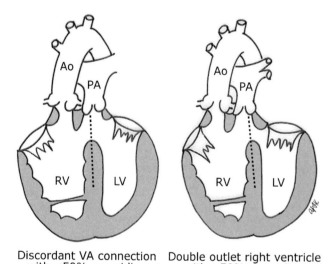

Discordant VA connection with <50% overriding pulmonary valve

Double outlet right ventricle with >50% overriding pulmonary valve

Fig. 2.14 Double-outlet versus concordant or discordant connection. When a ventriculoarterial valve overrides the ventricular septum, 50% rule is applied. RV, right ventricle; LV, left ventricle; Ao, ascending aorta; PA, pulmonary artery.

denotes the origin of both the aorta and the main pulmonary artery from the right or left ventricle. When one or both semilunar valves override the ventricular septum, a "50% rule" is applied: the valve is assigned to the ventricle that supports the greater part of its circumference (**Fig. 2.14**).

The great arterial relationship is described by defining the position of the aorta relative to the pulmonary artery at the semilunar valve level (**Fig. 2.15**).

When there is only one arterial trunk, it may be either a truncus arteriosus or a single arterial trunk (**Fig. 2.13**, right hand panels). Truncus arteriosus is defined as the arterial trunk that gives rise to the aorta, pulmonary arteries, and coronary arteries. In contrast, single arterial trunk denotes a condition in which one arterial trunk is absent. This condition occurs exclusively in the tetralogy of Fallot with pulmonary atresia in which the main pulmonary artery is not formed.

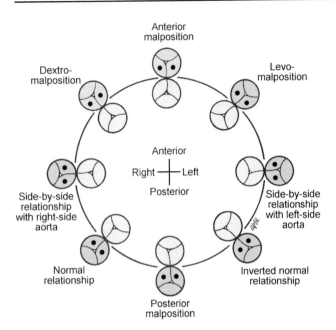

Fig. 2.15 Types of great arterial relationship. The position of the aortic valve relative to the pulmonary valve is described.

■ Evaluation of the Associated Anomalies at Each Segment

Once the segmental connections and relations have been determined, each cardiac chamber and each great artery should be examined to evaluate the associated anomalies. The systemic and pulmonary venous connections to the atria, the integrity of the atrial and ventricular septa, the presence of any obstructive lesion within the ventricles, the anatomy and function of the cardiac valves, and the patency of the pulmonary arteries and aortic arch should be catalogued.

References

1. Van Praagh R. The segmental approach to diagnosis in congenital heart disease. Birth Defects Orig Artic Ser 1972;8:4–23
2. Shinebourne EA, Macartney FJ, Anderson RH. Sequential chamber localization—logical approach to diagnosis in congenital heart disease. Br Heart J 1976;38(4):327–340
3. Stanger P, Rudolph AM, Edwards JE. Cardiac malpositions. An overview based on study of sixty-five necropsy specimens. Circulation 1977; 56(2):159–172
4. Van Praagh R. Terminology of congenital heart disease. Glossary and commentary. Circulation 1977;56(2):139–143
5. Anderson RH, Ho SY. Sequential segmental analysis—description and categorization for the millennium. Cardiol Young 1997;7: 98–116
6. Anderson RH. Terminology. In: Anderson RH, Baker EJ, Macartney FJ, Rigby ML, Shinebourne EA, Tynan M, eds. Paediatric Cardiology. 2nd ed. Edinburgh: Churchill Livingstone; 2002:19–36
7. Van Praagh R, Ongley PA, Swan HJ. Anatomic types of single or common ventricle in man. Morphologic and geometric aspects of 60 necropsied cases. Am J Cardiol 1964;13:367–386
8. Tonkin IL, Tonkin AK. Visceroatrial situs abnormalities: sonographic and computed tomographic appearance. AJR Am J Roentgenol 1982; 138(3):509–515
9. Huhta JC, Smallhorn JF, Macartney FJ. Two dimensional echocardiographic diagnosis of situs. Br Heart J 1982;48(2):97–108
10. Elliott LP, Cramer GG, Amplatz K. The anomalous relationship of the interior vena cava and abdominal aorta as a specific angiocardiographic sign in asplenia. Radiology 1966;87(5):859–863
11. Uemura H, Ho SY, Devine WA, Kilpatrick LL, Anderson RH. Atrial appendages and venoatrial connections in hearts from patients with visceral heterotaxy. Ann Thorac Surg 1995;60(3):561–569
12. Ho SY, Fagg N, Anderson RH, Cook A, Allan L. Disposition of the atrioventricular conduction tissues in the heart with isomerism of the atrial appendages: its relation to congenital complete heart block. J Am Coll Cardiol 1992;20(4):904–910
13. Seo J-W, Yoo S-J, Ho SY, Lee HJ, Anderson RH. Further morphological consideration on heart with twisted atrioventricular connection ("criss-cross hearts"). Cardiovasc Pathol 1991;1:211–217
14. Yoo S-J, Seo J-W, Lim T-H, et al. Hearts with twisted atrioventricular connections: findings at MR imaging. Radiology 1993;188(1):109–113
15. Van Praagh S, LaCorte M, Fellows KE, et al. Supero-inferior ventricles: anatomic and angiocardiographic findings in ten postmortem cases. In: Van Praagh R, Takao A, eds. Etiology and Morphogenesis of Congenital Heart Disease. Mount Kisco, NY: Futura,1980; 317–378
16. Anderson RH. Criss-cross hearts revisited. Pediatr Cardiol 1982;3(4): 305–313
17. Anderson RH, Smith A, Wilkinson JL. Disharmony between atrioventricular connections and segmental combinations: unusual variants of "crisscross" hearts. J Am Coll Cardiol 1987;10(6):1274–1277
18. Seo JW, Choe GY, Chi JG. An unusual ventricular loop associated with right juxtaposition of the atrial appendages. Int J Cardiol 1989;25(2): 219–228, discussion 229–233
19. Kim TH, Yoo S-J, Ho SY, Anderson RH. Twisted atrioventricular connections in double inlet right ventricle: evaluation by magnetic resonance imaging. Cardiol Young 2000;10(6):567–573

3 Basic Cardiac Function and Hemodynamics

Derek Wong and Shi-Joon Yoo

Correct anatomic diagnosis of specific congenital heart lesions is only the beginning of patient management. As important, if not more important, is the assessment of the patient's hemodynamic state and the status of their heart function. Such assessments are ongoing as these states can change with time, sometimes rapidly. A basic understanding of cardiac function and its applicability to various specific heart lesions is beyond the scope of this book. However, a basic understanding of cardiac function and the various modalities used in its assessment, their advantages, disadvantages and limitations, is vital toward communication with other health care professionals involved in the management of such complex patients.

■ The Cardiac Cycle

Traditionally, and for the purposes of this chapter, the cardiac cycle has been described for the function of the left ventricle, but similar events also occur within the right ventricle. The cardiac cycle typically is divided arbitrarily into two discrete phases – systole (the period during which there is ventricular contraction) and diastole (the period during which the ventricle is relaxing). The beginning of the cardiac cycle has been described from the onset of electrical activation of the ventricle, or ventricular depolarization (**Fig. 3.1**).

Systole itself is divided further into two stages. During early systole, the ventricle has begun the process of contraction. The pressure within the ventricle rises and increases beyond the pressure within the atrium, which causes the mitral valve to close. However, the pressure within the ventricle has not exceeded the aortic pressure and the aortic valve remains closed. As the ventricle continues to contract the pressure within the ventricle rises without any net movement of blood into or out of the ventricle. Therefore, the volume of the ventricle remains the same and this period of systole is referred to as isovolumetric contraction.

With further contraction, the pressure within the ventricle exceeds the aortic pressure and the aortic valve opens. The ventricular volume falls as the ventricle ejects blood into the aorta and this period of systole is referred to as ventricular ejection.

The onset of diastole is traditionally marked by the closure of the aortic valve and subsequent decrease in ventricular pressure. Diastole is also further divided into two stages. During early diastole, the pressure in the ventricle is less than the aortic pressure, but greater than the atrial pressure. Therefore, both the aortic and mitral valves remain closed as the ventricle relaxes and there is no net flow of blood into or out of the ventricle. This period of diastole is known as isovolumetric relaxation.

The next stage of diastole results in the filling of the ventricle with blood. As the ventricular pressure decreases below atrial pressure, the mitral valve opens. Filling of the ventricle occurs in two discrete phases. During the first phase, there is passive filling of the ventricle due to the pressure difference between the atrium and the ventricle. Blood flows into the ventricle, until the pressure difference across the mitral valve is eliminated. Following passive filling, there is atrial contraction, which raises the pressure in the atrium and allows for further filling of the ventricle. The blood flow waves through the mitral valve during passive filling and atrial systole are called E wave and A wave, respectively. Typically, two thirds of the ventricular stroke volume is filled during the passive filling stage, and one third with atrial contraction. When the heart rate is low, the mitral inflow ceases after the E wave until the atrium contracts to produce an A wave. This period is called diastasis. When the heart rate is high, the A wave starts before the E wave reaches the baseline and therefore a period of diastasis is not present. With a very high heart rate, the E and A waves may merge to produce a single peak. It is worthwhile to know that the cardiac cycle is shortened mostly at the expense of the diastolic filling period (**Fig. 3.2**).

After the atria contract, a new cardiac cycle is started with ventricular depolarization and initiation of ventricular contraction. Ventricular depolarization causes an influx of calcium ions into the myocyte from the sarcoplasmic reticulum. Calcium influx results in shortening of the actin–myosin cross-bridges and leads to myocardial contraction. During diastole, calcium is removed from the intracellular cytosol through an energy-dependent calcium pump and the decrease in intracellular calcium causes ventricular relaxation. Therefore, it should be noted that ventricular contraction and relaxation are both energy-dependent processes and that relaxation is not a passive process.

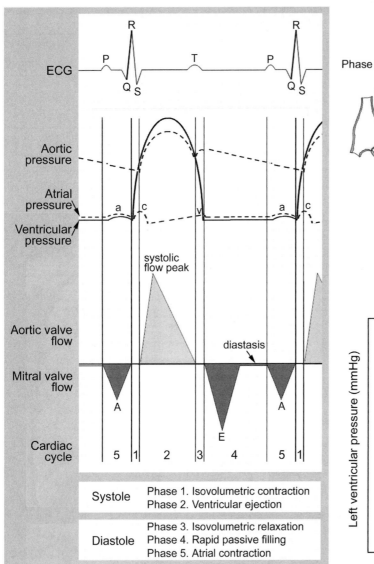

Fig. 3.1 Composite diagrams showing cardiac phases in pressure tracing, spectral Doppler flow curves, and a pressure-volume loop. In the atrial pressure wave, the a wave is due to atrial contraction, the c wave is associated with onset of ventricular systole, and the v wave is associated with atrial filling during systole. The blood flow through the atrioventricular valve consists of two peaks, E and A waves. The E wave is associated with early passive filling during ventricular relaxation, and the A wave is due to atrial contraction. When the heart rate is slow, the E and A waves are interposed by a period of cessation of blood flow, which is termed diastasis. The pressure–volume relationship shown in the diagram is a simplified representation of the normal left ventricular pressure–volume curve. Normal right ventricular pressure–volume relationship differs from that of the normal left ventricle. ECG, electrocardiogram, EDV, end–diastolic volume; ESV, end–systolic volume.

■ Determinants of Cardiac Output

The cardiac output is the product of the heart rate and the stroke volume. Stroke volume (i.e., how much blood is ejected with each heart beat) is affected by three variables: preload, afterload, and contractility.

- *Preload:* ventricular wall tension at end of diastole. In clinical terms, it is the stretch on the ventricular fibers just prior to contraction, often approximated by the end-diastolic volume or end-diastolic pressure.
- *Afterload:* ventricular wall tension during contraction. It is the systemic or pulmonary vascular resistance that must be overcome in order for the ventricle to eject its contents. It is often approximated by the systolic ventricular or arterial pressure.
- *Contractility:* Property of heart muscle that accounts for force of contraction, independent of the preload or afterload.

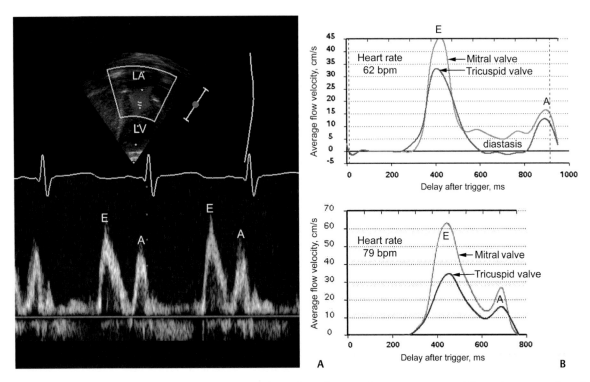

Fig. 3.2 Blood flow through the mitral valve. Ultrasound Doppler technique in the left panel traces the velocity spectrum, whereas phase-contrast velocity mapping at magnetic resonance in the right panel traces average velocity. E and A wave peaks are associated with early rapid filling during ventricular relaxation and atrial contraction, respectively.

MR flow tracings at two different heart rates show that the shortening of the cardiac phase with increased heart rate is mainly due to shortening of the diastolic phase. With a slower heart rate, the two peaks are interposed by a period of diastasis (right upper panel). LA, left atrium; LV, left ventricle.

For the sake of discussion, we will consider each individually, but it should be known that these factors work in concert, and there is a certain degree of interaction between these variables.

There is a direct relationship, known as the Frank–Starling relationship, between the stroke volume and the amount of preload in the ventricle (**Fig. 3.3**). According to this relationship, as the end-diastolic volume (i.e., the volume of the ventricle just prior to contraction) increases, the stroke volume of the ventricle also increases. In part, this is related to the fact that the amount of tension generated by individual myocardial fibers is proportional to the length to which the muscle is stretched. Microscopically, this is due to the degree of overlap between the actin and myosin filaments within the myofibrils of the cardiac myocyte. However, as the preload increases, the ventricle eventually becomes overdistended to a point that its ability to increase stroke volume becomes impaired. As a result, the increase in stroke volume per amount of preload plateaus and eventually, stroke volume begins to decrease.

The force with which the ventricle contracts is dependent on several factors – the degree of activity of the contractile proteins, the amount and sensitivity to

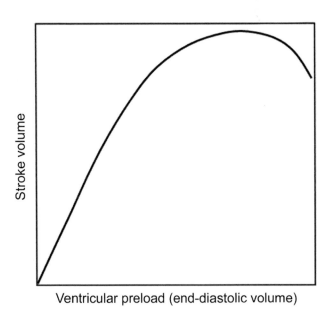

Fig. 3.3 Frank–Starling relationship between stroke volume and preload. The stroke volume increases proportional to increase in end-diastolic volume of the ventricle to the point where the ventricle fails.

intracellular calcium (calcium mediates myocardial contraction), the compliance of the ventricle, and the degree of actin–myosin cross-bridging.

The afterload of the heart is also dependent on several other factors – the pressure against which the ventricle pumps, the inertia of the blood, and the tension in the myocardial wall (also known as wall stress). There is an inverse relationship between the amount of afterload and the stroke volume. Practically, it is very difficult to quantify the total amount of afterload that a ventricle sees. Usually systemic vascular resistance is used as a surrogate for afterload.

Heart rate is another determinant of cardiac output. Younger infants are predominantly dependent on heart rate to maintain their cardiac output. If the stroke volume of the heart is held constant, increases in heart rate will result in proportionate increases in cardiac output, up to a point. As the heart rate increases, the diastolic period is shortened (**Fig. 3.2**). As a result, the amount of time allowed for filling decreases and cardiac output will subsequently decrease because of inadequate preload. Heart rate also affects the inherent contractility of the myocardium, through mechanisms that are still being determined. This relationship is known as the force-frequency relationship. As the heart rate increases, the force with which the myocardium contracts increases proportionally up to a point. It is felt that this response is related to calcium cycling within the myocyte as well as calcium sensitivity of the contractile elements of the myocyte.

However, despite describing these determinants separately, again, it must be kept in mind that there are interactions between these factors to help regulate cardiac output. The heart rate can influence the degree of contractility of the myocardium. The amount of preload can influence the degree of contractility. Within clinical situations, all of these forces are at work, and depending on the different situations, some factors may predominate over others.

■ Systolic Parameters of Ventricular Function

Initially, assessment of ventricular systolic function primarily focuses on evaluation of the "pumping" function of the ventricle. Classically, measures of left ventricular function have been easier to determine due to the ability to model the left ventricle after a prolated ellipse. Right ventricular systolic function has been more difficult to assess due to the crescent shape of the right ventricle, and the ability of its shape to change as a result of changes in the position of the interventricular septum. In addition to evaluation of various images, new techniques such as continuous wave Doppler, pulse wave Doppler, and tissue Doppler have allowed for assessment of hemodynamics, systolic, and more notably diastolic ventricular function.

Shortening Fraction

The shortening fraction represents the simplest and oldest method of assessing ventricular function. Basically, it is the percentage change in the measured ventricular dimension when looking at the ventricle in the short axis. The shortening fraction can be described as follows.

Percentage shortening fraction = (LVDD − LVSD)/LVDD × 100

where LVDD = left ventricular end-diastolic dimension, and LVSD = left ventricular end-systolic dimension. The normal shortening fraction ranges from 28 to 44% with a mean of 36%. The shortening fraction is dependent on the ventricular preload and afterload. The shortening fraction can be measured quite easily by either echocardiography or magnetic resonance imaging (MRI). The shortening fraction is primarily used for assessment of the left ventricle. The shortening fraction can be decreased in conditions with impaired myocardial contraction (i.e., ischemic heart disease, dilated cardiomyopathy). The shortening fraction can be increased if there is hyperdynamic function (i.e., hyperthyroidism, inotropic use, hypertrophic cardiomyopathy), but may be inaccurate if there are signs of regional wall motion abnormalities.

Ejection Fraction

The ejection fraction is the percentage of blood ejected from the left ventricle with each heart beat.

Ejection fraction = (EDV − ESV)/EDV × 100

where EDV = end-diastolic volume, and ESV = end-systolic volume. A normal ejection fraction varies from 55 to 70%. The ejection fraction can be measured either by echocardiography or MRI. Using echocardiography, the change in the ventricular dimensions as seen in the parasternal long axis are noted and using a prolated ellipse model of the left ventricle, the ejection fraction can be calculated. This method is valid only if there are no signs of regional wall motion abnormalities or uncoordinated ventricular motion because the mathematical model assumes all segments of the ventricle contract

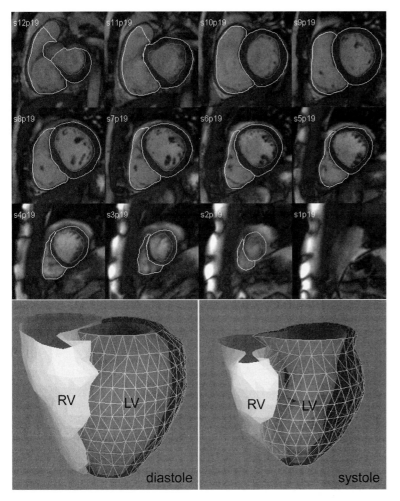

Fig. 3.4 Magnetic resonance imaging ventricular volume study. By using electrocardiogram-gated cine-imaging technique, the ventricles are sectioned into 10–12 short axis slices that are perpendicular to the long axis of the ventricles and parallel to the atrioventricular valve planes. The end-diastolic and end-systolic cavity volumes and myocardial mass (myocardial volume x myocardial tissue density [1.05]) are calculated from endocardial and epicardial traces. RV, right ventricle; LV, left ventricle.

toward the center. The left ventricular ejection fraction can be more accurately estimated through a method known as the biplane Simpson's method. With this method, the area of the left ventricle in both diastole and systole, as seen from two different echocardiographic views that are perpendicular to one another (i.e., the apical four-chamber view and the apical two-chamber view) are measured. Again, using mathematical modeling of the left ventricle, an ejection fraction can be calculated.

Cardiac magnetic resonance (MR) can provide a more sensitive method of calculating the ejection fraction (**Fig. 3.4**). A stack of equally divided and spaced short axis images of the entire ventricles are acquired by using a cine technique. The volumes of the ventricular cavities and myocardium of all slices at end-diastole and end-systole are calculated by multiplying the cross-sectional areas by the section thickness and then added. Cardiac MRI quantification of ventricular volumes does not involve any geometric assumption of the shape of the ventricles. Therefore, cardiac MRI is considered as the

gold standard for quantification of the left and right ventricular function. Quantification with MRI is more important when the ventricular cavity is not ellipsoid or there is regional wall motion abnormality.

Similar to the shortening fraction, the ejection fraction can be decreased in states of impaired myocardial contractility (i.e., ischemia, postoperative state, or cardiomyopathy), outflow tract obstruction, and regional wall motion abnormalities. The ejection fraction will also be increased, like the shortening fraction, in states of hyperdynamic function (i.e., hyperthyroidism, inotropic use, hypertrophic cardiomyopathy).

Stroke Volume and Cardiac Output

The stroke volume of the heart can be calculated from a ventricular volume study or quantification of the blood flow through the great arterial trunk. In a ventricular volume study, the stroke volume is the difference between the ventricular end-diastolic and end-systolic volumes. In flow assessment, the stroke volume can be calculated by multiplying the average blood velocity by the cross-sectional area of the arterial trunk. Although both echocardiography and MR can use either method to calculate stroke volume, MR is more accurate than echocardiography. Once the stroke volume is known, cardiac output and the cardiac index are calculated by using the following equations:

$$\text{Cardiac output (L/min)} = \text{stroke volume} \times \text{heart rate}$$
$$\text{Cardiac index (L/min/m}^2) = \text{cardiac output/body surface area}$$

Normal cardiac index ranges from 3.5 to 5.5 L/min/m^2.

Qualitative Measures of Systolic Ventricular Function

In addition to quantitative measures of systolic function, two-dimensional echocardiography and cardiac MR also allow for qualitative assessment of ventricular function. In particular, whether or not there is uncoordinated contraction of different segments of the myocardium, (also known as regional wall motion abnormalities) or overall "gestalt" impression of ventricular performance (i.e., normal, mildly, moderately, or severely reduced function) can be determined. Because these measures are qualitative in nature, they lack the robustness of other quantitative measures, but are nonetheless still important in an overall assessment of a patient's ventricular function.

■ Assessment of Ventricular Diastolic Function

Although in the past, measures of systolic function were in the forefront, it has recently been increasingly recognized that diastolic function plays as important, if not a more prominent role, in the management of patients with abnormal heart function. Diastolic dysfunction implies that there is an abnormality in the relaxation phase of diastole, or an abnormality in the inherent compliance of the myocardium. States that result in diastolic dysfunction include cardiomyopathy, poor ventricular function leading to increased ventricular end-diastolic pressures, ventricular hypertrophy, and pericardial disease.

Atrioventricular Valve Flow Patterns

As noted earlier in the chapter, during diastole, the ventricle fills through two phases—early passive filling and

atrial contraction. With the advent of echocardiography, and now with MRI, flow patterns across the atrioventricular valves can be assessed giving an estimate of diastolic function (**Fig. 3.2**). During early ventricular filling, there is initial flow into the ventricle that is recorded as the early (E) velocity. With atrial contraction, there is a second period of flow known as the atrial (A) velocity. With echocardiography, the pulse wave sample volume is placed at the tips of the atrioventricular valves using the apical four-chamber view and the velocities can be recorded (**Fig. 3.2A**). As with other

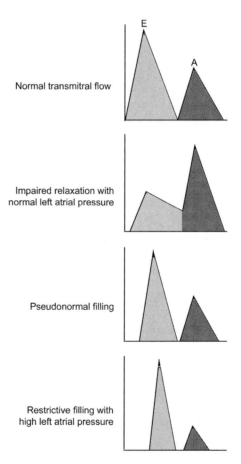

Fig. 3.5 Diagrammatic representation of the various stages of diastolic dysfunction seen in Doppler tracing of mitral valve flow. The normal mitral valve flow pattern is characterized by a larger E and a smaller A wave with an E/A ratio larger than 1. Impaired left ventricular relaxation or decreased left ventricular compliance is associated with a reversal of E/A ratio and prolongation of E-wave deceleration. Pseudonormalization of the E/A ratio can occur when increased left atrial pressure results in an increased driving pressure and a consequent increased E-wave velocity across the mitral valve into a noncompliant left ventricle. With severe diastolic dysfunction, the mitral valve inflow pattern can become restrictive, reflecting rapid equilibration of elevated left atrial and left ventricular diastolic pressures in the noncompliant left ventricle.

forms of Doppler echocardiography, accuracy depends on alignment with blood flow and placement of the sample volume in the correct position. MRI can also measure atrioventricular flow patterns through the use of phase contrast velocity mapping (**Fig. 3.2B**). Both atrioventricular valve orifices are cut in short axis, which allows comparison of simultaneous flow patterns through the two valves.

Various studies have tried to assess diastolic function by examining the E and A velocities, the ratio of E/A velocities, and the deceleration time (the time it takes the E velocity to return to baseline). From these studies, various patterns have been established to characterize the various forms of diastolic dysfunction (**Fig. 3.5**).

Pulmonary Vein Flow Patterns

Flow within the pulmonary veins has also been used to help characterize diastolic function. Normally during ventricular systole, the mitral valve is displaced downward creating a suction effect, causing the first phase of blood flow in the pulmonary veins, known as the S wave. When the mitral valve opens, blood drains out of the left atrium, into the ventricle. During this period of left atrial emptying into the left ventricle, a second phase of pulmonary vein flow occurs, which is known as the D wave. The left atrium then contracts and during this contraction, some blood will flow backward into the pulmonary vein producing a third phase of retrograde flow known as the A wave (**Fig. 3.6**).

Similar to atrioventricular flow patterns, pulmonary vein flow pattern changes with diastolic dysfunction. With increasing severity of diastolic dysfunction, the S wave becomes less prominent and the A wave reversal during atrial contraction increases in amplitude.

Isovolumetric Relaxation Time

Recall that the isovolumetric relaxation occurs when the ventricle begins to relax with both the mitral and aortic valves closed, resulting in a drop in the ventricular pressure without a change in volume. This can be estimated through the use of pulse wave Doppler echocardiography where the sample volume is placed at an intermediate position between the mitral and aortic valves. The isovolumetric relaxation time is the time between the end of aortic outflow and the beginning of mitral inflow. In hearts with diastolic dysfunction, the isovolumetric relaxation time will be prolonged due to impaired ventricular relaxation.

Tissue Doppler Patterns

Tissue Doppler represents a new echocardiographic technology that looks at the motion of tissue or muscle within the heart. With tissue Doppler, the velocities that are recorded are filtered in the range corresponding to the motion of the myocardium. During tissue Doppler, a pulse wave Doppler sample is placed at various points along the myocardium and the velocity of the myocardium is recorded. Typically, the sample volume is placed at the lateral portion of the mitral valve annulus, the basal portion of the interventricular septum, and the medial wall of the tricuspid valve annulus. During early passive filling of the ventricle, these portions of the heart will move upwards represented as the E' wave. Finally, during atrial contraction, these portions of the heart, move further upwards, denoted as the A wave (**Fig. 3.7**). Specific patterns of tissue Doppler have been used as indicators of diastolic dysfunction. One must keep in mind that tissue Doppler is inaccurate if the sample volume during pulse wave Doppler is not placed in the correct location or if there are regional wall motion abnormalities in different segments of the myocardium.

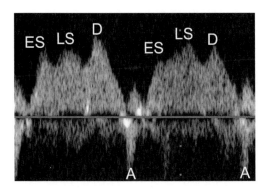
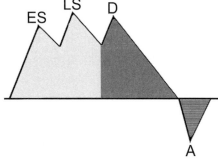

Fig. 3.6 Normal pulmonary venous Doppler tracing. The normal pulmonary venous flow is either biphasic or triphasic. Biphasic flow consists of systolic (S) and diastolic (D) peaks. Triphasic flow consists of early systolic (ES), late systolic (LS), and diastolic (D) flow peaks. Usually, a small reversed flow (A) can be seen during atrial contraction.

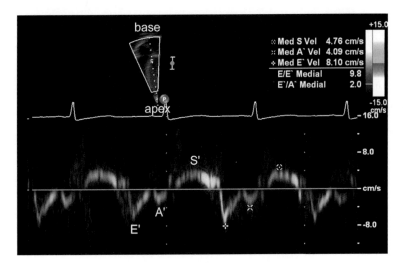

Fig. 3.7 Tissue Doppler tracing of the basal part of the interventricular septum. In systole, the myocardium moves toward the transducer placed on the apex causing an S' wave peak above the baseline. In diastole, the myocardium moves away from the transducer during the early filling phase causing an E' wave peak below the baseline. During atrial contraction, the myocardium moves further toward the base causing an A' wave peak.

■ Assessment of Combined Systolic and Diastolic Function

In the majority of patients with impaired cardiac function, systolic and diastolic dysfunction coexists. Myocardial performance index or Tei index is a Doppler index of combined systolic and diastolic function (**Fig. 3.8**). The index is calculated by the sum of isovolumetric contraction and isovolumetric relaxation time intervals divided by the ejection time of the ventricle.

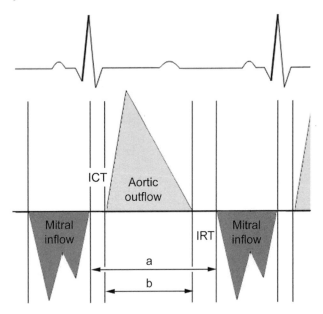

Tei (myocardial performance) index
= (ICT + IRT) / Ejection time
= (a-b) / b

Fig. 3.8 Calculation of the myocardial performance index or Tei index, where ICT is the isovolumetric contraction time, and IRT is the isovolumetric relaxation time.

■ Hemodynamic Parameters as Assessed by Cardiac Catheterization

Many measurements of cardiac hemodynamics have traditionally been measured through the use of invasive cardiac catheterization – and some measures can only be assessed by these means. Primarily cardiac catheterization allows for direct measurements of pressures and oxygen saturations, which can be later used to calculate such parameters as cardiac output, pulmonary and systemic blood flow, shunt fractions, and pulmonary and systemic vascular resistances (**Table 3.1**).

Cardiac catheterization involves obtaining vascular access and placement of fluid-filled catheters into various vascular structures allowing for direct blood sampling and pressure measurement.

Pressure Measurements

Measurements of pressure during cardiac catheterization provide information about vascular and ventricular compliance. It also allows direct measurement of the degree of obstruction across certain types of congenital heart defects (i.e., ventricular septal defect, atrial septal defect, valvular stenosis, arch obstruction, etc.) or the pressure present in either the left or right ventricles.

Pulmonary and Systemic Flow

Pulmonary and systemic blood flow can be determined through various methods in the cardiac catheterization laboratory (i.e., thermodilution or dye-based methods). The most common method is the Fick method. The amount of blood flow can be determined knowing the body's oxygen consumption (i.e., how much oxygen the body uses per minute indexed to body surface area), and the oxygen

Table 3.1 Normal Ranges of Commonly Used Hemodynamic Parameters

Parameters	Normal Ranges
Heart rate	60–120 beats/min
Right ventricular end-diastolic volume index	91 ± 16 mL/m^2
Right ventricular end-systolic volume index	36 ± 10 mL/m^2
Right ventricular ejection fraction	61 ± 6%
Right ventricular myocardial mass index	20.3 ± 3.6 g/m^2
Left ventricular end-diastolic volume index	80 ± 13 mL/m^2
Left ventricular end-systolic volume index	25 ± 7 mL/m^2
Left ventricular ejection fraction	69 ± 6%
Left ventricular myocardial mass index	59.2 ± 11 g/m^2
Stroke volume	70–130 mL/beat
Stroke volume index	30–60 mL/beat/m^2
Cardiac output (adult)	4–8 L/min
Cardiac index	2.8–4.2 L/min/ m^2
Mean right atrial pressure	0–8 mm Hg
a wave	2–10 mm Hg
v wave	2–10 mm Hg
Right ventricular systolic pressure	15–30 mm Hg
Right ventricular end diastolic pressure	0–8 mm Hg
Pulmonary artery systolic pressure	15–30 mm Hg
Pulmonary artery diastolic pressure	4–12 mm Hg
Mean pulmonary artery pressure	9–16 mm Hg
Mean pulmonary capillary wedge pressure	1–10 mm Hg
a wave	3–15 mm Hg
v wave	3–15 mm Hg
Mean left atrial pressure	5–10 mm Hg
a wave	3–12 mm Hg
v wave	5–15 mm Hg
Left ventricular systolic pressure	65–120 mm Hg
Left ventricular end diastolic pressure	3–10 mm Hg
Systemic arterial systolic pressure	90–140 mm Hg
Systemic arterial diastolic pressure	60–90 mm Hg
Mean systemic arterial pressure	70–105 mm Hg
Systemic vascular resistance	700–1500 dyne/ s per cm^{-5}
Pulmonary vascular resistance	20–120 dyne/ s per cm^{-5}
Systemic vascular resistance index	1700–2600 dyne/ s per cm^{-5}
Pulmonary vascular resistance index	70–200 dyne/ s per cm^{-5}

content proximally and distally to the vascular bed in question (i.e., pulmonary versus systemic vascular beds). It is described by using the following equation:

$$Q = \frac{VO_2}{\text{Distal } O_2 \text{ Content} - \text{Proximal } O_2 \text{ Content}}$$

where Q is the amount of blood flow, VO$_2$ is the oxygen consumption. The oxygen content is a combination of the amount of oxygen carried by hemoglobin, as well as that which is dissolved in the blood given by the following formula:

$$O_2 = \text{Content} =$$
$$O_2 \text{ Saturation} \times [\text{Hemoglobin}] \times 1.34 + P_aO_2 \times 0.0003$$

where [Hemoglobin] is the concentration of hemoglobin in the blood (g/L) and P_aO_2 is the partial pressure of oxygen dissolved in the blood. With this formula, the amount of blood flow to the pulmonary circulation (Q$_p$) can be calculated as the following:

$$Q_p = \frac{VO_2}{\text{Pulmonary Vein } O_2 \text{ Content} - \text{Pulmonary Artery } O_2 \text{ Content}}$$

Accordingly, the amount of systemic blood flow (Q$_S$) can also be similarly calculated:

$$Q_S = \frac{VO_2}{\text{Systemic Arterial } O_2 \text{ Content} - \text{Mixed Artery } O_2 \text{ Content}}$$

Finally, the ratio of pulmonary-to-systemic blood flow can be determined:

$$\frac{Q_P}{Q_S} = \frac{\text{Systemic Arterial } O_2 \text{ Content} - \text{Mixed Venous } O_2 \text{ Content}}{\text{Systemic Arterial } O_2 \text{ Content} - \text{Mixed Artery } O_2 \text{ Content}}$$

Vascular Resistance Measurements

The vascular resistance is a measure of the change in pressure related to the amount of blood flow as seen in the following equation:

$$R = \frac{\Delta \text{ Pressure}}{Q}$$

where R is the resistance, Δ Pressure is the change in pressure over the vascular bed in question, and Q is the amount of blood flow across the vascular bed in question. Usually, the pulmonary vascular resistance is the more important measure of resistance (the other being the systemic vascular resistance), as elevations in pulmonary vascular resistance can be associated with increased morbidity and mortality in certain types of congenital cardiac disease and may even be an absolute contraindication to surgical repair.

Suggested Reading

Boucek RJ Jr, Martinez R. Echocardiographic determination of right ventricular function. Cardiol Young 2005;15(Suppl 1):48–50

Fogel MA. Assessment of cardiac function by magnetic resonance imaging. Pediatr Cardiol 2000;21(1):59–69

Hudsmith LE, Petersen SE, Francis JM, Robson MD, Neubauer S. Normal human left and right ventricular and left atrial dimensions using steady state free precession magnetic resonance imaging. J Cardiovasc Magn Reson 2005;7(5):775–782

Myung Park. Pediatric Cardiology for Practitioners. 4th ed. Philadelphia: Mosby; 2002

Penny DJ. The basics of ventricular function. Cardiol Young 1999;9(2):210–223

Powell AJ, Geva T. Blood flow measurement by magnetic resonance imaging in congenital heart disease. Pediatr Cardiol 2000;21(1): 47–58

Quiñones MA. Assessment of diastolic function. Prog Cardiovasc Dis 2005;47(5):340–355

Redington AN, Gray HH, Hodson ME, Rigby ML, Oldershaw PJ. Characterisation of the normal right ventricular pressure-volume relation by biplane angiography and simultaneous micromanometer pressure measurements. Br Heart J 1988;59(1):23–30

Snider AR, Ritter SB, Serwer GA. Echocardiography in Pediatric Heart Disease. 2nd ed. Philadelphia: Mosby; 1997

Tei C, Ling LH, Hodge DO, et al. New index of combined systolic and diastolic myocardial performance: a simple and reproducible measure of cardiac function—a study in normals and dilated cardiomyopathy. J Cardiol 1995;26(6):357–366

Zile MR, Baicu CF, Bonnema DD. Diastolic heart failure: definitions and terminology. Prog Cardiovasc Dis 2005;47(5):307–313

4 Glossary of Pediatric Cardiovascular Surgical Procedures

Shi-Joon Yoo and Christopher A. Caldarone

As most congenital heart diseases are primarily structural defects, a surgical correction is required in the majority of the patients with a major defect. Surgery is performed when other forms of treatment cannot maintain adequate circulation or when the structural defect may result in damage to the heart, lungs, or other organs. Since Dr. Robert E. Gross performed the first surgical ligation of a patent ductus arteriosus in 1938,[1] a number of surgical procedures have been introduced for corrective or palliative treatment of various congenital heart diseases. Many physicians who interpret plain radiographs for patients with congenital heart disease are not as familiar with various cardiovascular surgical procedures as they should be. In this chapter, we intend to overcome this gap by providing an overview of congenital cardiac surgery and various associated surgical procedures using a glossary format.

◻ *Open-heart versus closed surgery.* In general, intracardiac defects require an open-heart surgical procedure, which is done with cardiopulmonary bypass. Extracardiac defects involving the aorta, pulmonary vessels, or ductus arteriosus can be repaired by a closed procedure without cardiopulmonary bypass.

◻ *Complete versus palliative surgery.* An ideal surgical procedure is a single-stage definitive corrective surgery. When the patient's condition or the complexity of the cardiovascular pathology does not allow complete repair, palliative procedures are performed. Palliative procedures are aimed to alter the hemodynamic physiology of the particular defect so that the complications of the defect are treated, delayed, or prevented. Palliative procedures may be performed as preparatory measures for a later definitive surgery or end-stage palliative procedures.

◻ *Biventricular versus univentricular repair.* Cardiovascular surgical procedures can be divided into biventricular and univentricular repairs. A biventricular repair is a surgical procedure that results in two separate ventricles pumping blood to the systemic and pulmonary circulations without any shunts. Univentricular repair refers to a surgical procedure in which the ventricle(s) are used exclusively for pumping blood to the systemic circulation, while the pulmonary blood flow is maintained with an aortopulmonary shunt, ventriculopulmonary shunt, or cavopulmonary shunt. Congenital heart diseases that require univentricular repair are called functionally single ventricle or univentricular heart diseases. They include double-inlet ventricles, tricuspid atresia, mitral atresia, hypoplastic left heart syndrome, critical aortic stenosis with hypoplastic left ventricle or severe endocardial fibroelastosis, and unbalanced atrioventricular septal defect. Additionally, hearts with two good-sized ventricles may be regarded as functionally single ventricular when the complex intracardiac anatomy precludes proper septation of the ventricles.

■ Glossary of Surgical Procedures

Atrial Switch Operation   Complete transposition of the great arteries requires switching of the abnormal circulation at one of three cardiac segment levels: the atrial, ventricular, or great arterial. Prior to the 1990s, the atrial switch operation had been the gold standard operation for complete transposition with intact ventricular septum or restrictive ventricular septal defect. Currently, the atrial switch has almost completely been replaced by the arterial switch operation in North American centers. Nevertheless, a large population of patients who underwent atrial switch procedures prior to the development of the arterial switch procedure are now adults and frequently present with long-term complications of the atrial switch including systemic venous baffle obstruction and systemic ventricular failure.

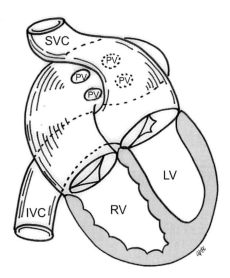

Fig. 4.1 Atrial switch operation. RV, right ventricle; LV, left ventricle; PV, pulmonary vein; SVC, superior vena cava; IVC, inferior vena cava.

An atrial switch operation consists of routing the systemic venous return to the left ventricle through the mitral valve and the pulmonary venous return to the right ventricle through the tricuspid valve by using an intraatrial baffle (**Fig. 4.1**). In the Senning operation, the atrial septum and atrial wall are used to construct the baffle.[2] In the Mustard operation, the atrial septum is removed and the baffle is constructed with autologous pericardium or synthetic material.[3] Although the atrial switch operation establishes a physiologic correction of the circulation, it leaves the right ventricle to support the systemic circulation, which is not desirable in the long term. In long-term follow-up, right ventricular failure, tricuspid regurgitation, and arrhythmias are common.[4] Today its use is limited to congenitally corrected transposition of the great arteries in which the atrial switch operation is performed in conjunction with an arterial switch operation (See Double-Switch Operation below).

Arterial Switch Operation (of Jatene) Complete transposition of the great arteries is now ideally repaired by an arterial switch operation pioneered in 1954 by Dr. William Mustard of Canada.[5] It was successfully performed for the first time in 1976 by Dr. Adib Jatene of Brazil.[6] As this operation restores the normal anatomic arrangement of the circulation, it has become the procedure of choice when the anatomy is appropriate.[4]

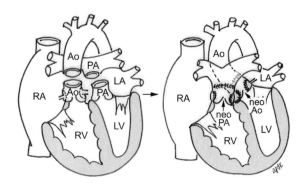

Fig. 4.2 Arterial switch operation using Lecompte maneuver. RA, right atrium; LA, left atrium; RV, right ventricle; LV, left ventricle; Ao, ascending aorta; PA, pulmonary artery.

The operation consists of transection of the great arteries above the sinuses and detachment of the coronary arteries along with a button of aortic sinus wall, followed by translocation of the dissected great arteries into their new positions and implantation of the coronary buttons to the neo-aorta (**Fig. 4.2**). Translocation of the great arteries that are anteroposteriorly related requires a Lecompte maneuver in which the transected pulmonary artery bifurcation is moved anterior to the aorta.[7] When the great arteries are related side-by-side (as in the Taussig–Bing anomaly), the Lecompte maneuver may not be necessary. In both cases, aortic and pulmonary artery continuity is restored and the procedure is completed.

Bidirectional Cavopulmonary (Bidirectional Glenn) Connection
Bidirectional Cavopulmonary (Bidirectional Glenn) Connection (BCPC) is used as an intermediate-stage palliation en route to a Fontan operation for patients with functionally single ventricle physiology.[8,9] It is performed as a primary procedure or as a second-stage operation following a prior systemic artery-to-pulmonary artery shunt or a pulmonary artery banding.

BCPC consists of dissection of the superior vena cava at its junction with the atrium and end-to-side anastomosis of the dissected superior vena cava to the ipsilateral pulmonary artery (**Fig. 4.3**).[8,9] In those patients with bilateral superior venae cavae, but without a bridging innominate vein, it is necessary to perform bilateral bidirectional cavopulmonary connections. It is usually performed at 3 to 6 months of age as a second-stage procedure. It may be performed earlier when it is performed as a primary surgery. Occasionally, it can be the final surgical procedure when high pulmonary vascular resistance does not allow a subsequent Fontan operation. This procedure has unique benefits. Compared with systemic artery-to-pulmonary arterial shunts, it avoids volume overload to the ventricle and prevents pulmonary vascular obstructive disease and distortion. In

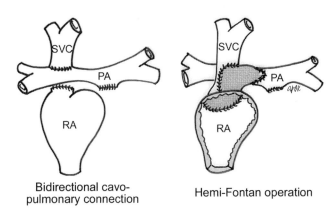

Fig. 4.3 Bidirectional cavopulmonary connection and hemi-Fontan operation. SVC, superior vena cava; PA, pulmonary artery; RA, right atrium.

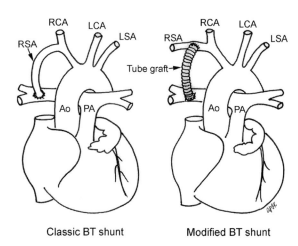

Classic BT shunt   Modified BT shunt

Fig. 4.4 Classic and modified Blalock–Taussig (BT) shunts. RSA, right subclavian artery; LSA, left subclavian artery; RCA, right coronary artery; LCA, left coronary artery; Ao, ascending aorta; PA, pulmonary artery.

addition, the volume of shunt flow increases with somatic growth. As the child ages, however, the relative body mass shifts disproportionately to larger lower body growth and relatively less upper body growth. Consequently, the ratio of blood passing through the superior vena cava and the inferior vena cava decreases. Because pulmonary blood flow is determined by superior vena caval flow after a BCPC, patients tend to develop progressive, deepening cyanosis as they enter late childhood. The hemi-Fontan operation (right panel in **Fig. 4.3**) is a variation of BCPC in which the continuity of the superior vena cava and right atrium is maintained when the superior vena cava is connected to the adjacent pulmonary artery.[10] A patch is sewn across the junction between the superior vena cava and the right atrium through the vertical incision extending along the medial aspect of the superior vena cava and the superior aspect of the right atrium. This allows easy excision of the patch at the time of completion of a Fontan operation and establishment of continuity between the inferior vena cava and the pulmonary arteries with a lateral tunnel procedure (See Fontan operation).

Blalock–Taussig Shunt   Blalock and Taussig introduced this landmark procedure in 1945 to treat patients with pulmonary stenosis or atresia by directing blood flow from a systemic artery to the pulmonary artery for oxygenation.[11] The Blalock–Taussig (BT) shunt has been widely used as a temporary procedure en route to corrective or further palliative surgery. Today the systemic artery-to-pulmonary arterial shunt is most commonly used in neonates with functionally single ventricle physiology as an intermediate procedure prior to a bidirectional cavopulmonary connection.

The original BT shunt, which is now called a "classic BT shunt," consisted of an end-to-side anastomosis of the subclavian artery to the ipsilateral pulmonary artery

(**Fig. 4.4**, left panel). Subsequently, various modifications have been introduced. The most commonly used modification is the modified BT shunt, in which an artificial tube graft with a diameter of 3 to 5 mm is interposed between the subclavian or common carotid artery and the ipsilateral pulmonary artery (**Fig. 4.4**, right panel).[12]

Direct connection of the aorta to the branch pulmonary arteries using a Potts shunt (between descending aorta and left pulmonary artery) or a Waterston shunt (between ascending aorta and right pulmonary artery) has been abandoned because of a high incidence of subsequent pulmonary hypertension and frequent pulmonary artery kinking/distortion along with preferential flow to one lung.[13]

The central shunt uses a short tube graft between the ascending aorta and main pulmonary artery (**Fig. 4.5**, left

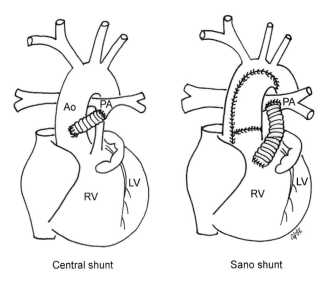

Central shunt   Sano shunt

Fig. 4.5 Central shunt and Sano shunt. RV, right ventricle; LV, left ventricle; Ao, ascending aorta; PA, pulmonary artery.

panel).[14] This procedure is used mainly for small neonates and young infants especially when the branch pulmonary arteries are very small. The Mee shunt is a direct central end-to-side anastomosis of the confluent pulmonary artery to the ascending aorta.[15] The Sano shunt is a right ventricle-to-pulmonary artery shunt using a tube graft (**Fig. 4.5**, right panel).[16] The major advantage of this procedure is maintenance of adequate diastolic pressure for coronary arterial perfusion in contrast to other arterial shunt procedures where systemic-to-pulmonary arterial run-off causes reduced aortic diastolic pressure that may contribute to coronary insufficiency.

Central Shunt   (See Blalock–Taussig shunt)

Cole's Procedure (Sutureless Pulmonary Vein Repair)   Surgery that involves pulmonary vein dissection is often complicated by subsequent stenosis of the suture sites on the repaired pulmonary veins. Cole's procedure was introduced to prevent postoperative stenosis of the pulmonary veins by avoiding direct suture of the pulmonary veins (**Fig. 4.6**).[17]

extended to the individual pulmonary veins. The pericardium is then sutured to the atrial wall with a suture line kept away from the divided edge of the pulmonary veins. This suture line contains the pulmonary venous effluent in a "controlled bleed" while avoiding any direct suturing of the pulmonary veins. A similar technique can also be used for total anomalous pulmonary venous connection.[17]

Damus–Kaye–Stansel Operation   In 1975, three different groups Damus–Kaye–Stansel (DKS) proposed a type of arterial repair for complex forms of complete transposition of the great arteries without coronary artery transfer.[18–21] The basic concept of this operation is to use the pulmonary and aortic valves as a dual source of systemic cardiac output and to reconstruct the pulmonary outflow tract using a conduit. With increased experience with the classic arterial switch operation in patients with complex patterns of coronary artery anatomy, this approach for complex transposition or Taussig–Bing anomaly has been largely abandoned.[22] Now, this procedure is typically used to relieve systemic ventricular outflow tract obstruction in a functionally single ventricle, such as tricuspid atresia or double-inlet left ventricle with subaortic stenosis.[23]

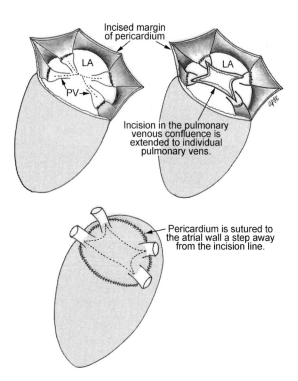

Fig. 4.6 Cole's procedure. LA, left atrium; PV, pulmonary veins.

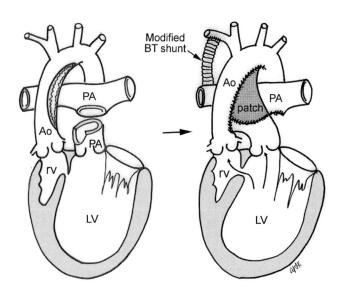

Fig. 4.7 Damus–Kaye–Stansel (DKS) operation. rv, rudimentary right ventricle; LV, left ventricle; Ao, ascending aorta; PA, pulmonary artery.

For patients with primary or postsurgical stenosis of pulmonary veins, the posterior wall of the left atrium and the pulmonary venous confluence are incised transversely. The incision on the pulmonary venous confluence is

This procedure consists of transection of the pulmonary artery, incision in the ascending aorta, end-to-side anastomosis of the proximal pulmonary arterial trunk to the ascending aorta, and augmentation of the anastomotic route by using an anterior patch (**Fig. 4.7**). The aortic valve and ventricular septal defect can be closed or left open. Pulmonary blood flow is reestablished by use of a modified BT or bidirectional cavopulmonary shunt depending on the patient's age and the pulmonary vascular anatomy and resistance.

Double-Switch Operation The standard surgical approach to congenitally corrected transposition of the great arteries is basically to treat the individual-associated abnormalities, such as repair or replacement of the dysplastic tricuspid valve, relief of pulmonary stenosis, and closure of a ventricular septal defect. However, the right ventricle may fail after a standard surgery because it supports the systemic circulation.

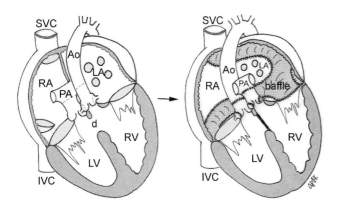

Fig. 4.8 Double-switch operation. RA, right atrium; LA, left atrium; RV, right ventricle; LV, left ventricle; Ao, ascending aorta; PA, pulmonary artery; SVC, superior vena cava; IVC, inferior vena cava; d, ventricular septal defect.

The double-switch operation consists of atrial and arterial switch procedures so that the left ventricle supports the systemic circulation (**Fig. 4.8**).[24] The atrial septum is removed and the superior and inferior vena caval flow is directed to the right ventricle on the left side using an intraatrial baffle. Then, an arterial switch procedure is performed as described in the section for arterial switch operation. When corrected transposition is associated with a ventricular septal defect and pulmonary outflow tract obstruction, an atrial switch operation can be combined with a Rastelli-type of operation, which is called an Ilbawi operation.[25,26] Both procedures certainly have a greater risk than other simple procedures, but a successful surgery results in better long-term outcome. Double switch is also needed in patients who have developed late complications of an atrial switch procedure for complete transposition. A previous atrial switch operation can be reversed with an arterial switch operation performed after a short period of left ventricular training by banding the main pulmonary artery.

Fontan Operation A Fontan circuit is the final goal for all hearts with a functionally single ventricle. This includes double-inlet left or right ventricles, tricuspid atresia, pulmonary atresia with intact ventricular septum and hypoplastic left heart syndrome, as well as other rare malformations that do not allow biventricular repair. The principle of the Fontan operation is to commit the functional single ventricle to support the systemic circulation and to let blood flow passively through the lungs without being pumped by a ventricle. This procedure normalizes systemic oxygen saturation and eliminates volume overload of the functioning ventricle (**Fig. 4.9**).

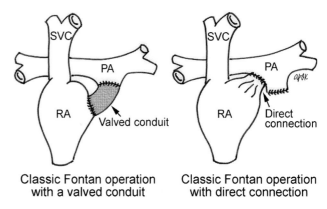

Classic Fontan operation with a valved conduit   **Classic Fontan operation with direct connection**

Fig. 4.9 Classic Fontan operation with or without valved conduit. SVC, superior vena cava; RA, right atrium; PA, pulmonary artery.

The classic Fontan operation consisted of connecting the right atrium to the pulmonary artery and closing the atrial septal defect so that the systemic venous return bypasses the ventricles.[27] Originally, a valved conduit was interposed between the right atrium and the pulmonary artery (**Fig. 4.9**, left panel).[27] Subsequently, a direct valveless connection was preferred (**Fig. 4.9**, right panel). This classic procedure was often complicated by marked dilatation of the right atrium causing arrhythmias and formation of mural thrombi, as well as high systemic venous pressure resulting in anasarca, ascites, pleural effusion, and protein-losing enteropathy.

A few variations of the Fontan operation have been introduced to improve the hemodynamic efficiency of the flow circuit and to minimize the postoperative complications. In most situations, a Fontan procedure requires an intermediate BCPC at 3 to 6 months of age to provide the pulmonary vascular bed an opportunity to mature. BCPC should be preceded by a systemic-to-pulmonary arterial shunt such as a modified BT shunt when the patient needs a shunt before the optimum age for a BCPC is reached. At 2 to 4 years of age, the inferior vena cava is connected to the pulmonary artery to complete the Fontan circuit. There are several variations of a Fontan operation named after how the inferior vena cava is routed to the pulmonary artery. Among these variations, the lateral tunnel and extracardiac techniques are the most widely used methods (**Fig. 4.10**).[28]

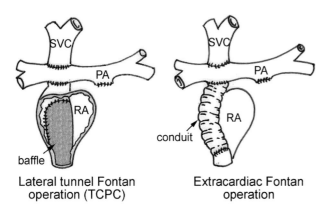

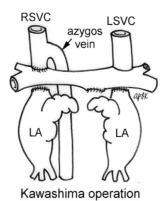

Fig. 4.10 Modifications of Fontan operation. SVC, superior vena cava; PA, pulmonary artery; RA, right atrium; RSVC, right superior vena cava; LSVC, left superior vena cava; LA, left atrium.

In the lateral tunnel method, a baffled tunnel is created within the atrium using a fabric patch (**Fig. 4.10**, upper left panel). The tunnel links the inferior vena caval orifice to the underside of the pulmonary artery that was already connected to the superior vena cava at the time of BCPC. The lateral tunnel can also be linked to the superior vena cava first and then to the pulmonary artery, which is termed a total cavopulmonary connection.[29] In the extracardiac method, a synthetic tube is grafted outside the heart to connect the dissected inferior vena cava to the underside of the pulmonary artery, avoiding an incision in the atrium (**Fig. 4.10**, upper right panel). In either method, a fenestration can be made between the higher-pressure systemic venous pathway and the lower-pressure atrium as a "safety pop-off" route when the systemic venous pressure is expected to be high. Blood passing through the fenestration will bypass the pulmonary vascular bed and, therefore, produce

some cyanosis. In general, the fenestration helps to maintain systemic cardiac output and the mild cyanosis is well tolerated. The fenestrations frequently close spontaneously and, if spontaneous closure does not occur, the fenestration can be closed by placing an occlusive device during catheterization when indicated. In patients with interruption of the inferior vena cava with azygos or hemiazygos continuation, connection of the superior vena cava to the pulmonary artery as in a BCPC diverts all but the hepatic venous blood flow into the pulmonary circulation (Kawashima operation) (**Fig. 4.10**, lower panel).[30] After the Kawashima operation is performed, patients are at risk of developing pulmonary arteriovenous fistulas and must have their hepatic venous flow connected to the pulmonary circulation either at the time of the Kawashima operation or soon thereafter.[31]

There is no doubt that the Fontan operation is an excellent solution for conditions with functionally single ventricle physiology. However, the Fontan operation carries significant late morbidity with development of supraventricular arrhythmias and systemic venous hypertension causing hepatic dysfunction, ascites, and protein-losing enteropathy.

A 1½ ventricular repair (partial biventricular repair) is a surgical option that can be used for patients with a hypoplastic or dysplastic right ventricle that precludes biventricular repair, though the right ventricle is able to deal with the blood flow returning from the inferior vena cava (**Fig. 4.11**). These conditions include Ebstein's malformation of the tricuspid valve, Uhl's anomaly of the right ventricle, atrioventricular septal defect with unfavorable anatomy for biventricular repair, double-outlet right ventricle with a remote ventricular septal defect or straddling atrioventricular valve, pulmonary atresia with intact ventricular septum, congenitally corrected transposition of the great arteries, and cardiac tumor encroaching on the right ventricular inlet or outlet.[32,33]

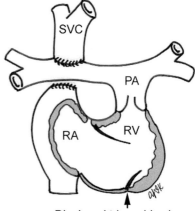

Fig. 4.11 One and a half ventricular repair. SVC, superior vena cava; RPA, right pulmonary artery; PA, pulmonary artery; RA, right atrium; RV, right ventricle.

The 1½ ventricular repair consists of a BCPC without isolation of the pulmonary artery from the pulmonary arterial trunk and intracardiac repair (**Fig. 4.11**). After the operation, the systemic venous return through the superior vena cava flows passively into the pulmonary artery through the BCPC and the systemic venous return from the inferior vena cava is pumped into the pulmonary artery by the ventricle. This procedure unloads the hypoplastic or dysplastic right ventricle, while pulsatile flow is maintained in the pulmonary circulation. In a limited number of cases, right ventricular growth after 1½ ventricle repair allows biventricular repair later in life.

Glenn Operation This procedure was invented as a palliative shunt procedure to increase pulmonary blood flow in cyanotic heart diseases.

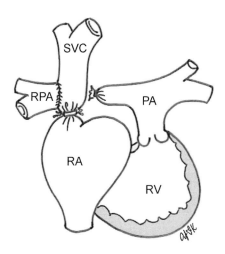

Fig. 4.12 Glenn operation. SVC, superior vena cava; PA, pulmonary artery; RA, right atrium; RV, right ventricle.

The procedure consists of ligation of the superior vena cava at its junction with the atrium, ligation of the azygos vein, end-to-side anastomosis of the dissected pulmonary artery to the superior vena cava, and ligation of the proximal part of the dissected pulmonary artery (**Fig. 4.12**).[34]

The Glenn operation did have advantages over systemic-to-pulmonary arterial shunt allowing growth parallel with somatic growth, and a lower incidence of pulmonary arterial distortion and pulmonary vascular obstructive disease. However, it has largely been abandoned because of a high risk for development of pulmonary arteriovenous fistulas and asymmetry of flow to the right and left lungs. A bidirectional cavopulmonary connection is commonly, but erroneously, referred to as a "bidirectional Glenn" procedure.

Hemi-Fontan Operation (See Bidirectional Cavopulmonary Connection)

Hybrid Procedure (See Norwood Operation)

Ilbawi Operation (Rastelli operation with atrial switch operation; see Double-Switch Operation)

Jatene Procedure (See Arterial Switch Operation)

Kawashima Operation in Single Ventricular Repair (See Fontan Operation)

Kawashima Procedure in Double-Outlet Right Ventricle Double-outlet right ventricle with subpulmonary ventricular septal defect can be repaired by either an arterial switch operation or intraventricular rerouting procedure. The arterial switch operation is considered optimal when the great arteries are anteroposteriorly related. When the great arteries have a side-by-side relationship, Kawashima intraventricular rerouting is required (**Fig. 4.13**).[35,36]

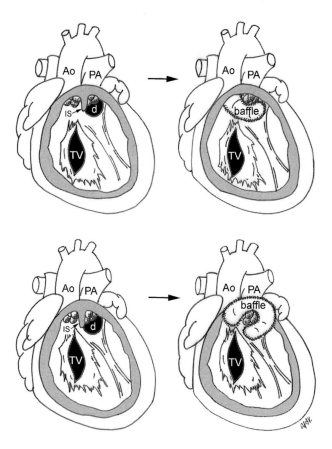

Fig. 4.13 Kawashima's rerouting procedures. Ao, ascending aorta; PA, pulmonary artery; d, ventricular septal defect; IS, infundibular septum; TV, tricuspid valve.

The Kawashima procedure consists of division of the right ventricular outflow tract into two parts, one for the systemic and the other for the pulmonary circulation. When the distance between the tricuspid valve and the pulmonary valve allows unobstructed intraventricular rerouting, the baffle can be placed between the two valves with resection of the infundibular septum (upper panel in **Fig. 4.13**). When the tricuspid and pulmonary valves are too close, the baffle needs to be placed around the antero-superior margin of the pulmonary valve (lower panel in **Fig. 4.13**). In some patients, the pulmonary valve cannot be spared during construction of the baffle between the ventricular septal defect and the aorta. In these cases, a right ventriculotomy is made and a conduit interposed between the right ventricle and the pulmonary arteries.

Konno–Rastan Operation (Aortoventriculoplasty) The Konno–Rastan operation is used in patients with severe aortic or subaortic stenosis where the obstruction is not amenable to simple valvotomy or resection of the obstructive lesion because of severe hypoplasia of the aortic valve and/or subaortic outflow tract.[37,38]

The operation involves enlargement of the left ventricular outflow tract by inserting a patch in the ventricular septum, aortic valve replacement, and enlargement of the aortic annulus and ascending aorta (**Fig. 4.14**). A vertical incision is made in the anterior wall of the aorta. The incision is extended into the anterior wall of the right ventricle (a-a'). The aortic incision is also extended through the ventricular septum (a-b). The outlet septum is excised and the margins of the excised ventricular septum and incised aorta are stretched open (**Fig. 4.14B**) and a prosthetic valve is placed in the enlarged annulus (**Fig. 4.14C**). The left ventricular outflow tract is augmented by applying a patch on the margin of the surgically created ventricular septal defect and the gap in the aorta. Finally, the right ventricular outflow tract patch is applied (**Fig. 4.14D**).

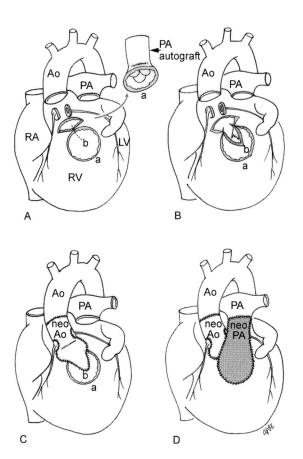

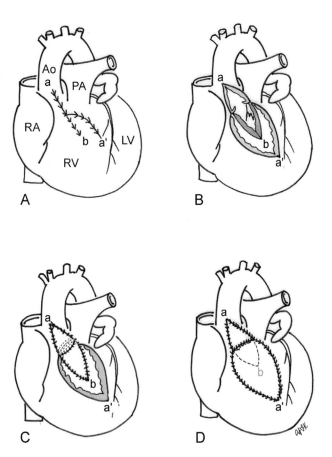

Fig. 4.14 Konno-Rastan operation. RA, right atrium; RV, right ventricle; LV, left ventricle; Ao, ascending aorta; PA, pulmonary artery; a, vertical incision in the anterior wall of the aorta; a-a', incision extended into the anterior wall of the right ventricle. a-b, incision extended into the ventircular septum.

Fig. 4.15 Ross–Konno operation. RA, right atrium; RV, right ventricle; LV, left ventricle; Ao, ascending aorta; PA, pulmonary artery; a, incised margin after harvest of the pulmonary homograft; b, incision made into the ventricular septum.

The Ross–Konno operation uses the patient's own pulmonary valve instead of an artificial prosthetic valve for aortic valve replacement (**Fig. 4.15**).[39] The aorta is divided above the valve and the valve tissue is excised (**Fig. 4.15A**). The coronary arteries are mobilized along with a button of aortic sinus. The pulmonary autograft is then harvested from the heart. An incision is made into the ventricular septum through the dissected right ventricular outflow tract and the aortic root (**Fig. 4.15B**). An obstructing lesion in the subaortic region is excised. The pulmonary autograft is then fit into the left ventricular outflow tract and the surgical gap in the ventricular septum is closed with a patch (**Fig. 4.15C**). The right ventricular outflow tract is reconstructed by placing a homograft (**Fig. 4.15D**).

Lateral Tunnel Procedure (See Fontan Operation)

Lecompte Maneuver (See Arterial Switch Operation)

Lecompte Operation (See Rastelli Operation)

Mee shunt (See Balock–Taussig Shunt)

Mustard Operation (See Atrial Switch Operation)

Nikaidoh Operation (See Rastelli Operation)

Norwood Operation The Norwood procedure is the most commonly performed initial palliative procedure for patients undergoing staged surgical palliation for hypoplastic left heart syndrome in the neonatal period (**Fig. 4.16**).[40,41]

The Norwood procedure consists of dissection of the distal pulmonary arterial trunk and closure of the pulmonary arterial side of the dissected pulmonary arterial trunk (**Fig. 4.16A**); division and complete excision of the ductus arteriosus; a large incision along the ascending aorta, aortic arch, and proximal descending aorta (**Fig. 4.16B**); and anastomosis of the pulmonary arterial trunk to the incised aorta by using a homograft patch (**Fig. 4.16C**). As pulmonary vascular resistance is high in the neonatal period, a modified BT (aortopulmonary) shunt or Sano shunt (ventriculopulmonary) shunt is constructed to provide a controlled source of pulmonary blood flow at the cost of volume loading the right ventricle. A second-stage procedure, the BCPC or hemi-Fontan procedure, is typically performed at 3 to 6 months of age. A third stage, usually performed at 2 to 4 years of age, is a Fontan procedure. This is performed to channel the remaining systemic venous return from the inferior vena cava to the pulmonary arteries.

The initial Norwood procedure is associated with rather high morbidity and mortality, which is at least partly related to cardiopulmonary bypass. In addition, suboptimal neurocognitive function among survivors after staged reconstruction has prompted the use of the hybrid procedure that avoids cardiopulmonary bypass and circulatory arrest in the neonatal period (**Fig. 4.17**).[41,42]

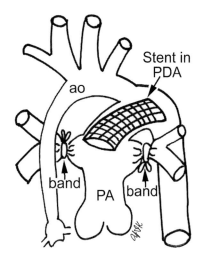

Fig. 4.17 Hybrid procedure for hypoplastic left heart syndrome. ao, aorta; PDA, patent ductus arteriosus; PA, pulmonary artery.

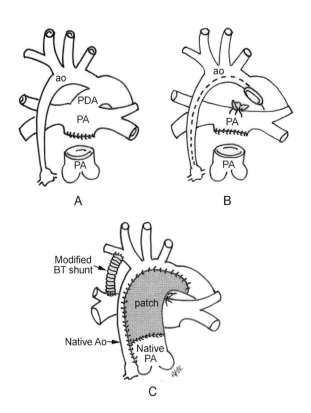

Fig. 4.16 Norwood operation. ao, aorta; PDA, patent ductus arteriosus; PA, pulmonary artery; BT, Blalock–Taussig.

The hybrid procedure is a combined surgical and interventional catheterization procedure to achieve bilateral branch pulmonary artery banding, enlargement or creation of an atrial septal defect, and stenting of the arterial duct as an alternative form of neonatal palliation for hypoplastic left heart syndrome (**Fig 4.17**). The second-stage reconstruction of the ascending aorta and arch is usually performed at 4 to 6 months of age and consists of stent removal, aortic arch reconstruction, and bidirectional cavopulmonary shunt.

One and a Half Ventricle Repair   (See Fontan Operation)

Potts Shunt   (See Blalock–Taussig Shunt)

Pulmonary Artery Banding The primary objective of performing pulmonary artery banding (PAB) is to reduce excessive pulmonary blood flow and protect the pulmonary vasculature from irreversible obstructive vascular disease causing pulmonary hypertension.[43] These bands commonly include a radiopaque marker and can be seen on chest radiographs.

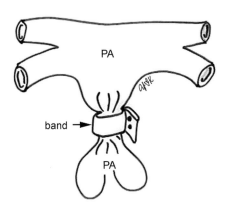

Fig. 4.18 Pulmonary artery (PA) banding.

The site of band placement is carefully selected in the midportion of the main pulmonary artery trunk, avoiding distortion or injury to the pulmonary valve or impingement of the branch pulmonary arteries (**Fig. 4.18**). This technique was widely used in the past as an initial surgical intervention for children born with a defect causing a large left-to-right shunt. With improvement of neonatal surgical techniques, early definitive intracardiac repair has largely replaced palliation with PAB.[44] However, it continues to maintain a role in certain subsets of patients with complex congenital heart disease that does not allow neonatal surgical treatment. PAB plays a role in the preparation and training of the left ventricle in patients with complete or corrected transposition of the great arteries for a delayed arterial switch procedure. Because there is potential for the band to encroach upon the lumen of either branch pulmonary artery, asymmetric appearance of pulmonary blood flow on chest radi-

ographs may be an important early sign of branch pulmonary artery stenosis.

Rastelli Operation The Rastelli operation was originally used for the repair of complete transposition of the great vessels with ventricular septal defect and pulmonary outflow tract obstruction.[45,46] It has subsequently been utilized for a variety of congenital heart defects characterized by two ventricles and overriding of the aorta with severe pulmonary stenosis or pulmonary atresia, such as double-outlet right ventricle with pulmonary stenosis or atresia and pulmonary atresia with ventricular septal defect.

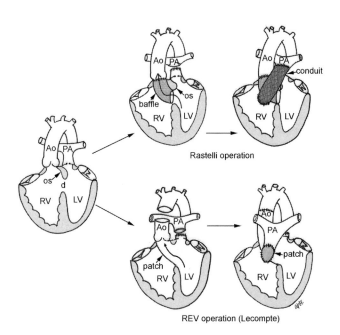

Fig. 4.19 Rastelli and REV ("Réparation à l'Etage ventriculaire") operations. RV, right ventricle; LV, left ventricle; Ao, ascending aorta; PA, pulmonary artery; os, outlet (infundibular) septum; d, ventricular septal defect.

The Rastelli operation consists of tunneling of the left ventricular outflow tract to the aorta by closing the ventricular septal defect with a baffle, division of the distal pulmonary arterial trunk, closure of the proximal arterial trunk, and reconstruction of the pulmonary outflow tract using a valved homograft conduit (upper panel in **Fig 4.19**).

The "Réparation à l'Etage ventriculaire" (REV) operation of Lecompte is a modification of the Rastelli operation.[46,47] The REV procedure consists of extensive excision of the outlet septum when present, anterior translocation of the pulmonary artery through the gap in the dissected ascending aorta, closure of the ventricular septal defect to the anterior wall of the aortic valve annulus, and direct anastomosis of the pulmonary artery to the right ventricle without a prosthetic conduit (lower panel in **Fig. 4.19**). The REV operation is less often complicated by aortic and pulmonary outflow tract obstruction compared with the Rastelli operation.

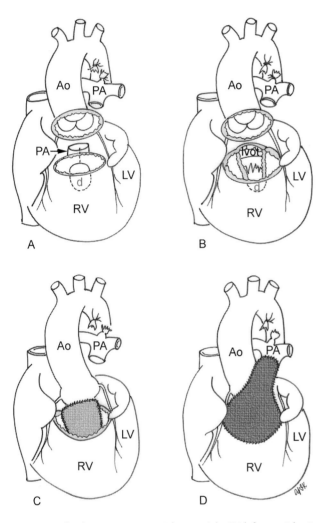

Fig. 4.20 Nikaido operation. RV, right ventricle; LV, left ventricle; Ao, ascending aorta; PA, pulmonary artery.

Another modification of the Rastelli operation is the Nikaidoh operation in which the aorta with its valve is translocated to the pulmonary position (**Fig. 4.20**).[48,49] This procedure consists of excision of the aortic root with the aortic valve from the right ventricular outflow tract without mobilization of the coronary arteries (**Fig. 4.20A**), division of the pulmonary annulus and excision of the outlet septum (**Fig. 4.20B**), implantation of the excised aortic root on the left ventricular outflow tract, patch closure of the ventricular septal defect along the anterior superior margin of the translocated aortic root (**Fig. 4.20C**), and reconstruction of the right ventricular outflow tract to the pulmonary artery with a homograft or outflow tract patch

(**Fig. 4.20D**). A recent study from a large center showed a favorable long-term outcome with a better anatomic result compared with Rastelli and REV operations.[50]

REV ("Réparation à l'Etage Ventriculaire") Operation (of Lecompte) (See Rastelli Operation)

Ross Operation Severe aortic stenosis or insufficiency requires replacement of the aortic valve with a mechanical or biologic valve. The patient with a mechanical valve needs lifelong anticoagulant therapy, whereas artificial biologic valves are less durable than mechanical valves. The Ross procedure utilizes the patient's own pulmonary valve (pulmonary autograft) for aortic valve replacement (**Fig. 4.21**).[51,52]

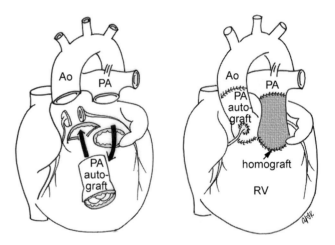

Fig. 4.21 Ross operation. Ao, ascending aorta; PA, pulmonary artery; RV, right ventricle.

The pulmonary valve is removed with the adjacent right ventricle and proximal pulmonary arterial trunk as a cylinder from the patient. The native aortic valve is then replaced by the removed cylinder of pulmonary autograft. The coronary arterial ostia are excised from the native aorta and reimplanted in the corresponding positions on the pulmonary autograft. The right ventricle-to-pulmonary artery connection is established with a homograft valve. As the pulmonary autograft grows with somatic growth, its longevity is excellent. The Ross procedure is the most ideal technique for small children and infants.[53] Furthermore, anticoagulation is not required following the procedure. Later replacement of the pulmonary valve homograft is generally required due to growth of the patient or degeneration of the homograft.

When there is intrinsic hypoplasia of the aortic outflow tract or aortic valve annulus, the Ross procedure can be combined with the Konno–Rastan type of operation, which is called a Ross–Konno operation (see Konno–Rastan Operation).[39]

Ross–Konno Operation   (See Konno–Rastan Operation)

Sano Shunt   (See Blalock–Taussig Shunt)

Senning Operation   (See Atrial Switch Operation)

Sutureless Pulmonary Vein Repair   (See Cole's Procedure)

Takeuchi Operation   An anomalous coronary artery arising from the pulmonary artery requires reimplan-tation of the anomalous coronary artery to the aorta using a technique similar to that used in an arterial switch operation for complete transposition of the great arteries.[54]

The Takeuchi operation is an intrapulmonary arterial baffling of the anomalous coronary artery that is used when the anomalous coronary artery cannot be mobilized for a coronary arterial translocation procedure (**Fig. 4.22**).[54,55]

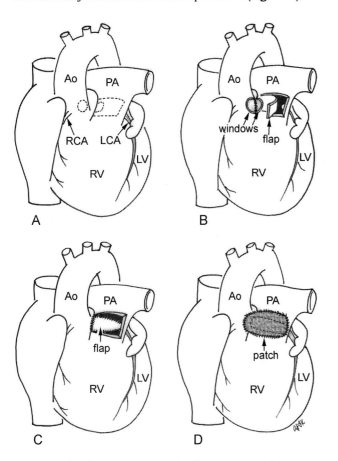

Fig. 4.22 Takeuchi operation. Ao, ascending aorta; PA, pulmonary artery; RV, right ventricle; LV, left ventricle; RCA, right coronary artery; LCA, left coronary artery.

The procedure consists of a round excision in the opposing walls of the aorta and pulmonary arterial trunks and transverse rectangular incision in the anterior wall of the pulmonary artery (**Fig. 4.22A**), creation of an aortopulmonary window (**Fig. 4.22B**), tunneling of the left coronary arterial route to the aorta within the pulmonary artery by using the flap from the pulmonary arterial wall (**Fig. 4.22C**), and patch graft of the anterior wall of the pulmonary artery (**Fig. 4.22D**).

Unifocalization of Pulmonary Arteries   In tetralogy of Fallot with pulmonary atresia, the pulmonary arterial blood flow is often supplied by multiple major aortopulmonary collateral arteries (upper panel in **Fig. 4.23**).

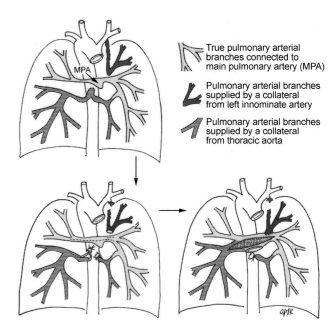

Fig. 4.23 Unifocalization of pulmonary arteries.

Corrective surgery in patients with multifocal pulmonary arterial blood flow involves so-called unifocalization in which the disconnected pulmonary arteries are bundled together into a single vessel or into the pulmonary artery when it is present (lower panels in **Fig 4.23**).[56,57] The unifocalized pulmonary artery is then connected to the right ventricle by using a homograft conduit. Depending on the anatomic status of the pulmonary arterial bed and pulmonary vascular resistance, the complete intracardiac repair can be performed simultaneously or later. Occasionally, complex

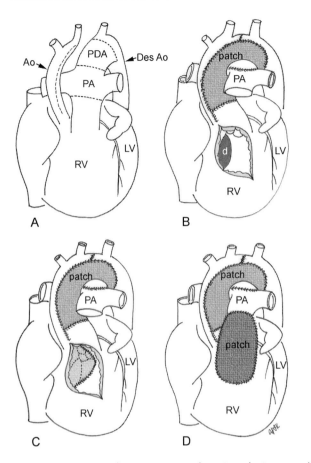

Fig. 4.24 Yasui procedure in interrupted aortic arch. Ao, ascending aorta; PDA, patent ductus arteriosus; Des Ao, descending aorta; PA, pulmonary artery; RV, right ventricle; LV, left ventricle.

pulmonary artery anatomy may require staged unifocalization of the pulmonary arteries followed by intracardiac repair.

Waterston Shunt (See Blalock–Taussig Shunt)

Yasui Procedure This procedure is used for primary biventricular repair of interruption or severe hypoplasia of the aortic arch and severe left ventricular outflow tract obstruction (**Fig. 4.24**).[58,59]

The procedure consists of an incision along the entire length of the ascending aorta, transaction of the distal main pulmonary artery, and complete removal of the ductus arteriosus (**Fig. 4.24A**); reconstruction of the ascending aorta and aortic arch (**Fig. 4.24B**); creation of dual outflow tracts for the left ventricle by baffling the ventricular septal defect to the pulmonary artery (**Fig. 4.24C**); and a new connection of the confluent pulmonary artery to the right ventricle (**Fig. 4.24D**). Aortic arch reconstruction is achieved by anastomosis of the proximal pulmonary trunk to the incised aortic arch with or without additional graft material depending on the severity of narrowing and availability of the native tissue. The patency of the left ventricular outflow tract is restored by baffling the ventricular septal defect to the pulmonary valve annulus and leaving the native left ventricular outflow tract untouched. The confluent pulmonary artery is connected to the right ventricle with or without using a valved conduit.

References

1. Gross RE. Surgical ligation of a patent ductus arteriosus: report of first successful case. JAMA 1939;112:729–731
2. Senning A. Surgical correction of transposition of the great vessels. Surgery 1959;45(6):966–980
3. Mustard WT. Successful two-stage correction of transposition of the great vessels. Surgery 1964;55:469–472
4. Warnes CA. Transposition of the great arteries. Circulation 2006;114(24):2699–2709
5. Mustard WT, Chute AL, Keith JD, Sivek A, Rowe RD, Vlad P. A surgical approach to transposition of the great vessels with extracorporeal circuit. Surgery 1954;36:39–51
6. Jatene AD, Fontes VF, Paulista PP, et al. Anatomic correction of transposition of the great vessels. J Thorac Cardiovasc Surg 1976; 72(3):364–370
7. Lecompte Y, Zannini L, Hazan E, et al. Anatomic correction of transposition of the great arteries. J Thorac Cardiovasc Surg 1981;82(4):629–631
8. Hopkins RA, Armstrong BE, Serwer GA, Peterson RJ, Oldham HN Jr. Physiological rationale for a bidirectional cavopulmonary shunt. A versatile complement to the Fontan principle. J Thorac Cardiovasc Surg 1985;90(3):391–398
9. Bridges ND, Jonas RA, Mayer JE, Flanagan MF, Keane JF, Castaneda AR. Bidirectional cavopulmonary anastomosis as interim palliation for high-risk Fontan candidates. Early results. Circulation 1990;82(5, Suppl):IV170–IV176
10. Jacobs ML, Pourmoghadam KK. The hemi-Fontan operation. Semin Thorac Cardiovasc Surg Pediatr Card Surg Annu 2003;6:90–97
11. Blalock A, Taussig HB. The surgical treatment of malformations of the heart in which there is pulmonary stenosis or pulmonary atresia. JAMA 1945;128:189–192
12. Gazzaniga AB, Elliott MP, Sperling DR, et al. Microporous expanded polytetrafluoroethylene arterial prosthesis for construction of aortopulmonary shunts: experimental and clinical results. Ann Thorac Surg 1976;21(4):322–327
13. Trusler GA, Miyamura H, Culham JAG, Fowler RS, Freedom RM, Williams WG. Pulmonary artery stenosis following aortopulmonary anastomoses. J Thorac Cardiovasc Surg 1981;82(3):398–404
14. Potapov EV, Alexi-Meskishvili VV, Dähnert I, Ivanitskaia EA, Lange PE, Hetzer R. Development of pulmonary arteries after central aortopulmonary shunt in newborns. Ann Thorac Surg 2001;71(3):899–905, discussion 905–906
15. Watterson KG, Wilkinson JL, Karl TR, Mee RB. Very small pulmonary arteries: central end-to-side shunt. Ann Thorac Surg 1991;52(5):1132–1137
16. Sano S, Ishino K, Kawada M, et al. Right ventricle-pulmonary artery shunt in first-stage palliation of hypoplastic left heart syndrome. J Thorac Cardiovasc Surg 2003;126(2):504–509, discussion 509–510
17. Yun TJ, Coles JG, Konstantinov IE, et al. Conventional and sutureless techniques for management of the pulmonary veins: evolution of indications

from postrepair pulmonary vein stenosis to primary pulmonary vein anomalies. J Thorac Cardiovasc Surg 2005;129(1):167–174

18. Damus PS. Letter to the editor. Ann Thorac Surg 1975;20:724–725
19. Kaye MP. Anatomic correction of transposition of great arteries. Mayo Clin Proc 1975;50(11):638–640
20. Stansel HC Jr. A new operation for D-loop transposition of the great vessels. Ann Thorac Surg 1975;19(5):565–567
21. Ceithaml EL, Puga FJ, Danielson GK, McGoon DC, Ritter DG. Results of the Damus-Stansel-Kaye procedure for transposition of the great arteries and for double-outlet right ventricle with subpulmonary ventricular septal defect. Ann Thorac Surg 1984;38(5):433–437
22. Lui RC, Williams WG, Trusler GA, et al. Experience with the Damus-Kaye-Stansel procedure for children with Taussig-Bing hearts or univentricular hearts with subaortic stenosis. Circulation 1993;88 (5 Pt 2):II170–II176
23. Masuda M, Tanoue Y, Ohno T, Tominaga R. Modified Damus-Kaye-Stansel procedure using aortic flap technique for systemic ventricular outflow tract obstruction in functionally univentricular heart. Eur J Cardiothorac Surg 2006;29(6):1056–1058
24. Imai Y, Sawatari K, Hoshino S, Ishihara K, Nakazawa M, Momma K. Ventricular function after anatomic repair in patients with atrioventricular discordance. J Thorac Cardiovasc Surg 1994;107(5):1272–1283
25. Ilbawi MN, DeLeon SY, Backer CL, et al. An alternative approach to the surgical management of physiologically corrected transposition with ventricular septal defect and pulmonary stenosis or atresia. J Thorac Cardiovasc Surg 1990;100(3):410–415
26. Hörer J, Haas F, Cleuziou J, et al. Intermediate-term results of the Senning or Mustard procedures combined with the Rastelli operation for patients with discordant atrioventricular connections associated with discordant ventriculoarterial connections or double outlet right ventricle. Cardiol Young 2007;17(2):158–165
27. Fontan F, Baudet E. Surgical repair of tricuspid atresia. Thorax 1971; 26(3):240–248
28. Vouhé PR. Fontan completion: intracardiac tunnel or extracardiac conduit? Thorac Cardiovasc Surg 2001;49(1):27–29
29. de Leval MR, Kilner P, Gewillig M, Bull C. Total cavopulmonary connection: a logical alternative to atriopulmonary connection for complex Fontan operations. Experimental studies and early clinical experience. J Thorac Cardiovasc Surg 1988;96(5):682–695
30. Kawashima Y, Kitamura S, Matsuda H, Shimazaki Y, Nakano S, Hirose H. Total cavopulmonary shunt operation in complex cardiac anomalies. A new operation. J Thorac Cardiovasc Surg 1984;87(1):74–81
31. McElhinney DB, Kreutzer J, Lang P, Mayer JE Jr, del Nido PJ, Lock JE. Incorporation of the hepatic veins into the cavopulmonary circulation in patients with heterotaxy and pulmonary arteriovenous malformations after a Kawashima procedure. Ann Thorac Surg 2005;80(5): 1597–1603
32. Billingsley AM, Laks H, Boyce SW, George B, Santulli T, Williams RG. Definitive repair in patients with pulmonary atresia and intact ventricular septum. J Thorac Cardiovasc Surg 1989;97(5):746–754
33. Chowdhury UK, Airan B, Talwar S, et al. One and one-half ventricle repair: results and concerns. Ann Thorac Surg 2005;80(6):2293–2300
34. Glenn WWL. Circulatory bypass of the right side of the heart. IV. Shunt between superior vena cava and distal right pulmonary artery; report of clinical application. N Engl J Med 1958;259(3):117–120
35. Kawashima Y, Fujita T, Miyamoto T, Manabe H. Intraventricular rerouting of blood for the correction of Taussig-Bing malformation. J Thorac Cardiovasc Surg 1971;62(5):825–829
36. Mavroudis C, Backer CL, Muster AJ, Rocchini AP, Rees AH, Gevitz M. Taussig-Bing anomaly: arterial switch versus Kawashima intraventricular repair. Ann Thorac Surg 1996;61(5):1330–1338
37. Konno S, Imai Y, Iida Y, Nakajima M, Tatsuno K. A new method for prosthetic valve replacement in congenital aortic stenosis associated with hypoplasia of the aortic valve ring. J Thorac Cardiovasc Surg 1975;70(5):909–917
38. Rastan H, Koncz J. Aortoventriculoplasty: a new technique for the treatment of left ventricular outflow tract obstruction. J Thorac Cardiovasc Surg 1976;71(6):920–927

39. Brown JW, Ruzmetov M, Vijay P, Rodefeld MD, Turrentine MW. The Ross-Konno procedure in children: outcomes, autograft and allograft function, and reoperations. Ann Thorac Surg 2006;82(4):1301–1306
40. Norwood WI, Kirklin JK, Sanders SP. Hypoplastic left heart syndrome: experience with palliative surgery. Am J Cardiol 1980;45(1):87–91
41. Alsoufi B, Bennetts J, Verma S, Caldarone CA. New developments in the treatment of hypoplastic left heart syndrome. Pediatrics 2007; 119(1):109–117
42. Gibbs JL, Wren C, Watterson KG, Hunter S, Hamilton JR. Stenting of the arterial duct combined with banding of the pulmonary arteries and atrial septectomy or septostomy: a new approach to palliation for the hypoplastic left heart syndrome. Br Heart J 1993;69(6):551–555
43. Muller WH Jr, Danimann JF Jr. The treatment of certain congenital malformations of the heart by the creation of pulmonic stenosis to reduce pulmonary hypertension and excessive pulmonary blood flow; a preliminary report. Surg Gynecol Obstet 1952;95(2):213–219
44. Takayama H, Sekiguchi A, Chikada M, Noma M, Ishizawa A, Takamoto S. Mortality of pulmonary artery banding in the current era: recent mortality of PA banding. Ann Thorac Surg 2002t;74(4):1219–1223, discussion 1223–1224
45. Rastelli GC, McGoon DC, Wallace RB. Anatomic correction of transposition of the great arteries with ventricular septal defect and subpulmonary stenosis. J Thorac Cardiovasc Surg 1969;58(4):545–552
46. Vouhé PR, Tamisier D, Leca F, Ouaknine R, Vernant F, Neveux JY. Transposition of the great arteries, ventricular septal defect, and pulmonary outflow tract obstruction. Rastelli or Lecompte procedure? J Thorac Cardiovasc Surg 1992;103(3):428–436
47. Lecompte Y. Reparation a l'etage ventriculaire: the REV procedure. Cardiol Young 1991;1:63–70
48. Nikaidoh H. Aortic translocation and biventricular outflow tract reconstruction. A new surgical repair for transposition of the great arteries associated with ventricular septal defect and pulmonary stenosis. J Thorac Cardiovasc Surg 1984;88(3):365–372
49. Yeh T Jr, Ramaciotti C, Leonard SR, Roy L, Nikaidoh H. The aortic translocation (Nikaidoh) procedure: midterm results superior to the Rastelli procedure. J Thorac Cardiovasc Surg 2007;133(2):461–469
50. Bautista-Hernandez V, Marx GR, Bacha EA, del Nido PJ. Aortic root translocation plus arterial switch for transposition of the great arteries with left ventricular outflow tract obstruction: intermediate-term results. J Am Coll Cardiol 2007;49(4):485–490
51. Ross DN. Replacement of aortic and mitral valves with a pulmonary autograft. Lancet 1967;2(7523):956–958
52. Ross DN. The pulmonary autograft: the Ross principle (or Ross procedural confusion). J Heart Valve Dis 2000;9(2):174–175
53. Pasquali SK, Shera D, Wernovsky G, et al. Midterm outcomes and predictors of reintervention after the Ross procedure in infants, children, and young adults. J Thorac Cardiovasc Surg 2007;133(4):893–899
54. Azakie A, Russell JL, McCrindle BW, et al. Anatomic repair of anomalous left coronary artery from the pulmonary artery by aortic reimplantation: early survival, patterns of ventricular recovery and late outcome. Ann Thorac Surg 2003;75(5):1535–1541
55. Takeuchi S, Imamura H, Katsumoto K, et al. New surgical method for repair of anomalous left coronary artery from pulmonary artery. J Thorac Cardiovasc Surg 1979;78(1):7–11
56. Sullivan ID, Wren C, Stark J, de Leval MR, Macartney FJ, Deanfield JE. Surgical unifocalization in pulmonary atresia and ventricular septal defect. A realistic goal? Circulation 1988;78(5 Pt 2):III5–III13
57. Reddy VM, McElhinney DB, Amin Z, et al. Early and intermediate outcomes after repair of pulmonary atresia with ventricular septal defect and major aortopulmonary collateral arteries: experience with 85 patients. Circulation 2000;101(15):1826–1832
58. Yasui H, Kado H, Nakano E, et al. Primary repair of interrupted aortic arch and severe aortic stenosis in neonates. J Thorac Cardiovasc Surg 1987;93(4):539–545
59. Nathan M, Rimmer D, del Nido PJ, et al. Aortic atresia or severe left ventricular outflow tract obstruction with ventricular septal defect: results of primary biventricular repair in neonates. Ann Thorac Surg 2006;82(6):2227–2232

5 The Best Radiographs with the Least Radiation

Ellen Charkot and Shi-Joon Yoo

Chest radiography is often the initial tool of investigation and detection of congenital heart disease in the pediatric age group. The production of good quality images is essential to accurately identify the condition and provide support to the clinical picture. To produce optimal images, the technologist must first consider issues of proper positioning and radiation dose, which are dependent on the age and condition of the particular child. There are substantial differences in approach between neonates, toddlers, and older children in terms of immobilization, positioning, and radiation protection, as well as taking the exposure at the appropriate moment of inspiration. In addition, there are considerations based on the type of technology available including film/screen radiography, computed radiography (CR), and digital radiography (DR). For well over a century, the standard for chest radiography was film/screen radiography, which produced excellent detail. In the last two decades, advances in computer technology have resulted in digital imaging receptors with increased sensitivity and a wide dynamic range. However, despite technology advances and changes, the skill of the technologist remains the most important factor in the acquisition of satisfactory diagnostic images in children with congenital heart disease.

■ Positioning Achieving Best Results at Different Age Groups

Chest radiographs should be obtained in the upright position. However, a study on a neonate or a child in intensive care is routinely performed in the supine position. Several factors need to be taken into consideration, regardless of whether the image obtained is upright or supine. Maximum inspiration, nonrotation of the patient, proper exposure factors, and collimation and correct side markers are essential in accurate interpretation. Images produced with poor inspiration or on expiration, and rotation (**Fig. 5.1**) are the most common causes of misinterpretation. At all times, the goal of the technologist is to produce the best image with the least radiation dose.

Neonates

The routine images obtained are AP (anteroposterior), supine, and lateral. When imaging a neonate, the technologist must be prepared ahead of time to work quickly. Neonates must be kept warm and appropriate infection control procedures must be followed. A neonate in an isolette frequently is connected to monitoring equipment, and may have tubes, leads, or lines obstructing the chest area. These should be disrupted as little as possible; however, the technologist should make every effort to clear the field of visualization prior to obtaining the image. This, as well as assisting with the proper positioning, should be accomplished in tandem with a nurse. The child's head and spine must be maintained in a straight position because the slightest shift to the left or right can result in a rotated image. However, when positioning a

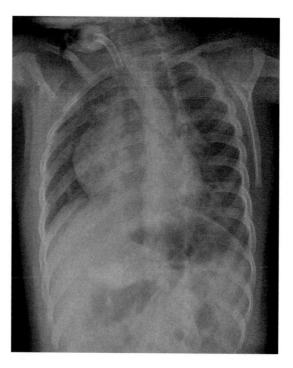

Fig. 5.1 Frontal chest radiograph obtained in a patient with atrial septal defect. It is nondiagnostic because of significant rotation. It is centered too low.

neonate with an endotracheal tube in situ, it is best to leave the head in its natural position, slightly turned to the side, to avoid dislodging the tube. One challenge facing the technologist is to obtain the image during full inspiration in a neonate with a rapid respiratory rate, which can be increased even further in congenital heart disease. Another challenge exists in choosing the correct exposure factors. For example, in an edematous neonate a higher exposure technique might be required. Limiting the field of exposure to the chest is not only necessary to produce a better quality image by reducing the scatter radiation, but it also plays an important role in reducing radiation exposure to the patient. This is further accomplished through the placement of a gonadal shield over the pelvis.

Babies Up to 2 Years Old

Immobilization of babies, a child up to 2 years of age, poses significant challenges for the technologist, particularly in acquiring images in the upright position. There are several techniques available, but the best results are achieved with the use of a Pigg-O-Stat (Modern Way Immobilizers, Inc., Clifton, TN) (**Fig. 5.2**). The Pigg-O-Stat is a form-fitting Plexiglas support, adjustable for patient size from infant to 2 years, easily manipulated from posteroanterior (PA) to lateral position and easily cleaned. With proper training, the technologist can ensure nonrotation and is able to monitor the breathing pattern before taking the exposure. Proper communication and explanation to the parent about using this device is essential as it can initially cause distress for a parent. It is important to explain the reason for the upright position and for a good inspiration, which is often aided by the patient crying.

Complete immobilization reduces the necessity for repeat exams and allows the technologist to work quickly at producing good quality images. The Pigg-O-Stat actually shortens the length of time spent conducting the study, thus reducing the impact on the child. Furthermore, as two people are required to position the child in the device properly, eliciting the parent's assistance can render the experience less traumatic for everyone.

The routine views taken for congenital heart disease in this age group are upright PA and lateral. The patient's gonads are protected by a lead shield. Often the child is crying because of the constraint, but this is helpful in achieving an inspiratory image. If the child is not crying, the Pigg-O-Stat's transparency allows the technologist to watch for the outlining of the ribs that indicates an inspiration; on the lateral view, the technologist can easily detect the expansive movement of the abdomen, which is typical in the breathing pattern of babies.

Toddlers and Young Children

This group is composed of children aged 3 to 7 years. Although immobilization is less of an issue, fidgeting can be a problem in this age group. To help them remain still throughout the study, the technologist should begin by explaining what is required, reassuring the child that there is no pain or discomfort involved. Practicing inspirations before beginning the exam, such as holding your breath under water or blowing out birthday candles, can be helpful. A younger child should be seated on a secure trolley or stool to help the child remain still while maintaining an upright nonrotated position. Routine views are upright PA and lateral. When taking a lateral exposure, a

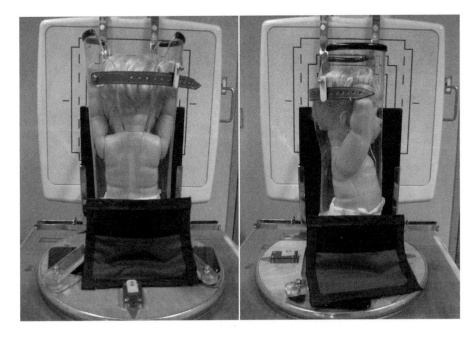

Fig. 5.2 Immobilization device (Pigg-O-Stat; Modern Way Immobilizers, Inc., Clifton, TN) used in babies up to 2 years of age. Transparency allows respiratory motion to be visible from outside.

parent can assist by holding the child's arms above its head as the child may be unsteady and have difficulty maintaining this position alone. A grid is used only in larger children to prevent scattered radiation from reaching the image receptors. Children less than 10 years of age do not need a grid for chest radiography. In terms of radiation protection, a gonadal shield is placed around the child's waist.

Older Children

Imaging children aged 8 to 18 years is less complicated. Beginning at 12 years of age, a grid is used during imaging to reduce the amount of scatter radiation to the image; thus, a higher exposure (120 kVp) is used in comparison with the younger age group. A radiation shield is used to cover the gonads. Immobilization is not required because the patients are usually cooperative and able to take directions, but proper positioning and good inspiration are still essential.

■ Assessing Resultant Image

Regardless of age the same principles apply to ensure that the resultant image is of diagnostic quality. To assess the image, a quick review should be performed.

Check that the patient is not rotated in the AP/PA projection by comparing the symmetric positions of the bony structures including bony ribs and clavicles (**Fig. 5.3**). The pairs of the anterior tips of the bony ribs should be mirror imaged with symmetric distances from the most lateral aspects of the bony thorax. Check that the image is taken in an inspiratory phase with the diaphragms seen at the level of the anterior tip of the 6th rib and slightly convexed upward. For a frontal chest radiograph, make sure that the arms are moved away from the chest wall. A lead marker should be visible to identify the correct side; this can be particularly important on initial images with dextrocardia or situs inversus (**Fig. 5.4**). For a lateral radiograph, the pairs of the costovertebral joints and ribs should be superimposed on each other and arms should be above the head to clearly visualize the apices.

■ Image Acquisition Methods

Plain chest radiography is acquired using either film/screen or digital technology, which consists of CR and DR. As with the conventional method of x-ray imaging using film and intensifying screens, CR requires a source of x-ray photons that interact with a subject to produce a latent image on an image plate. The difference between conventional technology and CR is that film/screen creates the latent image using light emitted by the intensifying screen and requires processing chemicals to develop the final film, whereas CR uses a photostimulable storage phosphor to produce a latent image. It is then scanned by a thin laser beam with

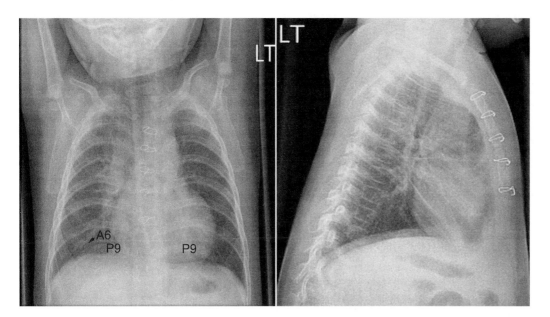

Fig. 5.3 Well-taken posteroanterior and left lateral chest radiographs in an infant who underwent open-heart surgery. It is well centered and not significantly rotated. The arms are stretched up and do not overlap on the chest. On frontal radiograph, both diaphragms are below the level of the posterior parts of the ninth ribs (P9) and the anterior tips of the sixth rib (A6), suggesting adequate depth of inspiration. Intervertebral spaces of the thoracic spine are faintly visible. On lateral radiograph, the sternum is well profiled and the posterior ribs are only slightly offset. The apices are cleared of the arms.

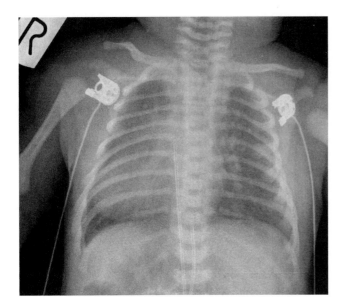

Fig. 5.4 Frontal chest radiograph shows dextrocardia. The abdominal situs is abnormal. Placement of correct lead marker is essential for correct diagnosis.

information converted to a digital format using an analog to digital (AD) converter. CR remains a cassette-based technology, making it useful for portable x-rays. DR uses a digital detector, which is an electronic device that directly converts x-ray energy to a digital format. DR that can be direct or indirect is a cassette-free technology making it generally more efficient, with higher resolution and more dose-efficient exposure. It is, however, much more expensive and is still in its early stages for use in portable x-rays. Because the images are digital, DR and CR are able to take advantage of postprocessing optimization. The ability to adjust and postprocess the image is especially advantageous in the chest area because of the high-contrast difference in the thoracic region between the low-density air-filled lungs and the high-density spine, mediastinum, and heart. The air-filled lungs are fully penetrated, whereas areas through the heart and mediastinum are obviously less so; with digital imaging, it is possible to manipulate the image to minimize the difference in density and better visualize the lung, heart, and mediastinum.

The introduction of digital technology (CR/DR) has had a significant impact on image acquisition, most notably in the reduction of repeat x-rays due to incorrect exposure factors. In film/screen exposure, errors of over- or underexposure can degrade the image quality and require a repeat image. CR/DR has wider latitude so incorrect exposure factors have less effect on the final quality, but it is still critical to choose the correct factors. Although digital technology can reduce repeats, the expertise of the technologist in positioning, coning, and capturing pediatric patients at full inspiration is by far the most critical factor

in reducing the overall radiation exposure to the patient. The wider dynamic range and latitude of CR/DR is an asset in the area of mobile radiography because these patients are more difficult to x-ray, and repeat images can be minimized. Digital technology has provided images for viewing and distribution hospital-wide.

Radiation Protection

Concerns of Exposure to Ionizing Radiation

The effects of ionizing radiation exposure are well documented and in the field of medicine, appropriate safeguards are standard procedure to minimize radiation dose. Chest radiography is considered a relatively low-dose exposure and the risks should be minimal. However, with regard to pediatric patients, because risk increases relative to longevity, and children are up to 10 times more sensitive to the effects of ionizing radiation, the professional responsibility of a technologist is to limit radiation dose during any image acquisition (see **Tables 5.1, 5.2,** typical exposure charts for various ages).

Achieving "ALARA"

ALARA is an acronym for "as low as reasonably achievable" and refers to the principle that radiation exposure during image acquisition should be kept to a minimum to all involved, while obtaining high quality images for diagnosis using the lowest possible radiation dose. To achieve this aim, there are several technical processes that are essential. First, good collimation is required, so that only the areas necessary for diagnosis are exposed. Second, correct exposure factors are essential; in addition, when using digital technology, proper reconstruction image algorithms must be used. A third factor involves positioning patients properly prior to taking exposures, using appropriate immobilization. Fourth, exposures should be taken on full inspiration to provide optimal diagnostic information. Finally, appropriate gonadal shielding is critical for all chest examinations.

The Ten Rules in Pediatric Chest Radiography

1. Proper nonrotated positioning is critical.
2. Choose correct exposure factors to optimize the image
3. Upright image is preferred whenever the patient's medical condition permits.
4. Ensure image exposure is at full inspiration

Table 5.1 Typical Examples of Technical Parameters for Supine Chest Radiography in Neonates Using a Portable Unit with 0.1 mm Cu Added

Neonate's Size	Projection	Exposure Factors	Distance	Skin Entrance Dose
Small neonate < 1.5 kg	PA	64 kVp @ 2 mAs	40 in	2.4 mR
	Lateral	70 kVp @ 2 mAs	40 in	3.1 mR
Large neonate > 2.5 kg	PA	64 kVp @ 2.5 mAs	40 in	3.3 mR
	Lateral	70 kVp @ 2.5 mAs	40 in	4.7 mR

Abbreviations: PA, posteroanterior; kg, kilogram; kVp, kilovolt peak; mAs, milliampare-second; in, inches; mR, milliroentgen.

Table 5.2 Representative Examples of Technical Parameters for Upright Chest Radiography in Children

Age Examples	Projection	Exposure Factors	Grid	Distance	Skin Entrance Dose
1 year	PA	86 kVp @ 2.5 mAs	No	72 in	4.1 mR
	Lateral	96 kVp @ 3.2 mAs	No	72 in	6.8 mR
5 year	PA	88 kVp @ 2.5 mAs	No	72 in	4.6 mR
	Lateral	96 kVp @ 4 mAs	No	72 in	8.9 mR
10 year	PA	88 kVp @ 2.5 mAs	No	72 in	4.9 mR
	Lateral	96 kVp @ 5 mAs	No	72 in	12 mR
12 year	PA	120 kVp @ 2.5 mAs	Yes	72 in	9 mR
	Lateral	120 kVp @ 5.0 mAs	Yes	72 in	14 mR

Abbreviations: PA, posteroanterior; kg, kilogram; kVp, kilovolt peak; mAs, milliampare-second; in, inches; mR, milliroentgen.

5. Correct lead side marker must be visible within the area of collimation.
6. Center image midway between C3 and the lower costal margin
7. Cone image from C3 to the lower costal margin
8. Lead shielding is required for gonadal protection.
9. Proper film placement at level of upper lip to ensure inclusion of airway
10. Use of a grid is not necessary for younger children.

Suggested Reading
Babyn P. Teaching Atlas of Pediatric Imaging. New York: Thieme Medical Publishers; 2006

Balinger PW, Frank ED, ed. Merrill's Atlas of Radiographic Positions and Radiologic Procedures. (10th ed.). St. Louis: Mosby Publishers; 2003

Freedom RM, Benson LN, Smallhorn JF, eds. Neonatal Heart Disease. New York: Springer Verlag;1992

Hall EJ. Lessons we have learned from our children: cancer risks from diagnostic radiology. Pediatr Radiol 2002;32(10):700–706

Wilmot DM, Sharko GA, eds. Pediatric Imaging for the Technologist. New York: Springer-Verlag; 1987

II Systematic Approach to Chest Radiographs

Chest radiographs provide abstract information regarding the patient's cardiovascular status and associated abnormalities in the extracardiac structures. Some abnormal findings can be easily appreciated, whereas other subtle findings can be recognized only by meticulous search. Therefore, it is important to assess the chest radiographs systematically in a step-by-step fashion. This section introduces a six-step systematic approach to the assessment of chest radiographs in children with cardiac problems:

1. Identification, clinical history, and radiographic techniques
2. Visceral situs, heart position, and aortic arch position
3. Heart size, overall configuration, and specific chamber enlargement
4. Pulmonary vascularity
5. Aorta and systemic veins
6. Airways, lungs, pleurae, mediastinum, diaphragm, and chest wall

6 Identification, Clinical History, and Radiographic Techniques

Before starting analysis of the radiographic findings, one should ascertain (1) the identification of the patient, including the name, medical record number, age, and gender; (2) the clinical information; (3) the right and left sides of the patient on the radiograph; and (4) the radiographic projection and exposure.

■ Identification

The patient's identification should always be checked every time the radiographs are reviewed. Putting an incorrect identification on a radiograph or taking radiographs from the wrong patient is a serious mistake that should be avoided, although it does happen. Recognition of incorrect labeling is easy when previous studies are available for comparison. The patient's age, gender, and clinical information may provide clues in discovering incorrect identifications. The age of the patient should also be taken into consideration in radiographic interpretation, as normal radiographic findings vary with age.

■ Clinical Information

The clinical information given in the request for radiographs may include the clinical diagnosis, the patient's major symptoms and signs, and the medical or surgical interventions. The radiographic findings at first should be reviewed blindly to avoid a potential bias, and then with the clinical information taken into consideration. The radiographic findings should be assessed as to whether or not they are in accordance with the given clinical information, the severity of the radiographic manifestations, and the patient's diagnosis or condition. The findings should also be reviewed for any additional unrecognized or unsuspected features.

■ Right/Left Sides of the Patient on Radiographs

Incorrect labeling of the right/left side of the chest is rare. But there are a few pitfall conditions that may lead the radiographic technologist to make this mistake. For example, at our hospital we were unable to place in the supine position a newborn with a meningomyelocele, so all radiographs were taken in the prone position. But the radiographs were incorrectly labeled with a side marker in the same way as for patients whose radiographs are routinely obtained in a supine position. We also had a patient with situs inversus and dextrocardia on whose radiograph the side of the chest was initially labeled with a proper side marker but later it was replaced with an incorrect marker when the technologist thought that there had been a mistake.

■ Radiographic Projection and Exposure

Chest radiographs are usually obtained with the patient upright and in deep inspiration, using a posteroanterior projection for a frontal view and a right-to-left projection for a lateral view. These projections allow full expansions of the lungs for optimal assessment and minimize magnification of the cardiac silhouette. There are occasions when these standard projections are not possible. In particular, newborns and critically ill patients in the intensive care unit require imaging in a supine position, which is routinely performed using an anteroposterior projection. A large cardiac silhouette and indistinct cardiac borders result from both supine positioning of the patient and the anteroposterior projection (**Fig. 6.1**).

An oblique radiographic projection to the right or left is not uncommon in pediatric patients. The configuration and size of the cardiovascular silhouette may appear

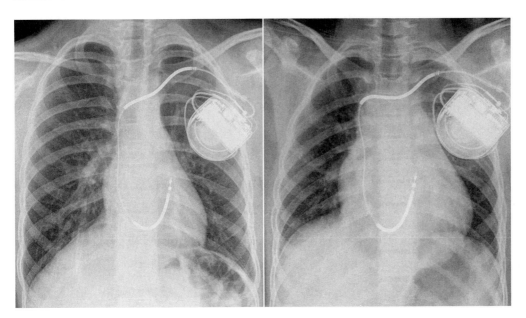

Fig. 6.1 Frontal chest radiographs in posteroanterior *(left panel)* and anteroposterior *(right panel)* projections from a 10-year-old patient with left ventricular myocardial noncompaction and an intracardiac defibrillator complex in place. The scapulas are nicely positioned without significant overlap over the lungs on posteroanterior view, but larger parts of the scapulas are superimposed on the lungs on anteroposterior view. The cardiac silhouette appears larger and more globular on anteroposterior view than on posteroanterior view.

significantly different in oblique views (**Fig. 6.2**). An oblique projection can be easily identified by comparing the positions of the anterior tips of the bony ribs. When a frontal chest radiograph is obtained in a left anterior or right posterior oblique view, the tips of the right ribs are aligned far outward along the lateral boundary of the right thorax, whereas the tips of the left ribs are projected inward (**Fig. 6.2**, left panel). When a frontal chest radiograph is obtained in the right anterior or left posterior oblique view, the tips of the left ribs are aligned far outward, whereas the tips of the right ribs are projected inward (**Fig. 6.2**, right panel). When there is levocardia, the cardiac silhouette is smaller in the left anterior or right posterior oblique view than in the straight frontal view

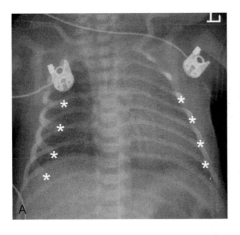
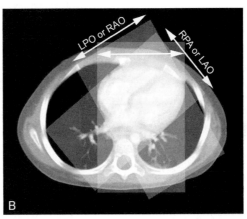

Fig. 6.2 (A) Oblique projections in an infant with levocardia. An oblique projection can be easily identified by comparing the positions of the anterior tips *(asterisks)* of the right and left bony ribs. On the left posterior or right anterior oblique (LPO or RAO) view *(left panel)*, the tips of the right ribs are projected medially and those of the left ribs are projected laterally. On the right posterior or left anterior oblique (RPO or LAO) view *(right panel)*, the tips of the right ribs are projected laterally and those of the left ribs are projected medially. Note that the cardiac silhouette is larger on the left posterior or right anterior oblique view, whereas it is smaller on the right posterior or left anterior oblique view when compared with a straight frontal view *(middle panel)*. **(B)** Axial computed tomography (CT) image at the four-chamber level showing an oblique orientation of the cardiac long axis relative to the orthogonal body axes, which explains the cardiac size differences in oblique and straight frontal projections.

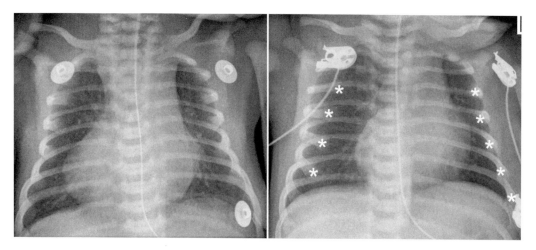

Fig. 6.3 Oblique projection in a patient with dextrocardia. Radiograph of a proper straight frontal view *(left panel)* shows dextrocardia. Radiograph of a left posterior oblique view *(right panel)*. Note that the anterior tips *(asterisks)* of the left bony ribs are projected lateral to the outer boundary of the left thorax, whereas those of the right ribs are projected medially. More than two thirds of the cardiac silhouette appears in the left thorax in this left posterior oblique view.

because the short axis of the heart is projected toward the radiographic screen in the former. In contrast, the cardiac silhouette is larger in the right anterior or left posterior oblique view because the long axis of the heart is projected toward the screen. When there is dextrocardia, this relationship between size and obliquity is reversed (**Fig. 6.3**).

A frontal chest radiograph may be obtained with a cranial or caudal angulation of the radiographic beam (**Figs. 6.4, 6.5**). When the beam is cranially angulated in an AP

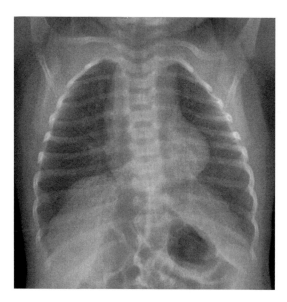

Fig. 6.4 Anteroposterior lordotic view. The chest frontal view obtained with the patient in a supine position, leaning back during the x-ray exposure, creates a lordotic image. The clavicles are above the first ribs and the anterior parts of the first five ribs are projected above their posterior parts. The cardiac apex is uplifted from the diaphragm and rounded, having a configuration similar to that seen in tetralogy of Fallot.

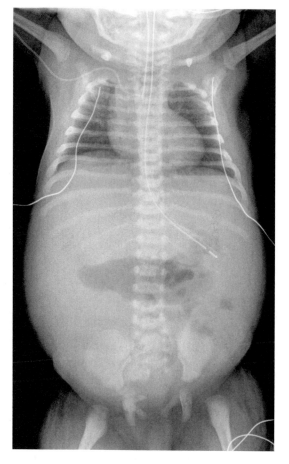

Fig. 6.5 Frontal radiograph of the chest and abdomen obtained with the patient in the supine position. The thorax is projected cranially because the radiographic beam is centered on the upper abdomen. The clavicles are seen above the lungs, and the anterior parts of the upper five ribs are projected above their posterior parts. The cardiac apex is well above the left diaphragmatic contour.

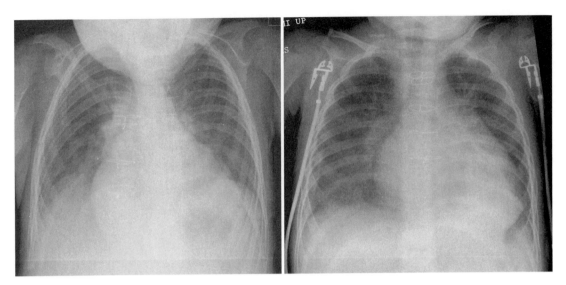

Fig. 6.6 Anteroposterior kyphotic view. The frontal chest radiograph *(left panel)* is obtained with the patient in the supine position with caudal angulation. The shape of the thoracic cage and the cardiac contour are different from those seen in a straight frontal view *(right panel)* from the same patient. Caudal angulation results in a kyphotic view of the chest. The clavicles are projected over the upper lungs, and approximately one third of the cardiac silhouette is seen below the diaphragmatic domes. The ribs are more vertically aligned in a kyphotic view.

view or caudally angulated in a PA view, the clavicles are projected superiorly above the first ribs, clearing the lung apices as in the so-called AP lordotic view that has been used for assessment of the lesions in the apices of the lungs (**Fig. 6.4**). This projection brings the cardiac silhouette above the dome of the diaphragm, and the cardiac apex appears elevated and rounded. In addition, the pulmonary vascularity may falsely appear diminished because a larger lung volume is projected on the radiographic screen. As a result, the findings may mimic those seen in tetralogy of Fallot. This projection is particularly common in infants and young children who tend to lean back when they are placed supine on the radiographic cassette, especially when a proper immobilization device is not used. A similar effect is also seen when a radiograph of the chest and abdomen is obtained in the supine position as a single view, because the radiographic beam is centered at the upper abdomen and therefore is cranially angled toward the chest (**Fig. 6.5**). When the radiographic beam is caudally angulated in an AP view or cranially angulated in a PA view, the clavicles are projected downward on the upper or middle lung zones (**Fig. 6.6**). This projection brings a large part of the cardiac silhouette below the dome of the diaphragm.

A lateral chest radiograph also can be obtained in an oblique projection. Obliquity of the lateral view can be assessed by observing the corresponding levels of the right and left ribs and the contours of the spinal bodies. In a well-taken lateral view, the most anterior and posterior parts of the right and left ribs are nicely superimposed on one another with only slight offset, the contours of the

spinal bodies are square and clearly defined by a single cortical line, and the cardiac silhouette is in direct contact with the most anterior part of the bony thorax. In an oblique lateral view, the cardiac silhouette is closer to or superimposed on the spinal column, and therefore the heart may falsely appear enlarged. Additionally, the anteriormost part of one lung is interposed between the anteriormost part of the chest cage and the cardiac silhouette.

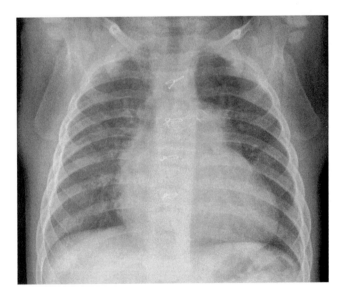

Fig. 6.7 Frontal chest radiograph with asymmetric radiographic exposure. The left lung is slightly more lucent than the right lung, which may suggest right lung or pleural disease. Note however, that the soft tissue is also denser in the right thorax.

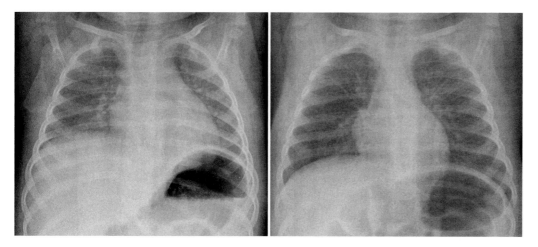

Fig. 6.8 Effect of respiration. The cardiac silhouette appears larger and more globular, and the pulmonary vascular markings more prominent in a radiograph obtained in an expiration phase *(left panel)* than in one obtained in an inspiration phase *(right panel)*.

Uncommonly, the right and left sides of the thorax show different radiographic densities. This may be due to an abnormality in a lung, a unilateral pleural lesion, or an asymmetric chest wall or breast. However, one should be aware that asymmetric blackness of a frontal chest radiograph is often due to an oblique projection or less commonly an asymmetric radiographic exposure (**Fig. 6.7**).

Finally, the depth of inspiration should also be taken into consideration. With deep inspiration, the cardiac silhouette appears slender and elongated, and the lungs appear hyperlucent. With incomplete inspiration or expiration, the cardiac silhouette is globular and appears enlarged, and the lungs appear hazy with prominent vascular markings (**Fig. 6.8**). The level of inspiration can be assessed by counting the ribs. During moderate inspiration, the diaphragmatic domes are at the level of the sixth ribs anteriorly and tenth ribs posteriorly. Because it is the anterior part of the diaphragm that domes on chest radiographs, counting of the anterior ribs is preferred.

Pearls

- Before analyzing the radiographs, the patient's name, age, and sex should always be checked, and the clinical history and radiographic techniques should be reviewed.

- The cardiac silhouette appears larger in a frontal radiograph obtained by an AP projection than in one obtained by a PA projection.

- The degree of obliquity in frontal chest radiographs can be easily assessed by comparing the positions of the anterior tips of the bony ribs.

- When there is levocardia, the cardiac silhouette is smaller on a right posterior or left anterior oblique view and larger on a left posterior or right anterior oblique view when compared with a straight frontal view.

- The cardiac silhouette is projected upward above the diaphragmatic dome on a lordotic view, and downward below the dome on a kyphotic view.

- The cardiac silhouette appears larger and more globular on a radiograph obtained in expiration than on a radiograph obtained in inspiration.

7 Visceral Situs, Heart Position, and Aortic Arch Position

The second step in interpretation of a chest radiograph obtained in a new patient is to ascertain visceral situs, the heart position, and the position of the aortic arch relative to the trachea. For example, the radiographic report may start with this sentence: *"The radiograph shows situs solitus, levocardia and a left aortic arch."*

■ Visceral Situs

Visceral situs refers to the pattern of arrangement of the body organs relative to the midline. There are four types of visceral situs: situs solitus, situs inversus, heterotaxy with thoracic right isomerism, and heterotaxy with thoracic left isomerism (**Fig. 7.1**).[1–4] Visceral heterotaxy has also been described as situs ambiguus, which means uncertain situs. This term should be abandoned because the situs is not uncertain but rather needs more words to describe it precisely. The structures that are helpful in determination of the situs include (1) the gastric air bubble, (2) the larger lobe of the liver, (3) the tip of the spleen, (4) the bronchi and pulmonary arteries, (5) the minor fissure,

and (6) the azygos vein. The basic concepts regarding visceral situs is discussed in detail in Chapter 2.

In situs solitus, the gastric air bubble is on the left side, and the larger lobe of the liver is on the right side (**Fig. 7.2**). The splenic tip can often be identified when the stomach and adjacent bowel loops are filled with air. When the bronchial air column can be traced, an asymmetric bronchial branching pattern with a short right and a long left main bronchus can be appreciated on the frontal radiograph. Normally the left main bronchus is 1.5 to 2 times longer than the right main bronchus. At the pulmonary hilum, the left pulmonary artery is seen slightly higher than the right pulmonary artery. The left pulmonary artery is seen above the left upper lobe bronchus, whereas the right pulmonary artery (in fact, its descending branch) is seen below the right upper lobe bronchus. An asymmetric branching pattern of the bronchi and pulmonary arteries is also evident on the lateral radiograph. As the upper lobe bronchi normally have horizontal courses, they are seen as two round lucencies arranged superoinferiorly in the middle mediastinum. The right upper lobe bronchus is located approximately one vertebral height above the left upper lobe bronchus. The right

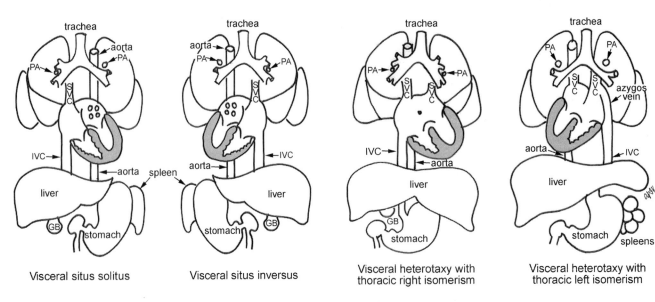

Fig. 7.1 Four types of visceral situs. GB, gallbladder; IVC, inferior vena cava; PA, pulmonary artery; SVC, superior vena cava.

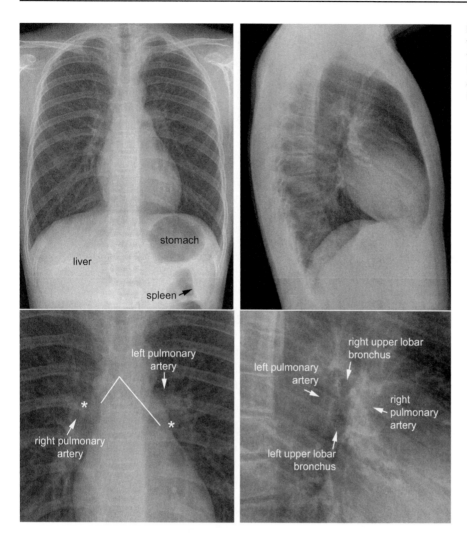

Fig. 7.2 Situs solitus. Magnified views of the hilar anatomy (*lower panels*). *Asterisks* on the magnified frontal view mark the upper lobe bronchi. The left main bronchus is twice as long as the right main bronchus in this individual (*solid lines*).

pulmonary artery lies anterior and slightly inferior to the right upper lobe bronchus. The left pulmonary artery lies posterior and superior to the left upper lobe bronchus. In short, the right upper lobe bronchus lies higher than the left, and the left pulmonary artery lies higher than and posterior to the right pulmonary artery. The minor fissure may cast a horizontal linear shadow over the midzone of a trilobed right lung.

Situs inversus is characterized by a mirror-image arrangement of the visceral organs (**Fig. 7.3**). The gastric bubble is on the right and the larger lobe of the liver on the left. However, it is important to understand that the situs should not be called "situs inversus" solely because of the inverted positions of the gastric bubble and hepatic shadow. Plain film diagnosis of situs inversus can only be made when an inverted bronchial and pulmonary arterial branching pattern is clear. A lateral radiograph is helpful in differentiating the lateralized situs (i.e., situs solitus and inversus) from the symmetric situs (i.e., right isomerism or left isomerism). Normal hilar arrangement of the upper lobe bronchi and branch pulmonary arteries on the lateral view with a right-sided gastric bubble on the frontal view is highly suggestive of situs inversus even if the splenic shadow is not identified.

In right isomerism, the hepatic shadow usually extends across the upper abdomen (**Fig. 7.4**). The gastric bubble can be seen on either side but tends to be closer to the midline. Interestingly, about 15% of patients with right isomerism have a hiatal hernia (**Fig. 7.5**).[5] Hiatal hernia can be regarded as a manifestation of visceral heterotaxy. Bilaterally short bronchi can be appreciated in a well-taken frontal radiograph (**Fig. 7.6**). However, this feature is often unclear in infants. On the lateral radiograph, the end-on shadows of the upper lobe bronchi are seen at the same or similar horizontal level, and the pulmonary arterial shadow is seen mostly in front of the bronchi (**Fig. 7.4**). The presence of bilateral minor fissures indicates right isomerism (**Fig. 7.7**). In fact the diagnosis of right isomerism can be entertained when the minor fissure is present on the same side as the stomach even when a minor fissure is identified only on one side (**Fig. 7.4**, left panel). This is because the minor fissure and stomach cannot be

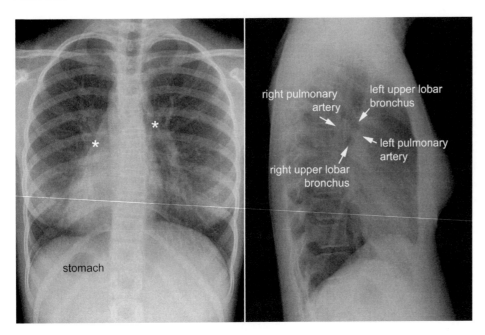

Fig. 7.3 Situs inversus. The frontal view shows mirror-image arrangement of the bronchial and pulmonary arterial trees. *Asterisks* mark the upper lobe bronchi. The lateral view appears identical to that seen in situs solitus (**Fig. 7.2**) but note the difference in labeling. This patient had Kartagener's syndrome with subtle pulmonary infiltrates in the right lower lung.

on the same side in either situs solitus or situs inversus, and no minor fissure is present in either lung in left isomerism. However, a potential pitfall is the presence of an accessory fissure, which can simulate a horizontal fissure (**Fig. 7.8**).[6,7] Right isomerism is associated with complex congenital heart disease in almost all cases. We have not seen any single case of right isomerism without complex congenital heart disease. As pulmonary atresia or stenosis is present in the majority of cases, the pulmonary vascularity is usually reduced (**Figs. 7.4, 7.5, 7.6, 7.7**).

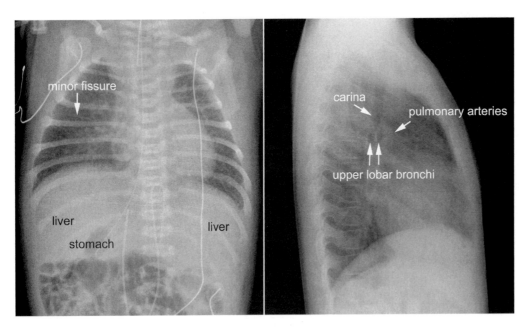

Fig. 7.4 Heterotaxy with thoracic right isomerism. The hepatic silhouette extends symmetrically across the upper abdomen. The stomach with a nasogastric tube in place is on the right side, lying somewhat close to the midline. A minor fissure is visible in the right lung. The presence of a minor fissure on the same side of the stomach is conclusive evidence of right isomerism. On the lateral view, the similar length of the right and left main bronchi results in the upper lobe bronchi being projected at a similar horizontal level. The right and left pulmonary arteries are projected mostly in front of the upper lobe bronchi.

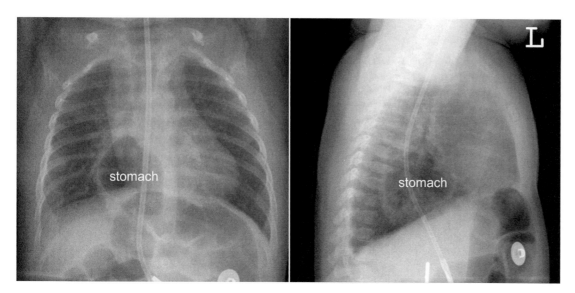

Fig. 7.5 Ectopic location of a part of the stomach in the thorax, which is often described as hiatal hernia, in a neonate with abdominal heterotaxy and thoracic right isomerism.

Left isomerism is also characterized by a symmetric visceral arrangement. However, the hepatic shadow in left isomerism is usually less symmetric than in right isomerism, and it is not uncommon for the hepatic shadow to be indistinguishable from that seen in situs solitus or inversus (**Fig. 7.9**). The gastric bubble can be on either side. The splenic shadow can be identified along the greater curvature of the stomach. On the frontal radiograph, bilaterally long bronchi can often be appreciated (**Fig. 7.9**, right panels). On the lateral radiograph, the upper lobe bronchi cast end-on shadows at the same or similar horizontal level, and the pulmonary arterial shadow is mostly seen behind the bronchi. The presence of a minor fissure in either lung excludes the

Fig. 7.6 Symmetrically short main bronchi are shown in this frontal radiograph in a child with right isomerism. This feature is not usually as apparent in neonates and small children. *Asterisks* indicate the origins of the upper lobar bronchi.

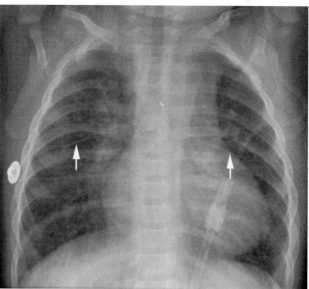

Fig. 7.7 Bilateral minor fissures (*arrows*) in a neonate with right isomerism.

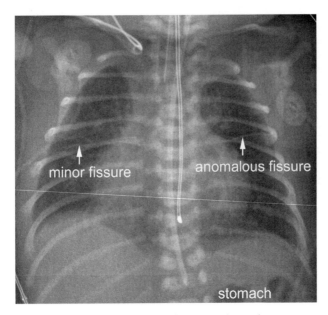

Fig. 7.8 Accessory left anomalous fissure simulating the appearance of bilateral minor fissures in an infant with situs solitus and hypoplastic left heart syndrome. Right isomerism was suspected, but there was a situs solitus arrangement of the other organs. An accessory left minor fissure is not an uncommon normal variant.[6,7]

diagnosis of left isomerism. In approximately 80% of cases, left isomerism is associated with interruption of the inferior vena cava with azygos or hemiazygos venous continuation.[8] In this situation, the dilated azygos vein can be identified in the area of the tracheobronchial angle (**Fig. 7.9,** left panels). Absence of the inferior vena caval shadow on the lateral radiograph has also been described in patients with an interrupted inferior vena cava. We find this feature unreliable. As interruption involves the postrenal prehepatic segment of the inferior vena cava, the posthepatic segment of the inferior vena cava is present and collects the hepatic veins. Therefore, a web-like shadow, albeit somewhat smaller than normal, can be identified in the lateral radiograph. In addition, the inferior vena caval shadow can be hidden by the posteriorly enlarged heart. In contrast to right isomerism, left isomerism is not always associated with congenital heart disease. Left isomerism may be seen as an incidental finding in otherwise normal individuals or in patients with an arrhythmia or biliary atresia.[9]

It should be remembered that there are exceptions, although rare, to these rules, as discussed in Chapter 2.

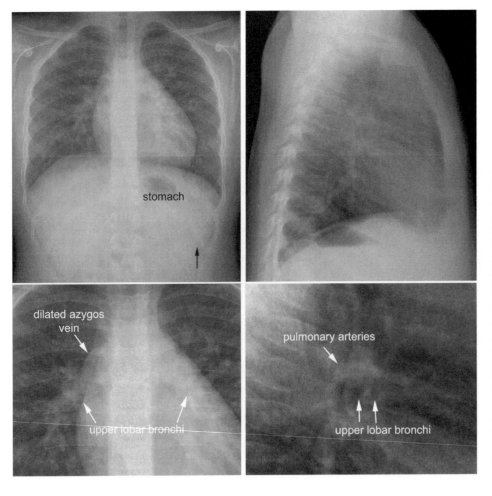

Fig. 7.9 Heterotaxy with left isomerism. Magnified views of the hilar anatomy (*lower panels*). The hepatic silhouette is not as asymmetric as it is in situs solitus or situs inversus, but is not as symmetric as it is in right isomerism. The splenic silhouette is barely visible lateral to the stomach (*arrow*). Symmetric bronchial branching can be appreciated on the frontal radiograph. The dilated azygos vein is seen above the right tracheobronchial angle. The trachea is mildly bent to the right by the left aortic arch. The lateral view shows the upper lobe bronchi at a similar horizontal level because of a similar length of the right and left main bronchi. The right and left pulmonary arteries cast a shadow mostly behind and above the upper lobe bronchi. The inferior vena caval shadow is not obvious on the lateral view.

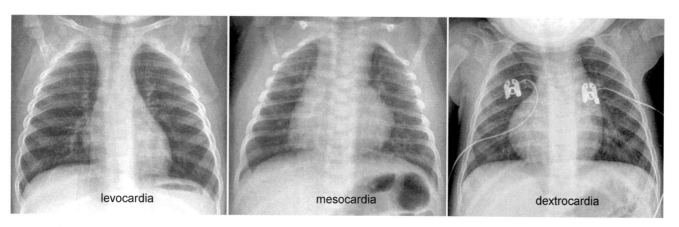

Fig. 7.10 Three cardiac positions defined by the location of the main part of the heart relative to the midline.

■ Heart Position

The cardiac position is described by using the terms *levocardia, dextrocardia,* and *mesocardia* (**Fig. 7.10**), which describe where the main part of the heart is located within the thorax. These terms are not used when the heart is displaced to one or the other side due to extracardiac pathology, such as hypoplasia of a lung or deformity of the thoracic cage (**Fig. 7.11**). When the heart is partially or completely outside the thorax, it is called ectopia cordis. Usually the cardiac apex points toward the side where the main part of the heart is positioned. However, there are exceptions where the cardiac position and the base-apex orientation are not matched.

When defining the position of the heart on a chest radiograph, it is important to check whether there is any obliquity of radiographic projection. A subtle obliquity may bring the cardiac silhouette to the other side of the thorax (see **Fig. 6.2**). In general, the cardiac silhouette is brought to the right when the radiograph is obtained in a left anterior or right posterior oblique projection, whereas it is brought to the left when the radiograph is obtained in a right anterior or left posterior oblique projection.

Although there are many exceptions, levocardia tends to have the right-sided right ventricle and the left-sided left ventricle (so-called D-loop ventricles), whereas dextrocardia tends to have the left ventricle on the right and the right ventricle on the left (so-called L-loop ventricles). This tendency explains why congenitally corrected transposition

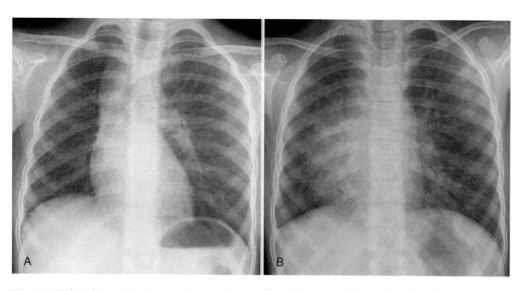

Fig. 7.11 **(A)** Rightward displacement of the heart due to right lung hypoplasia in a patient with absence of the right pulmonary artery in the mediastinum and **(B)** in another patient with scimitar syndrome.

The displaced cardiac position in scimitar syndrome is often called *dextroposition*, which is a confusing term.

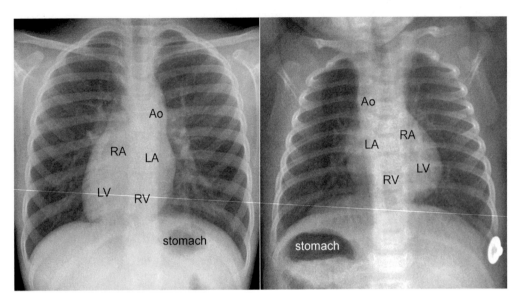

Fig. 7.12 Discordant visceral situs and heart position. Situs solitus and dextrocardia (*left panel*). Situs inversus and levocardia (*right panel*). Both cases had congenitally corrected transposition of the great arteries.

Ao, ascending aorta; LA, left atrium; LV, left ventricle; RA, right atrium; RV, right ventricle.

of the great arteries is the most common diagnosis when there is discordance between the heart position and visceral situs, such as dextrocardia with situs solitus (**Fig. 7.12**, left panel) and situs inversus with levocardia (**Fig. 7.12**, right panel).

■ Position of the Aortic Arch

The reference structures used for the determination of the left- or right-sidedness of the aortic arch are the trachea and main bronchi.[10] The left aortic arch courses backward on the left side of the trachea and above the left main bronchus, whereas the right aortic arch courses backward on the right side of the trachea and above the right main bronchus.

Chest radiographic determination of the aortic arch position depends largely on the indentation of the tracheal air column. A left aortic arch indents and bends the trachea to the right side, whereas a right arch indents and bends the trachea to the left (**Fig. 7.13**). In almost all cases, the aortic arch continues with the proximal descending aorta on the same side, which is usually identifiable as a vertical stripe along the spine. The rare exceptions are the so-called circumflex retroesophageal aortic arches in which the distal segment of the aortic arch crosses the midline behind the esophagus to connect to the descending aorta on the opposite side[10,11] (**Fig. 7.14**). When there

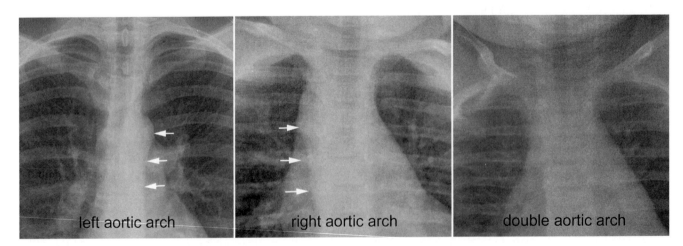

Fig. 7.13 Aortic arch positions relative to the trachea. The trachea normally shows indentation on the side of the aortic arch. The most proximal part of the descending aorta (*arrows*) can be traced on the same side of the aortic arch. Bilateral indentation is typically seen in double aortic arch but other forms of vascular ring cannot be excluded.

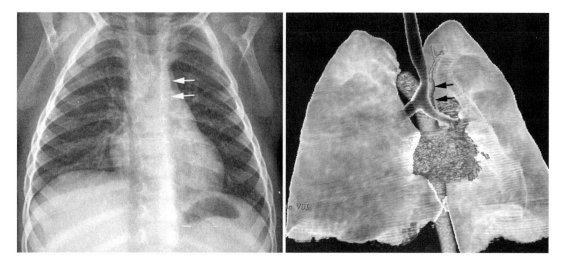

Fig. 7.14 Circumflex retroesophageal right aortic arch (right aortic arch with a left descending aorta). The proximal aortic arch is on the right side, whereas the distal arch has a retroesophageal course to con-nect to the descending aorta on the left side of the spine. The tracheal indentation is on the right side with the descending aorta seen on the left (*arrows*).

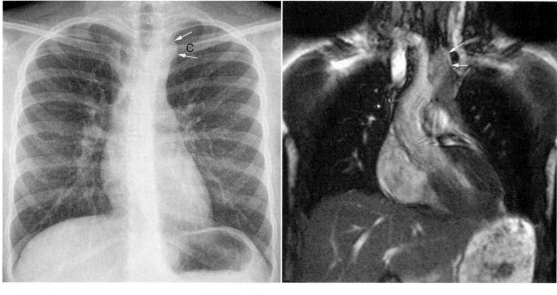

A

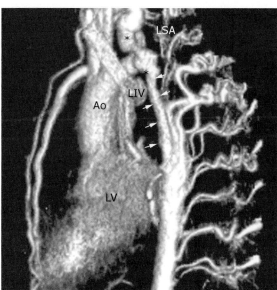

B

Fig. 7.15 Cervical left aortic arch in a 14-year-old patient. **(A)** Chest radiograph and coronal magnetic resonance (MR) image show the aortic arch (*arrows*) reaching the upper thorax above the level of the clavicle (C). **(B)** Contrast-enhanced MR angiogram seen from the left side shows a tortuous aortic arch, aneurysmal dilatation (*asterisks*) in the distal aortic arch and left subclavian artery (LSA) and severe long segment narrowing of the proximal descending aorta. Dilated intercostal arteries are seen as collateral channels. As an incidental finding the left innominate vein (LIV) takes a retroaortic course. Ao, ascending aorta; LV, left ventricle.

is double aortic arch, the trachea is bent to neither side or bent only slightly to the side of the smaller aortic arch. The trachea may show bilateral indentations with concentric narrowing of its lumen (**Fig. 7.14**). The descending aorta can be seen on either side, although a left-sided descending aorta is more frequent. The aortic arch can be unusually high, its apex reaching above the level of the clavicle (**Fig. 7.15**). This condition is called a cervical aortic arch.[10,12] It occurs more commonly with a right aortic arch, often taking a retroesophageal course. It is commonly associated with tortuosity, aneurysmal dilatation, and narrowing.

Pearls

- The situs can be accurately defined when the bronchial branching pattern is clearly shown.

- A right-sided gastric air bubble is not a specific sign for situs inversus, as it can also be seen with right and left isomerism. A right-sided gastric air bubble simply means that the situs is not normal.

- The presence of a minor fissure in both lungs is a definitive sign for right isomerism. However, its absence means nothing.

- The presence of a minor fissure on the same side of the stomach is a definitive sign of right isomerism.

- Symmetry of the right and left lobes of the liver is highly suggestive of right isomerism, especially when the heart is not enlarged and the pulmonary vascularity is diminished.

- A dilated azygos vein on either side is highly suggestive of left isomerism, but can be seen in other conditions such as superior or inferior vena caval obstruction.

- Cardiac position has nothing to do with the type of visceral and atrial situs.

- Levocardia tends to occur with D-loop ventricles (right ventricle on the right), and dextrocardia with L-loop ventricles (right ventricle on the left), but there are many exceptions.

- A left aortic arch indents the left side of the trachea, and a right aortic arch indents the right side of the trachea.

- The stripe of the descending aorta is seen on the same side as the aortic arch in most cases.

- In double aortic arch, the trachea bends to neither side if the arches are symmetric in size. When the arches are asymmetric in size, the trachea may bend to the side of the smaller arch. The descending aorta can be seen on either side.

References

1. Stanger P, Rudolph AM, Edwards JE. Cardiac malpositions. An overview based on study of sixty-five necropsy specimens. Circulation 1977; 56:159–172
2. Van Praagh R. Terminology of congenital heart disease. Glossary and commentary. Circulation 1977;56:139–143
3. Uemura H, Ho SY, Devine WA, Anderson RH. Analysis of visceral heterotaxy according to splenic status, appendage morphology, or both. Am J Cardiol 1995;76:846–849
4. Nagel BHP, Williams H, Stewart L, Paul J, Stümper O. Splenic state in surviving patients with visceral heterotaxy. Cardiol Young 2005;15: 469–473
5. Hsu JY, Chen SJ, Wang JK, Ni YH, Chang MH, Wu MH. Clinical implication of hiatal hernia in patients with right isomerism. Acta Paediatr 2005;94:1248–1252
6. Abiru H, Ashizawa K, Hashmi R, Hayashi K. Normal radiographic anatomy of thoracic structures: analysis of 1000 chest radiographs in Japanese population. Br J Radiol 2005;78:398–404
7. Gesase AP. The morphological features of major and accessory fissures observed in different lung specimens. Morphologie 2006;90:26–32
8. Applegate KE, Goske MJ, Pierce G, Murphy D. Situs revisited: imaging of the heterotaxy syndrome. Radiographics 1999;19:837–852, discussion 853–854
9. Gilljam T, McCrindle BW, Smallhorn JF, Williams WG, Freedom RM. Outcomes of left atrial isomerism over a 28-year period at a single institution. J Am Coll Cardiol 2000;36:908–916
10. Yoo SJ, Bradley TJ. Vascular rings, pulmonary artery sling and related conditions. In: Anderson RH, Edward JB, Penny D, Redington AN, Rigby ML, Wernovsky G, eds. Pediatric Cardiology, 3rd ed. Philadelphia: Elsevier, 2009, in press
11. Philip S, Chen SY, Wu MH, Wang JK, Lue HC. Retroesophageal aortic arch: diagnostic and therapeutic implications of a rare vascular ring. Int J Cardiol 2001;79:133–141
12. Baravelli M, Borghi A, Rogiani S, et al. Clinical, anatomopathological and genetic pattern of 10 patients with cervical aortic arch. Int J Cardiol 2007;114:236–240

8 Heart Size, Overall Configuration, and Specific Chamber Enlargement

The third step of the chest radiographic interpretation is to assess the overall heart size and configuration, and search for signs of specific chamber enlargement. For example, this part of the radiographic report can read as follows: *"The heart is enlarged with a cardiothoracic ratio of 70% and shows an egg-on-side configuration. There are signs of right atrial enlargement that include increased height and outward bulge of the right atrial segment of the right cardiac contour on the frontal chest radiograph."*

■ Heart Size

The heart size is estimated by comparing the transverse diameter of the cardiac silhouette with the transverse diameter of the thoracic cage seen on the frontal radiograph. It can be estimated either qualitatively or by calculating the cardiothoracic (CT) ratio as a percentage (**Fig. 8.1**). On a well-taken straight posteroanterior view, the CT ratio is less than 50% in normal adults and large children. The CT

ratio can be up to 60% in newborns and diminishes to 50% within a year or two (**Fig. 8.2**).[1] Assessment of the heart size may be difficult in young infants with a large thymus that overlies the heart on the frontal radiograph. The increased CT ratio in infants is partly due to a more circular configuration of the thoracic cage as compared with the adult chest (**Fig. 8.3**). In the first few days of life, volume overload secondary to excessive cord stripping may result in a transient increase in heart size.

The lateral radiograph can also be used for heart size assessment. The tracheal air column is a useful landmark. Normally the posterior margin of the cardiac silhouette does not extend beyond the line that is drawn downward along the anterior wall of the trachea (**Fig. 8.4A**).[2] The heart can be regarded as enlarged if its posterior part is seen beyond this line with or without evidence of posterior displacement of a bronchus or bronchi (**Fig. 8.4B**). An enlarged heart encroaches on the retrosternal precardiac or retrocardiac prespinal clear space. It should be noted, however, that the CT ratio on the lateral view is significantly affected by the depth of the thorax.

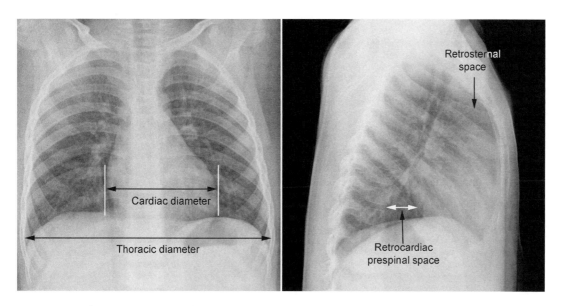

Fig. 8.1 Normal posteroanterior and lateral radiographs of the chest from a 4-year-old child. Cardiothoracic ratio is the ratio between the transverse diameter of the cardiac silhouette and the maximum inner diameter of the thoracic cage seen on the frontal chest radiograph. It is important to be familiar with the extent of the normal retrosternal and retrocardiac prespinal spaces.

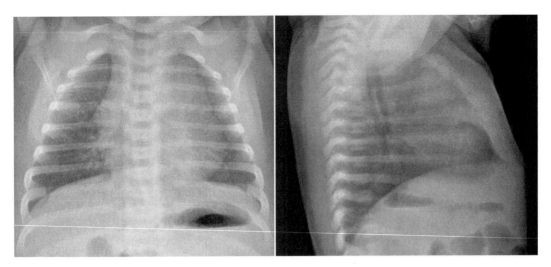

Fig. 8.2 Normal posteroanterior and lateral chest radiographs from a 16-day-old neonate. The cardiothoracic ratio is larger than that is seen in **Fig. 8.1**. The normal thymus overlies the upper part of the heart, showing a sail sign on the right side and multiple thymic waves on the left side. The retrosternal space is filled with the thymus. The frontal chest radiograph is obtained with a slight caudal angulation, resulting in a lordotic view.

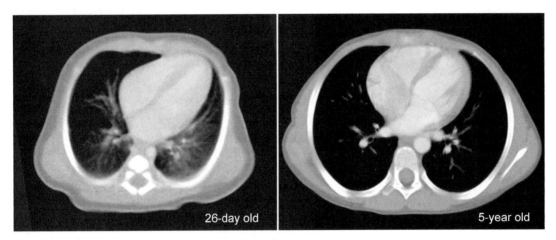

26-day old   5-year old

Fig. 8.3 Difference in the shape of the thoracic cage between a neonate and a young child. The neonate shows a more circular configuration of the thoracic cage when compared with a 5-year-old child.

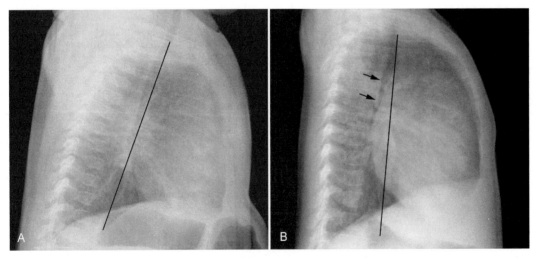

Fig. 8.4 (A) Lateral chest radiographs from a normal infant and **(B)** from an infant with a ventricular septal defect. Lines are drawn along the anterior wall of the trachea and extended downward. The posterior margin of the normal heart in **A** does not extend beyond this limit, whereas the enlarged heart with a ventricular septal defect in **B** shows a prominent posterior margin bulging beyond the line. The bronchi (*arrows*) are displaced backward by the enlarged heart.

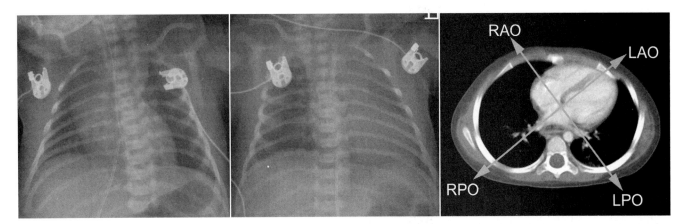

Fig. 8.5 Right and left posterior oblique chest radiographs obtained from a newborn with levocardia. The cardiac silhouette is small on the right posterior oblique view (*left panel*) because the short axis of the heart is projected toward the screen, whereas it is larger on the left posterior oblique view (*middle panel*) because the long axis of the heart is projected toward the screen. *Right panel* shows that the right posterior oblique (RPO) and left anterior oblique (LAO) views project the short axis of the heart toward the screen, whereas the left posterior oblique (LPO) and right anterior oblique (RAO) views project the long axis of the heart toward the screen.

In assessing heart size, it should be taken into consideration that the heart size can appear larger or smaller than it really is depending on the degree of inspiration and the radiographic projection. The transverse diameter of the cardiac silhouette becomes large with a high diaphragmatic position that can be due to incomplete inspiration, obesity, or abdominal pathology. The cardiac silhouette is more magnified on the anteroposterior view than on the posteroanterior view because the heart is located in the anterior part of the thorax. Subtle oblique projection may cause a significant difference in heart size and configuration. The heart in levocardia casts a smaller silhouette in the left anterior or right posterior oblique view than in a straight frontal view, whereas it casts a larger silhouette in the right anterior or left posterior oblique view (**Fig. 8.5**). The shape of the thoracic cage also influences the cardiac silhouette seen on the frontal radiograph. The heart appears large with an increased CT ratio in individuals who have a small overall thoracic cage or a circular thorax configuration as in newborns. The heart can be compressed and therefore casts a larger silhouette in a frontal radiograph, if the thorax has a decreased depth as in pectus excavatum and straight back syndrome or flat chest. The CT ratio may be less than 50% when there is overinflation of the lungs.

Although CT ratio is more objective in assessing the heart size, subjective grading into borderline, mild but obvious, moderate, and severe cardiomegaly is more practical. It should be emphasized that the heart may maintain its normal size on radiographs until it is significantly enlarged (**Figs. 8.6, 9.7A**). Changes in overall heart size and configuration on radiographs are rather insensitive parameters of disease processes.

■ Volume Versus Pressure Overload and Heart Size

Heart diseases can be grouped into two categories according to the loading condition: those with volume overload and those with pressure overload (**Table 8.1**). Isolated volume overload conditions include congenital heart diseases with left-to-right or left-to-left shunts, congenital and acquired lesions with valvular regurgitation, ventricular failure with stagnation of blood volume, large extracardiac vascular malformations such as vein of Galen malformation and hepatic hemangioendothelioma, and high cardiac output status such as severe anemia and thyrotoxicosis. Pressure overload conditions include congenital and acquired lesions with obstruction in the blood pathway that include outlet of a cardiac chamber, major arterial root, or peripheral vascular beds. For instance, valvular stenosis, coarctation of the aorta, peripheral pulmonary artery stenosis, obstructive pulmonary vascular disease, pulmonary venous obstruction, and systemic hypertension are all pressure overload lesions. Congenital heart diseases with right-to-left shunt, such as tetralogy of Fallot, are also pressure overload lesions.

When there is a volume overload lesion, the overloaded chambers dilate with or without associated myocardial hypertrophy. Therefore, the radiographs show the signs of

Table 8.1   Volume Versus Pressure Overload to the Cardiac Chamber

	Volume Overload	Pressure Overload
Pathology	Left-to-right shunt	Right-to-left shunt
	Valvular regurgitation	Intracardiac or extracardiac obstructive lesions
	Ventricular failure	Pulmonary vein stenosis
	Large vascular malformation	Pulmonary hypertension
	Hyperdynamic circulation	Systemic hypertension
Response of the involved cardiac chamber	Dilatation with or without hypertrophy	Hypertrophy
Compliance of the involved cardiac chamber	Mildly reduced	Severely reduced
Radiographic findings	Enlargement of the involved cardiac chambers proportional to volume overload	Contour changes with minimal changes in size

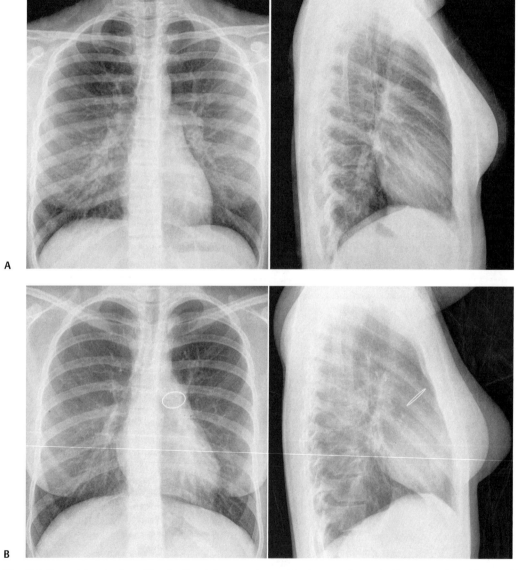

A

B

Fig. 8.6 Normal heart size with significant increase in ventricular volumes. **(A)** Atrial septal defect in a 15-year-old patient with pulmonary-to-systemic blood flow ratio (Qp/Qs) of 2.2 and right ventricular end-diastolic volume index of 151 mL/m² of body surface area. **(B)** Moderately severe pulmonary regurgitation in a 16-year-old patient who previously underwent a Ross operation with an artificial pulmonary valve implantation for aortic stenosis. Magnetic resonance imaging (MRI) flow and ventricular volume assessment showed a pulmonary regurgitant fraction of 31% and right ventricular volume index of 119 mL/m² of body surface area. The implanted pulmonary valve is calcified.

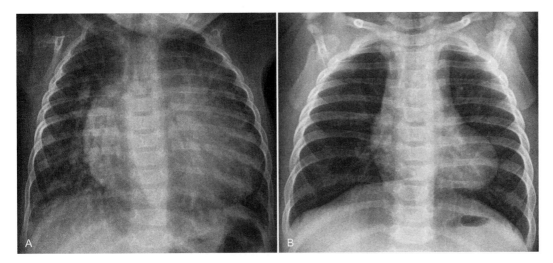

Fig. 8.7 Volume versus pressure overload lesions. **(A)** Volume overload lesion. Frontal chest radiograph from a 4-month-old infant with a large ventricular septal defect shows marked cardiomegaly and increased pulmonary vascularity. **(B)** Pressure overload lesion. Frontal chest radiograph from a 5-month-old infant with tetralogy of Fallot shows normal heart size. The cardiac apex is rounded and elevated. The pulmonary vascularity is mildly reduced.

chamber enlargement that is proportional to the amount of the volume overload (**Fig. 8.7A**). The pressure overload lesions result in myocardial hypertrophy without dilatation of the cavity. As hypertrophy is both outward and inward, the external size of the hypertrophied chamber is only mildly increased whereas the cavity volume can be reduced. Therefore, hypertrophy results in only mild changes in chamber size on radiographs. Hypertrophy should be severe to cause significant enlargement of the cardiac silhouette. On the other hand, hypertrophy usually causes significant contour changes (**Fig. 8.7B**). When there is a pure right-to-left shunt without any valvular regurgitation, radiographic cardiomegaly is not seen because the intracardiac blood volume is reduced. Hypertrophy causes reduced compliance of the chamber and therefore impaired filling.

■ Overall Cardiac Configuration

The overall cardiac configuration is often highly suggestive of a specific cardiac disease. One may be able to make a confident diagnosis of the specific disease based on the radiographic findings in conjunction with clinical symptoms and signs. Chest radiographs may provide clues to the diagnosis that may be missed by clinical or even echocardiographic investigation. This section introduces a few well-recognized named cardiac configurations, including boot-shaped heart, egg-on-side appearance, snowman appearance, triangular heart, cascade right heart border, and water-bottle appearance. Scimitar syndrome is discussed in Chapter 11.

Boot-Shaped Heart (Coeur en Sabot)

A boot-shaped heart is a well-known configuration of the heart that is most commonly seen in tetralogy of Fallot and tetralogy of Fallot with pulmonary atresia (pulmonary atresia with ventricular septal defect), and less commonly truncus arteriosus (**Figs. 8.8, 8.9**).[3,4] The boot-shaped heart is characterized by a round and elevated cardiac apex and concave pulmonary arterial segment. Elevation and rounding of the cardiac apex are due to counterclockwise and leftward rotation of the heart as seen from front and below, respectively. As a result, both ventricular long axes lie more horizontally than normal, and the cardiac apical contour in the frontal view is formed by the elevated right or left ventricular apex. In extreme cases with a severely hypertrophied right ventricle, the ventricular apex can be higher than the base of the ventricles. The boot-shape with upturned cardiac apex is usually ascribed to concentric right ventricular hypertrophy. However, this appearance is not seen in patients with acquired right ventricular hypertrophy or in patients with severe pulmonary valve stenosis or pulmonary atresia and intact ventricular septum.[4] The appearance, therefore, may represent the primary morphologic abnormality rather than right ventricular hypertrophy. The concave pulmonary arterial segment is due to hypoplasia of the right ventricular outflow tract and main pulmonary artery as well as an abnormal orientation of the main pulmonary artery coursing more rightward than normal. A boot-shaped heart can be seen without cardiomegaly in classic tetralogy of Fallot with predominant right-to-left shunt (**Fig. 8.8A**). A boot-shaped heart without significant cardiomegaly is also seen in pulmonary atresia with ventricular septal defect when the

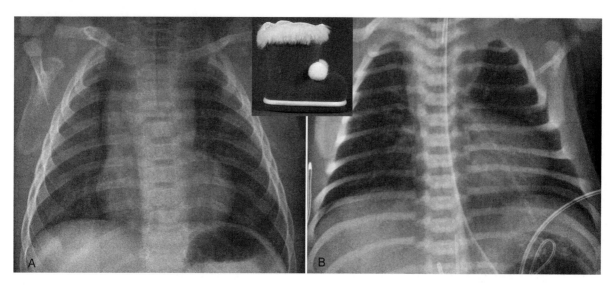

Fig. 8.8 Examples of small boots. **(A)** Tetralogy of Fallot in a 4-month-old infant. **(B)** Tetralogy of Fallot with pulmonary atresia and patent ductus arteriosus in a newborn. Both cases show an upturned and rounded cardiac apex. A large thymus hides the concave pulmonary arterial segment in **A**. The concave pulmonary arterial segment of the left heart border is uncovered in **B** because of thymic hypoplasia. This patient had microdeletion of chromosome 22q11.

pulmonary blood supply is through a small patent ductus or stenotic systemic collateral arteries (**Fig. 8.8B**). When pulmonary atresia is associated with unobstructed collaterals, a boot-shaped heart is associated with dilated left-sided chambers, causing an enlarged cardiac silhouette (**Fig. 8.9A**). A large boot-shaped heart is also seen in truncus arteriosus (**Fig. 8.9B**).

Egg-on-Side Appearance

An egg-on-side appearance is classically seen in complete transposition of the great arteries (**Fig. 8.10A**).[3] This configuration is mainly due to rightward displacement of the right ventricular outflow tract. Normally the right ventricular outflow tract is a left-sided structure and contributes

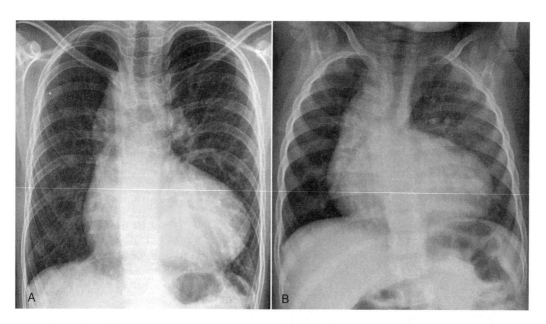

Fig. 8.9 Examples of large boots. **(A)** Pulmonary atresia with ventricular septal defect and multiple major aortopulmonary collateral arteries in a 14-year-old patient. The left lung is supplied by larger collateral arteries. **(B)** Truncus arteriosus in a 3-year-old patient. Both cases show a large boot-shaped heart. Cardiomegaly in both cases is due to volume overload with increased pulmonary blood flow.

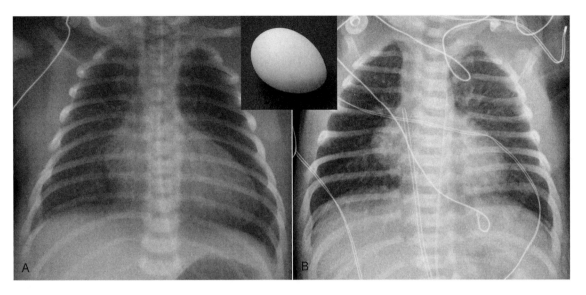

Fig. 8.10 Egg-on-side appearance. **(A)** Uncomplicated complete transposition of the great arteries in a 3-day-old neonate. **(B)** Double outlet right ventricle with subpulmonary ventricular septal defect and overriding pulmonary valve (so-called Taussig-Bing malformation) in a 2-day-old neonate. Both patients show a flattened left heart border below the pulmonary arterial segment. As shown in **Fig. 8.11**, this configuration in these two cases is due to rightward displacement of the right ventricular outflow tract. In both conditions, the great arteries have a parallel course with an anteroposterior relationship, showing a narrow superior mediastinum on the frontal view, in the majority of cases. The narrow vascular pedicle results from involuted thymus due to postnatal stress.

to the mild convexity of the left midcardiac contour below the pulmonary arterial segment in the frontal view, although it is not border forming (**Fig. 8.11**, left panel). Therefore, the right ventricular outflow tract is partly responsible for the bulk of the left upper heart border. In complete transposition, the right ventricular outflow tract is a right-sided structure as it supports the ascending aorta that is located anterior to and rightward of the pulmonary trunk (**Fig. 8.11**, right panel). As a consequence, the left upper cardiac contour is flattened in complete transposition. The egg-on-side appearance may not be obvious on the first day of life when a large thymus obscures the cardiac

contour. However, the cardiac contour is usually unveiled within a day or a few days as the thymus becomes smaller in coping with a postnatal critical condition. A similar feature is also seen in the so-called Taussig-Bing malformation, in which a double outlet right ventricle is associated with a subpulmonary ventricular septal defect (**Fig. 8.10B**). Complete transposition often shows a narrow superior mediastinum because of a parallel anteroposterior relationship of the great arteries.

Truncus arteriosus may also show an egg-on-side appearance (**Fig. 8.12A**). In truncus arteriosus, a concave pulmonary arterial segment on the frontal view is due to

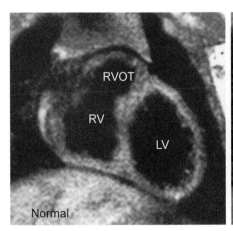

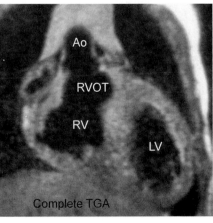

Fig. 8.11 Why the egg-on-side appearance in complete transposition of the great arteries (TGA)? Coronal T1-weighted MR images show a different location of the right ventricular outflow tract. Normally, the right ventricular outflow tract is located on the left connecting with the left-sided pulmonary trunk and forms a bulk underneath the left atrial appendage segment of the left heart border. In complete transposition (TGA), the right ventricular outflow tract is displaced rightward and the left upper heart border is flat. Ao, ascending aorta; LV, left ventricle; RV, right ventricle; RVOT, right ventricular outflow tract.

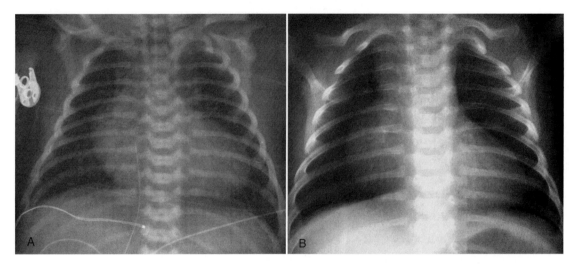

Fig. 8.12 Egg-on-side appearance in newborns with **(A)** truncus arteriosus and **(B)** pulmonary atresia with intact ventricular septum. In truncus arteriosus, the right ventricular outflow tract connects to the common arterial trunk. The left upper heart border is flat because there is no right ventricular outflow tract leading to the pulmonary artery. In pulmonary atresia with intact ventricular septum, the right ventricular outflow tract is hypoplastic, whereas the right atrium is dilated because of tricuspid regurgitation.

absence of a pulmonary outflow tract. As in complete transposition, the thymus can be small due to a poor clinical condition. In addition, the thymus can be small or absent in association with DiGeorge or chromosome 22q11 microdeletion syndrome. In contrast to complete transposition, truncus arteriosus is associated with more significant cardiac enlargement, and typically there is increased pulmonary vascularity from the newborn period.

The egg-on-side appearance is also seen in pulmonary atresia with intact ventricular septum (**Fig. 8.12B**). The "egg" in this condition is typically large. The blunt side of the egg opposite to the apex is formed by an enlarged right atrium. The left upper heart border is flat because the right ventricular outflow tract is underdeveloped. The superior mediastinum is narrow because of the small size of the pulmonary arterial trunk and a small thymus. The pulmonary vascularity is typically diminished. A large heart with an egg-on-side appearance, right atrial enlargement, and decreased pulmonary vascularity in a cyanotic newborn is typical of pulmonary atresia or critical pulmonary stenosis with intact ventricular septum.

Snowman or Figure-of-8 Configuration

When it is seen with increased pulmonary vascularity, a snowman or figure-of-8 configuration is highly suggestive of total anomalous pulmonary venous connection to the innominate vein (**Fig. 8.13A**). The upper part is formed by the vertical vein that drains the pulmonary venous return

on the left and the dilated superior vena cava on the right. The lower part is formed by the enlarged heart. However, this well-known sign is rarely apparent in infancy and therefore rarely encountered in developed countries, as a surgical correction is typically undertaken in the early neonatal period.[5,6] As a caution particularly in infancy, a normal thymus can be globular in shape, and the cardiothymic silhouette can be similar to that of total anomalous pulmonary venous connection to the innominate vein on the frontal radiograph. On the lateral radiograph, a vertical band-like density can be seen along the anterior aspect of the trachea.[5] We have experienced similar findings in a patient with a severe form of cor triatriatum, with the proximal chamber of the left atrium decompressed to the left innominate vein through a channel called a levoatriocardinal vein (**Fig. 8.13B**).[7]

Triangular Heart

The triangular cardiac silhouette is characterized by a straight left heart border (**Fig. 8.14**). The straightening is due to enlargement of the left atrium and prominence of the pulmonary arterial segment. With left atrial enlargement, the normally concave segment of the left heart border formed by the left atrial appendage straightens or even bulges outward in a convex shape. The pulmonary arterial segment is prominent because of elevation of the pulmonary arterial pressure. When rheumatic fever was a common etiology of acquired heart disease, a triangular heart was typically seen with mitral valvular disease. A predominantly stenotic lesion of the mitral valve is not

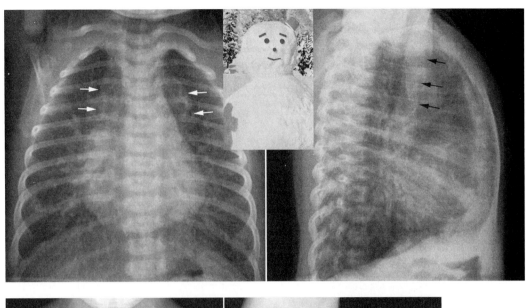

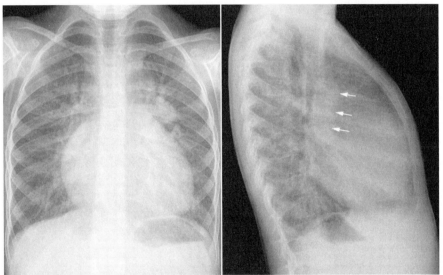

Fig. 8.13 (A) Snowman or figure of-8 appearance in total anomalous pulmonary venous connection to the left innominate vein. This finding is rarely seen in infancy. The upper part of the snowman is formed by the dilated vertical vein and right superior vena cava (*white arrows*). The vertical veins and superior vena cava are superimposed on one another and seen as a band of haziness (*black arrows*) in the pretracheal region, which differentiates it from thymus located in the retrosternal clear space on the lateral radiograph. **(B)** Snowman or figure of-8 appearance in a 5-year-old child with cor triatriatum. The proximal chamber of the left atrium was decompressed through a levoatriocardinal vein that connected the left upper pulmonary vein to the left innominate vein. Chest radiographs show moderate cardiomegaly, increased pulmonary vascularity, and findings of mild pulmonary venous hypertension. Both left and right upper mediastinal borders are convex, formed by the dilated levoatriocardinal vein and right superior vena cava, respectively. Note a pretrachial haziness (*arrows*) on the lateral view.

associated with overt cardiomegaly on chest radiographs, whereas a predominantly regurgitant lesion shows cardiomegaly because of volume overload to the left atrium and left ventricle. Congenital mitral stenosis is rare and is due to a parachute mitral valve or mitral arcade. Congenital mitral regurgitation is even rarer. Now, more common causes of a triangular heart include dilated cardiomyopathy in which left-sided heart failure results in enlargement of both the left atrium and left ventricle

with or without mitral regurgitation (**Fig. 8.14B**). Although rare, left-sided heart failure can also be due to anomalous origin of the left or, less commonly, the right coronary artery from the pulmonary trunk, which causes myocardial ischemia in early life (**Fig. 8.15**).[8] When a triangular heart is seen with pulmonary venous hypertension in a newborn or young infant, it is important to suggest this entity, as this diagnosis can be delayed if not suspected.

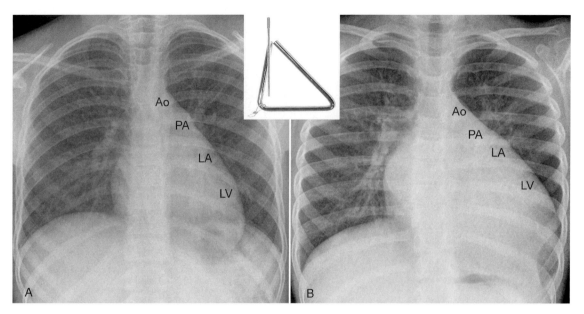

Fig. 8.14 Triangular hearts. **(A)** Congenital mitral regurgitation in a 12-year-old patient. **(B)** Dilated cardiomyopathy in a 4-year-old patient. The left heart border is straightened due to a prominent pulmonary arterial (PA) segment and enlarged left atrium (LA). The left ventricular (LV) segment is elongated due to dilatation in both cases. Ao, ascending aorta.

Regardless of the underlying etiology, the triangular heart is associated with pulmonary venous hypertension and a degree of pulmonary arterial hypertension.

Cascade Right Lower Heart Border

Normally, the upper half of the right heart border is straight or only slightly convex, whereas the lower half is convex. In young children, a normal thymus can overlie and obscure the upper heart borders. The convexity of the lower half of the right heart border is formed by the right atrial appendage. Rarely, the right lower heart border is slightly concave, giving rise to a *cascade* configuration. A cascade right lower heart border is highly suggestive of left juxtaposition of the atrial appendages (**Fig. 8.16**). Juxtaposition of the atrial appendage is a rare condition in which the appendage of one atrium is displaced to the other side and lies above the other atrial

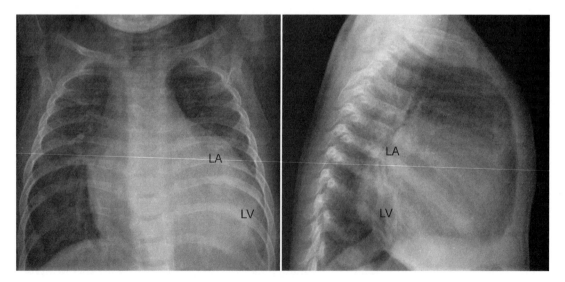

Fig. 8.15 Anomalous origin of the left coronary artery from the pulmonary artery in a 5-month-old infant. The left atrium (LA) and left ventricle (LV) are markedly enlarged. The left atrial border on the frontal view shows a large convexity. The enlarged left ventricle obliterates the retrocardiac prespinal clear space on the lateral radiograph.

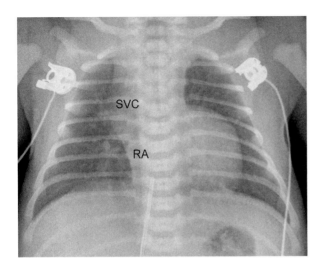

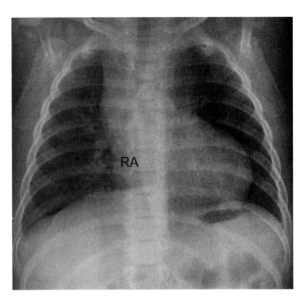

Fig. 8.17 Left juxtaposition of the atrial appendages in a 5-month-old patient with complex double outlet right ventricle. The concavity of the right lower heart border is subtle. The right superior mediastinum shows a double contour related to the curved superior vena cava and the overlying thymic margin. RA, right atrium.

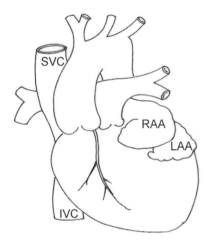

Fig. 8.16 Cascade right lower heart border in a newborn with left juxtaposition of the atrial appendages. The patient had tricuspid atresia and double outlet right ventricle. The right lower heart border is characteristically concave due to leftward displacement of the right atrial appendage. The right upper mediastinum shows an outward convexity because of the curved downward course of the superior vena cava (SVC) to connect to the displaced right atrium (RA). Altogether the right heart border shows an elongated sigmoid configuration. The left mid-heart border where the atrial appendages are juxtaposed is prominent and squared. IVC, inferior vena cava; LAA, left atrial appendage; RAA, right atrial appendage.

appendage. The displacement is through the transverse sinus of the pericardial sac, which is the space behind the great arterial roots. Juxtaposition to the left side is more frequent than juxtaposition to the right.[9,10] In situs solitus, left juxtaposition of the right atrial appendage is usually associated with right atrial outlet obstruction such as tricuspid atresia, right ventricular hypoplasia, or abnormal development of the ventricular outflow tracts

such as double outlet right ventricle. In contrast, right juxtaposition of the left atrial appendage is usually associated with obstruction to the left atrial outlet, left ventricular hypoplasia, and a normally developed ventricular outlet. When there is left juxtaposition in a situs solitus patient, the right lower heart border appears concave on the frontal radiograph because the right atrial appendage forming this part of the cardiac silhouette is displaced. The right upper mediastinal border is often convex outward because of a curved course of the superior vena cava. In addition, the juxtaposed atrial appendages cause a convex or a squared bulge of the atrial appendage segment of the left heart border. These radiographic findings can be less obvious in infants (**Fig. 8.17**).

Water-Bottle Appearance

The bottle referred to in "water-bottle appearance" is not a glass bottle but a leather bottle. This configuration refers to an enlarged cardiac silhouette with a disproportionate enlargement of the lower part of the cardiac silhouette above the diaphragm compared with the upper part (**Fig. 8.18**).[11] Usually, the enlargement is toward both sides. Classically it is seen on the erect frontal chest radiograph of the patient with a gradual collection of a large amount of pericardial effusion. It is worth noting that an acute collection of a large amount of pericardial fluid results in cardiac tamponade with

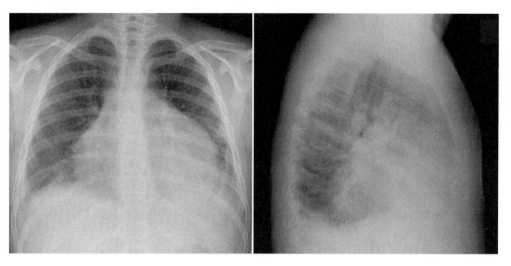

Fig. 8.18 Leather water-bottle appearance. There is disproportionate enlargement of the lower part of the cardiac silhouette. Bilateral pleural effusions are present.

less obvious enlargement of the cardiac silhouette and more compression of the cardiac chambers. In addition to the water-bottle appearance, the cardiac silhouette is sharp and smooth because the cardiac pulsation is reduced and the pericardium outlines the pericardial fluid rather than the undulated heart margin. When there is an abundant amount of epicardial fat, a lucent stripe of fat can be seen some distance inside the cardiac silhouette, outlining the outer surface of the heart. This "epicardial fat pad sign" is more commonly seen on the lateral view.[11] Pericardial effusion is often associated with pleural effusion, particularly in the left thorax.[12] Pulmonary vascularity is reduced when there is a large amount of pericardial effusion. The water-bottle appearance may also be seen with heart failure because of ventricular dilatation and reduced pulsatility of the heart. However, heart failure is associated with a pulmonary venous hypertension pattern of pulmonary vascularity, and the pleural effusion seen in heart failure is more frequently right-sided than left-sided.[12]

■ Specific Chamber Enlargement

The radiographic signs of enlargement of each cardiac chamber have been well described in many standard radiographic textbooks. However, these well-known radiographic signs are often not evident in children, especially in infants. This is partly because of the presence of a large thymus that overlies the upper part of the cardiac silhouette on the frontal view and obliterates the

retrosternal clear space on the lateral view. Occasionally, a large thymus can extend to the level of diaphragm. Radiographic evaluation of specific chamber enlargement is less important now than it was a few decades ago when plain chest radiography played an important role in the diagnosis of congenital heart disease. Now, plain chest radiographs are obtained to evaluate the overview of the cardiovascular status rather than specific chamber enlargement. However, it is still worthwhile to understand the radiographic signs of chamber enlargement. In general, radiographic signs of left-side chamber enlargement are easier to recognize and perhaps more sensitive to disease processes than are the signs of right-side chamber enlargement. It should be noted that the following descriptions are for cases with situs solitus and levocardia.

Right Atrial Enlargement

The enlarged right atrium produces convex bulging of the right lower heart border on the frontal view. When the vertical line, tangential to the right atrial border, extends beyond the medial one third of the right thorax, the right atrium can safely be considered enlarged (**Figs. 8.12B, 8.19**). It can also be considered enlarged when the right atrial border occupies more than half of the vertical distance between the medial end of the right clavicle and the dome of the right hemidiaphragm (**Figs. 8.12B, 8.20**). However, slight enlargement of the right atrium is usually not perceived, as there are hardly any abnormal radiographic findings. For

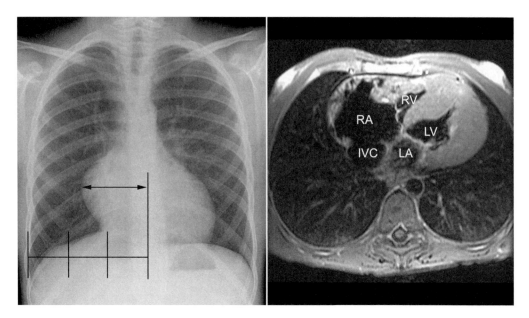

Fig. 8.19 Right atrial enlargement in hypertrophic cardiomyopathy with restrictive physiology. The right atrial border extends beyond the medial one third of the right thorax. On magnetic resonance imaging the right atrium (RA) and inferior vena cava (IVC) are markedly dilated. The right and left ventricles (RV and LV) are hypertrophied. LA, left atrium.

instance, right atrial enlargement is not evident on chest radiographs in most patients with an atrial septal defect. In a significant number of cases with an atrial septal defect, the right atrial border is even flatter than normal (**Fig. 8.21,** right panel). The superior vena cava and or azygos venous arch at the right tracheobronchial angle can be seen enlarged with right atrial enlargement in right-sided heart failure (**Fig. 8.22**). Right atrial enlargement can be mistakenly considered when the right atrium is displaced rightward due to enlargement of another part of the heart. **Table 8.2** lists the causes of right atrial enlargement.

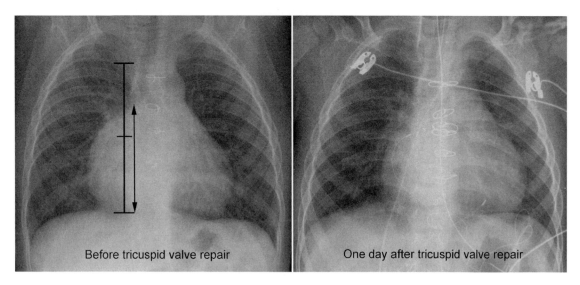

Before tricuspid valve repair

One day after tricuspid valve repair

Fig. 8.20 Right atrial enlargement due to tricuspid regurgitation in a 2-year-old patient who underwent a Norwood operation and bidirectional cavopulmonary anastomosis (*left panel*). The height of the right atrial margin extends above the limit of the lower half of the distance between the right clavicle and right hemidiaphragm. The lateral margin of the right atrium extends beyond the medial one third of the right thorax. The right atrium shows marked reduction in its size after tricuspid valve repair at the time of a modified Fontan operation (*right panel*).

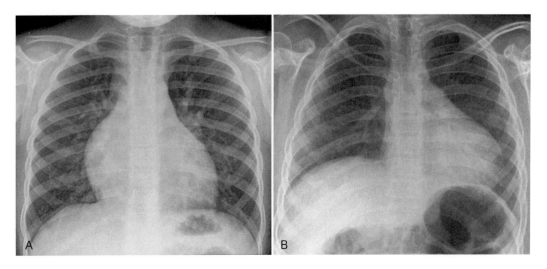

Fig. 8.21 Two patients with a secundum atrial septal defect. A 5-year-old patient **(A)** shows an overt evidence of right atrial enlargement. A 15-year-old patient **(B)** shows no radiologic evidence of right atrial enlargement. The right atrial border is unusually flat.

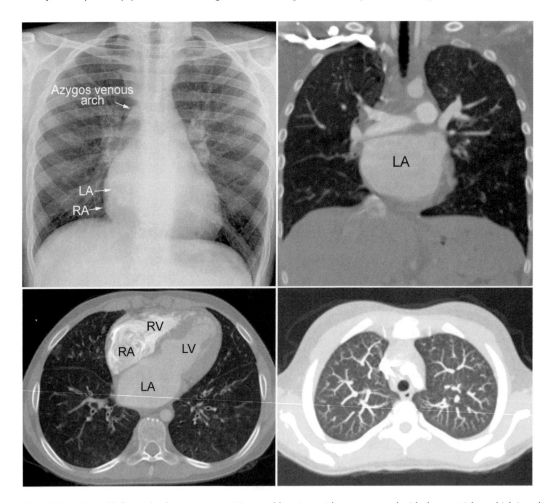

Fig. 8.22 Right and left atrial enlargement in a 12-year-old patient with restrictive cardiomyopathy. Frontal chest radiograph shows a mildly prominent right atrial (RA) border and double contour of an enlarged left atrium (LA) inside the right atrial border. The azygos venous arch at the right tracheobronchial angle is prominent. Contrast-enhanced computed tomography (CT) image (left lower panel) shows a so-called spade-shaped heart due to disproportionate dilatation of the atrial cavities as compared with the ventricles, which is a classic finding of restrictive cardiomyopathy. There is generalized increase in interstitial markings with redistribution of pulmonary vascularity to the upper lungs, suggesting pulmonary venous hypertension. Note thickened bronchial walls (*right upper and left lower panel*). CT image with lung setting (*right lower panel*) shows prominent vessels in the upper lungs with interstitial markings extending to the pleural surfaces. LV, left ventricle; RV, right ventricle.

Table 8.2 Causes of Right Atrial Enlargement

Shunt into right atrium

Atrial septal defect

Anomalous pulmonary venous connections

Left ventricle-to-right atrial shunt

Ruptured aortic sinus into right atrium

Coronary artery fistula to right atrium or coronary sinus

Tricuspid regurgitation/stenosis

Ebstein malformation of the tricuspid valve

Dysplastic tricuspid valve

Uhl's abnormality

Tricuspid stenosis

Right atrial tumor

Pulmonary atresia/critical stenosis with intact ventricular septum

Secondary to right ventricular hypertension

Pulmonary atresia/critical stenosis with intact ventricular septum

Pulmonary hypertension

Right ventricular failure

Hypertrophic cardiomyopathy

Dilated cardiomyopathy

Restrictive cardiomyopathy

Left Atrial Enlargement

Although only the tip of the appendage of the left atrium forms a short straight border on the left on the frontal view, left atrial enlargement produces several useful radiographic signs. The left atrium can enlarge posteriorly, superiorly, inferiorly, to the right, to the left, or in any combination of these. Posterior enlargement increases the radiographic opacity causing double density in the central part of the cardiac silhouette below the carina on the frontal view (**Figs. 8.22, 8.23, 8.24**). The double density of the left atrium can be delineated by a circular line producing a double contour. However, as a caution a double contour can be seen in normal hearts. Backward and upward displacement of the left main bronchus can be appreciated on the lateral view. With upward enlargement of the left atrium, the carinal angle is widened (**Figs. 8.24, 8.25**). Normally the carinal angle does not exceed 90 degrees. The enlarged left atrium flattens the left heart border by filling the concave segment of the left atrial appendage between the pulmonary arterial and left ventricular segments (**Fig. 8.14A**). With further enlargement, the left atrial segment produces a convexity (**Figs. 8.14B, 8.24B, 8.25**). The enlarged left atrium can extend toward the

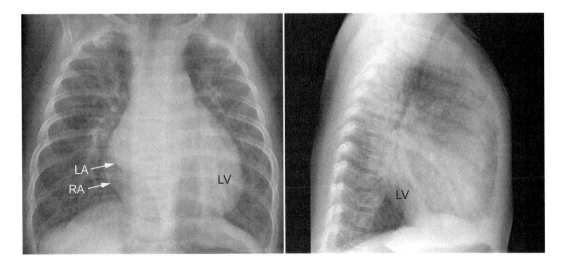

Fig. 8.23 Left atrial enlargement forming a double contour in a 3-month-old patient with ventricular septal defect. The right margin of the enlarged left atrium (LA) is seen inside the lateral margin of the right atrium (RA). There is biventricular enlargement obliterating both retrosternal and retrocardiac spaces. LV, left ventricle.

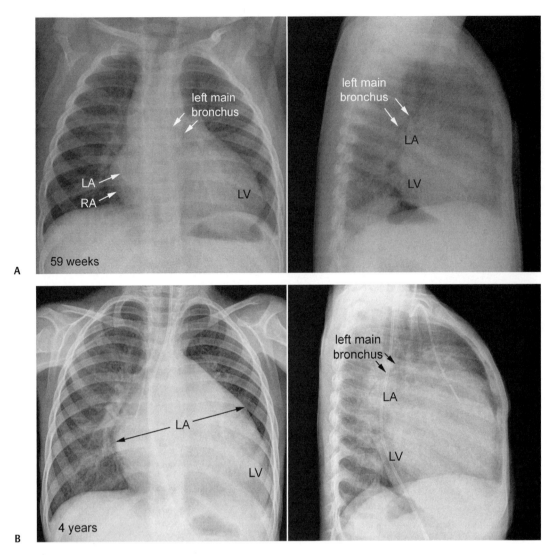

Fig. 8.24 Dilated cardiomyopathy showing interval change in chamber size between 59 weeks and 4 years of age. **(A)** At 59 weeks, the left main bronchus is displaced upward and backward. The carinal angle is increased on the frontal view. The left atrial margin (LA) is seen medial to the right atrial margin, whereas the left atrial segment of the left heart border is still concave. **(B)** At 4 years of age, the left atrium (LA) is markedly dilated. The left atrial segment is convex and the left atrium touches the right heart border. The left main bronchus is displaced further upward on the lateral view. Note that the nasogastric tube is displaced to the right and backward by the enlarged left atrium. LV, left ventricle; RA, right atrium.

right side and form the right heart border (**Fig. 8.26**). Enlargement of the left atrium and ventricle is often associated with left lower lobe collapse. The lingular segment of the left upper lobe can also be collapsed. The enlarged left atrium displaces the esophagus backward and usually to the right and less frequently to the left (**Fig. 8.24B**). The descending aorta can be displaced to the left by the enlarged left atrium. **Table 8.3** lists the causes of left atrial enlargement. Differential diagnosis of bulging of the left atrial segment is a partial pericardial defect involving this area (**Fig. 8.27**).

Right Ventricular Enlargement

Traditionally a rounded and elevated cardiac apex has been considered as the hallmark of right ventricular hypertrophy (**Figs. 8.8, 8.9**). This feature is characteristically seen in tetralogy of Fallot, tetralogy with pulmonary atresia, and truncus arteriosus, as discussed earlier in this chapter. The rounded and elevated contour is produced by leftward and superior deviation of the cardiac axis. With superior deviation of the cardiac axis, the cardiac apex is uplifted, producing a rounded apical contour shown above

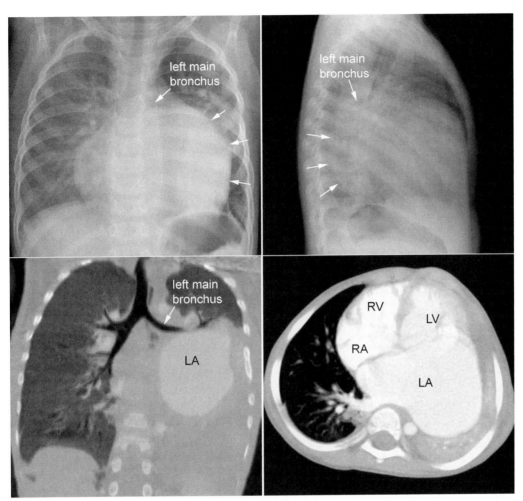

Fig. 8.25 Left atrium enlarged mainly to the left. There is a square bulge of the left mid-heart border on the frontal view (*arrows*). The left heart overlies the spinal column on the lateral view (*arrows*). Computed tomography (CT) angiogram shows that this segment is the dilated left atrium (LA). The left atrium does not extend rightwards to produce a double contour. The left main bronchus is markedly elevated on both views. The left lower lobe and lingular segment of the left upper lobe are collapsed on CT. Note that the cardiac axis is rotated to the right due to the leftward enlargement of the left atrium. LV, left ventricle; RA, right atrium; RV, right ventricle.

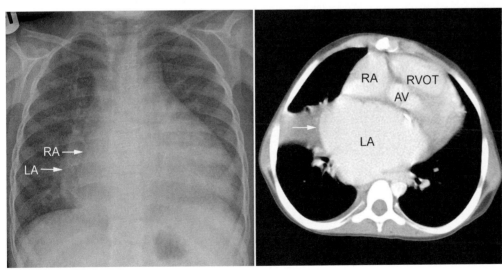

Fig. 8.26 Left atrium (LA) enlarged mainly to the right. The right heart border has a double contour. Computed tomography (CT) angiogram shows that the outer contour is the left atrial margin, whereas the anterior inner contour is the right atrial margin. AV, aortic valve; RA, right atrium; RVOT, right ventricular outflow tract.

Table 8.3 Causes of Left Atrial Enlargement

Left-to-right shunts
Ventricular septal defect
Ruptured aortic sinus
Coronary artery fistula
Aortopulmonary window
Patent ductus arteriosus

Mitral stenosis
Parachute mitral valve
Mitral arcade
Commissural fusion: congenital or rheumatic
Left atrial tumor
Acquired mitral stenosis (rheumatic origin)

Mitral regurgitation
Congenital
Traumatic rupture of the tension apparatus of the mitral valve
Rheumatic or other causes of myocarditis
Rheumatic mitral valve disease
Ischemic myocardial or papillary muscle injury of the left ventricle

Secondary to left ventricular hypertension
Severe aortic stenosis
Hypertrophic obstructive cardiomyopathy
Severe systemic hypertension

Secondary to left ventricular failure
Hypertrophic cardiomyopathy
Dilated cardiomyopathy
Restrictive cardiomyopathy
Ischemic cardiomyopathy
    Anomalous origin of a coronary artery from pulmonary artery
    Kawasaki disease sequelae

the diaphragmatic silhouette on the frontal view. With leftward deviation of the cardiac axis, the right ventricular apex is brought to the left, forming the apical silhouette. Although it is regarded as a distinct configuration, the rounded apex may vary significantly in its shape (**Fig. 8.28**). As a radiographic pitfall, lordotic positioning of the patient relative to the radiographic beam projects the cardiac apex above the diaphragmatic silhouette, causing a false impression of right ventricular hypertrophy with a rounded and elevated cardiac apex (**Fig. 8.29;** also see **Fig. 6.3**). This is a common situation in infants and small children who usually lean back when being positioned for a radiograph. When the chest and abdomen are included in the same exposure in a supine position, the chest is also projected above the diaphragmatic silhouette because of the low radiographic center. The cardiac apex is also projected above the diaphragm when it is displaced downward due to hyperinflation of the lungs, which is not uncommon in patients with congenital heart diseases with markedly increased pulmonary vascularity, severe interstitial edema, or severe cyanosis.

However, a rounded and elevated cardiac apex is not usually seen in right ventricular enlargement from other causes, such as pulmonary hypertension, atrial septal defect, pulmonary valve stenosis, and Ebstein's malformation of the tricuspid valve (**Figs. 8.30, 8.31**).[4] Normally, the right ventricle forms the anterior margin on the lateral view, whereas it is not border forming on the frontal view. The right ventricular outflow tract and main pulmonary artery are demarcated by the lungs behind the sternum, which is called the retrosternal clear space. The

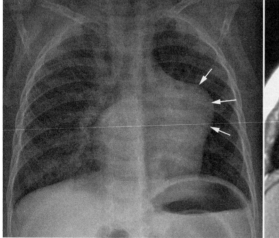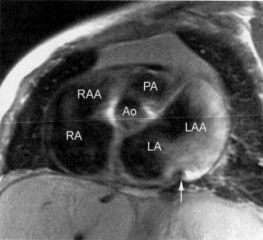

Fig. 8.27 Partial pericardial eventuration in the region at and around the left atrial appendage. There is a very unusual bulge of the left mid-heart border. Chest radiographic differential diagnosis included partial pericardial defect, cardiac tumor, and left juxtaposition of the atrial appendages. T1-weighted magnetic resonance image shows marked dilatation of the left atrial appendage (LAA). There is a sharp indentation (*arrow*) at the junction of the left atrium and appendage (LAA). At operation, the pericardium overlying this region was not deficient but markedly thinned. Ao, ascending aorta; LA, left atrium; PA, pulmonary artery; RA, right atrium; RAA, right atrial appendage.

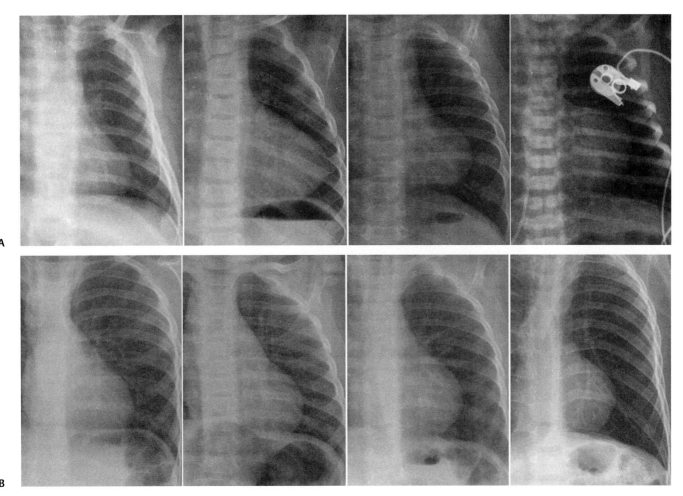

Fig. 8.28 Various shapes of the cardiac apex in tetralogy of Fallot. **(A)** Four different cases with tetralogy showing mild to severe degrees of elevation of the cardiac apex with a rounded configuration. **(B)** Four different cases with tetralogy of Fallot showing mild to severe degrees of elevation of the cardiac apex with a less obvious rounded configuration.

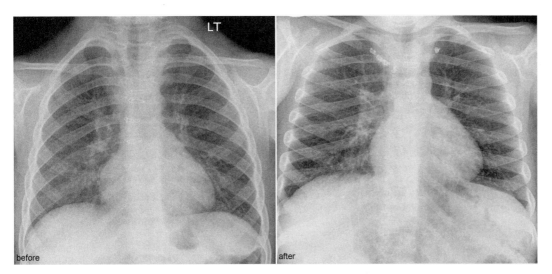

Fig. 8.29 Effect of lordotic view on the shape of the cardiac apex in a patient with hypoplastic left heart syndrome after Norwood and Fontan operation. The chest radiographs were obtained before and after coil embolization of the internal mammary arteries because of florid systemic arterial collateral circulation to the lungs. A lordotic view (*right panel*) shows the clavicles at the level of the first ribs and the cardiac silhouette above the diaphragmatic silhouette. The apex appears uplifted and round. LT, left.

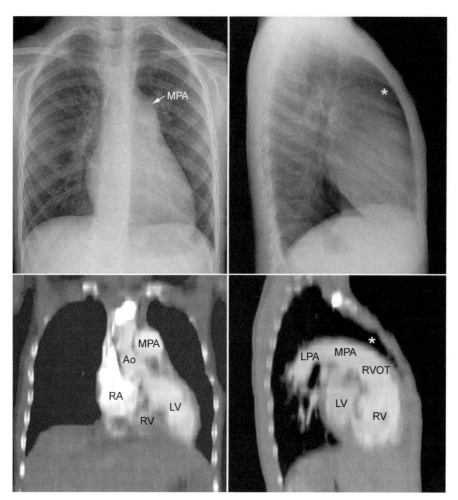

Fig. 8.30 Right ventricular hypertrophy in a 5-year-old patient with idiopathic pulmonary hypertension. The left lower heart contour on the frontal view is formed by the left ventricle (LV) as shown in a coronal CT image. The left heart border is similar to the normal configuration except that the left ventricle is laterally displaced by the hypertrophied right ventricle (RV). The retrosternal space (*asterisk*) is encroached on by the dilated right ventricular outflow tract (RVOT) and main pulmonary artery (MPA) from below and behind. The pulmonary arterial segment of the left heart border shows a convex bulge due to dilatation of the main pulmonary artery. Ao, ascending aorta; LPA, left pulmonary artery; RA, righ atrium.

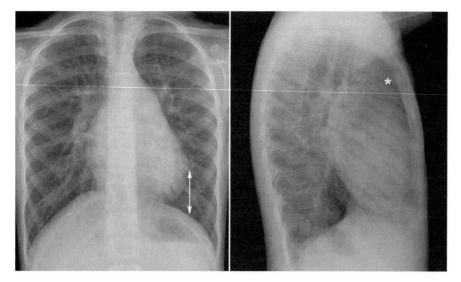

Fig. 8.31 Right ventricular enlargement in an 8-year-old patient with a secundum atrial septal defect. The apex is elevated (*double-headed arrow*) on the frontal view. The retrosternal space (*asterisk*) is encroached on as in **Fig. 8.30**. The configuration is different from the elevated and rounded contours in **Fig. 8.28**.

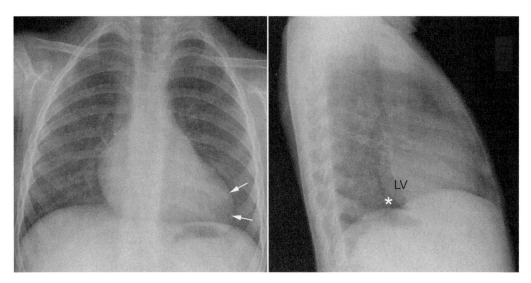

Fig. 8.32 Right ventricular enlargement in a 3-year-old child with Ebstein's malformation of the tricuspid valve showing radiographic findings similar to left ventricular enlargement shown in **Figs. 8.34** and **8.35**. The heart is rotated to the left displacing the left ventricle (LV) and obliterating the retrocardiac prespinal space (*asterisk*) on the lateral view. Note that the cardiac apex (*arrows*) is displaced outward and downward on the frontal view.

enlarged right ventricle and main pulmonary artery encroaches on this space with increased contact of the right ventricle to the anterior chest wall (**Figs. 8.30, 8.31**). However, this radiographic sign cannot be applied when the thymus is large. On the frontal view, the left ventricle can be uplifted by the enlarged right ventricle, causing some elevation of the cardiac apex above the diaphragmatic silhouette (**Fig. 8.31,** left panel). However, the apex is often normal looking on the frontal view (**Fig. 8.30,** left panel). When the heart with right ventricular enlargement is rotated to the left, the radiographic features may be similar to those of left ventricular enlargement (**Fig. 8.32**).

As the right ventricular outflow tract is immediately underneath the pulmonary arterial segment and medial to the left atrial appendage segment on the frontal radiograph, its enlargement may produce a contour change in the left heart border. In Ebstein's malformation of the tricuspid valve, the right ventricular outflow tract is dilated and may produce a focal bulge of the left midcardiac border that is normally occupied by the pulmonary arterial and left atrial appendage segments (**Fig. 8.33**). A similar

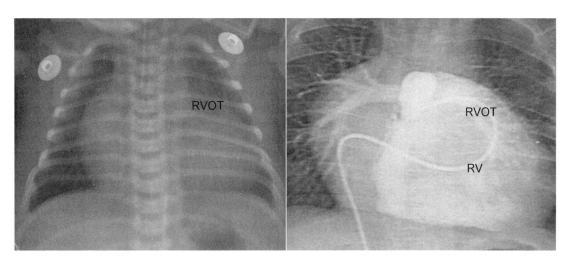

Fig. 8.33 Marked dilatation of the right ventricular outflow tract (RVOT) forming the left upper heart border in a 3-day-old neonate with Ebstein's malformation of the tricuspid valve. Note the aneurys-mally dilated right ventricular outflow tract on the right ventriculo-gram. RV, right ventricle.

Table 8.4 Causes of Right Ventricular Enlargement

Tricuspid regurgitation

Ebstein malformation of the tricuspid valve

Dysplastic tricuspid valve

Uhl's abnormality

Pulmonary regurgitation

Congenital pulmonary regurgitation

After right ventricular outflow tract repair

    For tetralogy of Fallot with or without pulmonary atresia

    For severe pulmonary stenosis or atresia with intact ventricular septum

    For truncus arteriosus

Right ventricular outflow tract obstruction

Pulmonary stenosis

Tetralogy of Fallot with or without pulmonary atresia

Other pathologies causing tetralogy-like hemodynamics

Pulmonary hypertension

Idiopathic pulmonary hypertension

Pulmonary thromboembolism

Complicating left-to-right shunt lesion

Secondary to pulmonary venous hypertension

Left-to-right shunt with volume overload to right ventricle

Atrial septal defect

Atrioventricular septal defect

Ventricular septal defect

Ruptured aortic sinus rupture into right ventricle

Coronary artery fistula to right atrium or right ventricle

but less obvious feature can also be seen in an atrial septal defect. **Table 8.4** lists the causes of right ventricular enlargement.

Left Ventricular Enlargement

The left ventricle enlarges leftward, posteriorly, and inferiorly. Left ventricular enlargement produces elongation of the left heart border with leftward and downward displacement of the cardiac apex on the frontal view (**Figs. 8.24, 8.34, 8.35**). The displaced cardiac apex can be seen below the diaphragmatic contour through the gastric air bubble. On the lateral view, the enlarged left ventricle encroaches on the retrocardiac prespinal clear space (**Figs. 8.24, 8.34, 8.35**). Left ventricular hypertrophy causes changes in the contour of the apex with or without actual enlargement (**Fig. 8.36**). The cardiac apex tends to be more rounded or squared (**Fig. 8.36**). The apex, however, is not elevated. **Table 8.5** lists the causes of left ventricular enlargement.

■ Additional Features

Convex Pulmonary Arterial Segment

The second segment of the left heart border is formed by the distal main pulmonary arterial trunk. Usually it is straight or slightly convex. Less often, especially in healthy young girls, this segment shows considerable

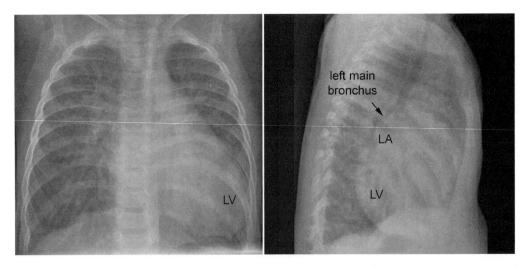

Fig. 8.34 Left ventricular enlargement in an 8-month-old infant with patent ductus arteriosus. Frontal view shows elongation of the left heart border and outward displacement of the cardiac apex. On the lateral view, the retrocardiac prespinal space is obliterated by the enlarged left ventricle (LV). The enlarged left atrium (LA) displaces the left main bronchus upward and backward.

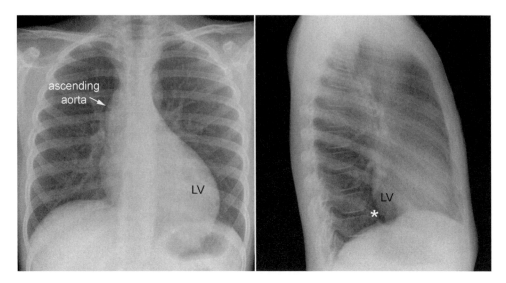

Fig. 8.35 Left ventricular enlargement in aortic stenosis/insufficiency. The left lower heart border is elongated and the cardiac apex is displaced outward and downward on the frontal view. The retrocardiac prespinal space (*asterisk*) is encroached on by the enlarged left ventricle (LV). The dilated ascending aorta forms a round border of the right upper mediastinum.

convexity (**Fig. 8.37** left upper panel). Significant convexity of this segment due to dilatation of the main pulmonary artery is seen in pulmonary valve stenosis, pulmonary regurgitation, pulmonary hypertension of any cause, and congenital heart disease with a left-to-right shunt with or without pulmonary hypertension (**Fig. 8.37**).

Table 8.5 Causes of Left Ventricular Enlargement

Mitral regurgitation
Congenital
Traumatic rupture of the tension apparatus of the mitral valve
Rheumatic or other causes of myocarditis
Rheumatic mitral valve disease
Ischemic myocardial or papillary muscle injury of the left ventricle
Aortic regurgitation
Congenital aortic regurgitation
Aorto-left ventricular tunnel
Aortic valve prolapse
Marfan's syndrome
Left ventricular outflow tract obstruction
Aortic valve stenosis
Subaortic stenosis
Supravalvar aortic stenosis
Obstructive lesions of the aortic arch
Systemic hypertension
Left-to-right shunt with volume overload to left ventricle
Ventricular septal defect
Ruptured aortic sinus rupture
Coronary artery fistula
Aortopulmonary window
Patent ductus arteriosus
Left heart failure
Myocarditis
Cardiomyopathies
Myocardial ischemia

Fig. 8.36 Left ventricular (LV) hypertrophy in a 3-month-old infant with hypertrophic cardiomyopathy. There is severe cardiomegaly. The cardiac apex is squarer in configuration as compared with the cases shown in **Figs. 8.33, 8.34**.

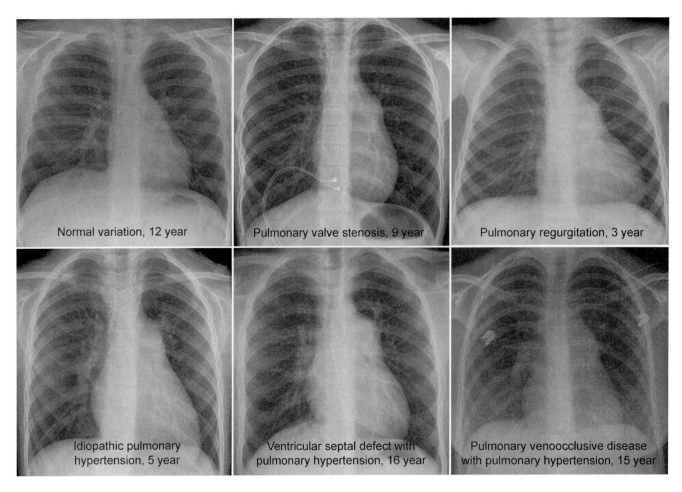

Fig. 8.37 Convex pulmonary arterial segment of the left heart border in various listed conditions.

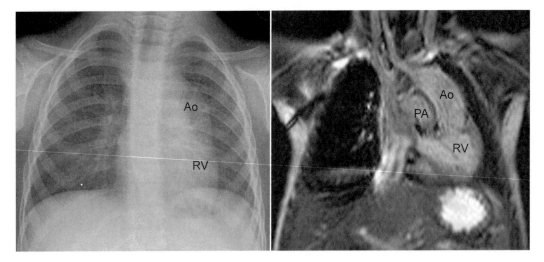

Fig. 8.38 Convex left upper mediastinal border due to a left-sided ascending aorta in a 3-year-old child with congenitally corrected transposition of the great arteries, straddling left atrioventricular valve, and pulmonary stenosis. The morphologically right ventricle (RV) is on the same side as the ascending aorta (Ao). This tendency is described as "aortic localization of the morphologically right ventricle." PA, pulmonary artery.

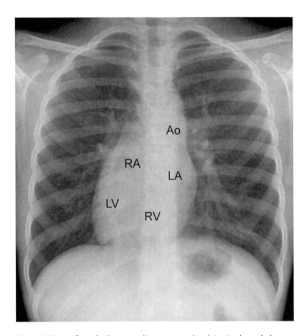

Fig. 8.39 Left-sided ascending aorta (Ao) in isolated dextrocardia. Mild convexity of the left upper mediastinum is due to a left-sided ascending aorta. The combination of situs solitus, dextrocardia, and left-sided ascending aorta is strongly suggestive of congenitally corrected transposition of the great arteries. Note that the morphologically right ventricle (RV) is on the same side as the ascending aorta as in **Fig. 8.38**. LA, left atrium; LV, left ventricle; RA, right atrium.

Left-Sided Ascending Aorta

Normally, the ascending aorta is located to the right of and posterior to the main pulmonary artery. It courses upward obliquely toward the right upper thorax and makes a rounded turn to the aortic arch. Unless it is dilated, it is not seen on the plain chest radiographs. The left upper mediastinum may show a straight or rounded bulge when the aorta ascends on the left side of the main pulmonary artery (**Fig. 8.38**). This is typically seen in a congenitally corrected transposition of the great arteries and double inlet right-sided left ventricle with discordant ventriculoarterial connection. Isolated dextrocardia with left-sided ascending aorta is strongly suggestive of a congenitally corrected transposition of the great arteries (**Fig. 8.39**).

Unexplainable Abnormal Cardiac Contour

Rarely a cardiac contour is abnormal but hard to explain by any specific pathology or any chamber enlargement. An unexplainable cardiac contour change may occur with a large cardiac tumor such as fibroma, rhabdomyoma, teratoma, and lipoma (**Fig. 8.40**). The cardiac contour can also be very abnormal when there is a pericardial defect (**Fig. 8.27**).

Rapid Change in Size of Cardiac Silhouette

When the cardiac silhouette shows unexplained enlargement on a follow-up study in an acutely ill patient, pericardial effusion or acute development of congestive heart failure should be considered (**Fig. 8.41**).

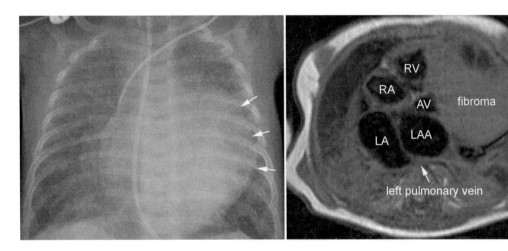

Fig. 8.40 Unusual cardiac configuration with a large bulge (*arrows*) in the left mid-heart border. T1-weighted image (*right panel*) shows that the bulge is produced by a large fibroma. The left atrium is markedly dilated due to left atrial outlet obstruction by the mass. The lungs on chest radiograph show severe pulmonary edema. The partition between the left atrium proper (LA) and left atrial appendage (LAA) is a fold in the roof of the dilated left atrium. Note that the left pulmonary vein is severely compressed between the large heart and the spine. AV, aortic valve; RA, right atrium; RV, right ventricle.

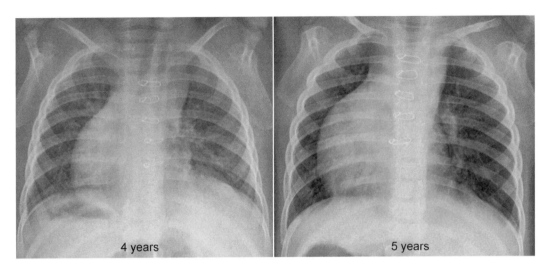

4 years

5 years

Fig. 8.41 Pericardial effusion showing change in heart size in a 5-year-old child with left atrial isomerism and dextrocardia who underwent Kawashima operation for double outlet right ventricle. The patient developed asthma-like symptoms. Chest radiographs show interval enlargement of cardiac silhouette with an unusual pencil-sharp cardiac contour. Echocardiography confirmed moderate amount of pericardial effusion.

Pearls

- The cardiothoracic ratio in the frontal chest radiograph is less than 50% in children over 5 years of age, and it can be as large as 60% in newborns.
- The heart diseases can be classified into volume overload lesions and pressure overload lesions. Volume overload lesions enlarge the silhouettes of the overloaded chambers, whereas pressure overload lesions change the contour of the affected chamber with or without silhouette enlargement.
- The heart may maintain its normal size on radiographs until it is significantly enlarged. Changes in overall heart size and configuration on radiographs are rather insensitive parameters of disease processes.
- Overall configuration of the heart may provide the clues to the diagnosis. Helpful named cardiac configurations include boot-shaped heart, egg-on-side appearance, triangular heart, cascade right heart border, and water-bottle appearance.
- In general, radiographic signs of left-sided chamber enlargement are easier to recognize and perhaps more sensitive to disease processes than the signs of right-side chamber enlargement.

- The signs of obvious right atrial enlargement include extension of the right atrial border beyond the limit of the medial one third of the right thorax, and increased height of the right atrial border occupying more than half of the vertical distance between the medial end of the right clavicle and the dome of the right hemidiaphragm on the frontal view. Right atrial enlargement, however, is often not obvious on radiographs. The right heart border can even be flat with significant right atrial enlargement due to leftward rotation of the heart.
- The signs of left atrial enlargement include double density or double contour within the cardiac silhouette, elevation or posterior displacement of the left main bronchus, and flattening or bulging of the left atrial appendage segment of the left heart border.
- The signs of right ventricular enlargement include elevation or rounding of the cardiac apex on the frontal view, and bulkiness of the anterior part of the heart with obliteration of the retrosternal clear space on the lateral view. The typical boot-shaped configuration is seen only in congenital lesions such as tetralogy of Fallot

with or without pulmonary atresia and truncus arteriosus. Severe right ventricular enlargement with leftward rotation of the heart can cause radiographic findings similar to left ventricular enlargement.

▫ The signs of left ventricular enlargement include elongation of the left heart border and downward lateral displacement of the cardiac apex on the frontal view, and posterior displacement of the lower heart border obliterating the retrocardiac prespinal clear space on the lateral view.

▫ Prominent pulmonary arterial segment of the left heart border is seen in pulmonary valve stenosis, pulmonary regurgitation, pulmonary hypertension of any cause, and congenital heart disease with a left-to-right shunt. Mildly convex pulmonary arterial segment may occasionally be seen as a normal variation.

▫ Prominent left upper mediastinum due to a left-sided ascending aorta in situs solitus is seen in a congenitally corrected transposition of the great arteries and double inlet right-sided left ventricle with discordant ventriculoarterial connection.

▫ Unexplainable change in cardiac contour suggests a cardiac tumor or pericardial defect.

▫ Unexplained rapid change in cardiac silhouette size suggests pericardial effusion or acute development of congestive heart failure.

References

1. Taybi H. Roentgen evaluation of cardiomegaly in the newborn period and early infancy. Pediatr Clin North Am 1971;18:1031–1058
2. Strife JL, Bisset GS III, Burrows PE. Cardiovascular system. In: Kirks DR, Griscom NT, eds. Practical Pediatric Imaging. Diagnostic Radiology of Infants and Children, 3rd ed. Philadelphia: Lippincott-Raven, 1998:511–618
3. Ferguson EC, Krishnamurthy R, Oldham SA. Classic imaging signs of congenital cardiovascular abnormalities. Radiographics 2007;27: 1323–1334
4. Haider EA. The boot-shaped heart sign. Radiology 2008;246:328–329
5. Weaver MD, Chen JT, Anderson PA, Lester RG. Total anomalous pulmonary venous connection to the left vertical vein. A plain-film sign useful in early diagnosis. Radiology 1976;118:679–683
6. Genz T, Locher D, Genz S, Schumacher G, Bühlmeyer K. Chest X-ray film patterns in children with isolated total anomalous pulmonary vein connection. Eur J Pediatr 1990;150:14–18
7. Amoretti F, Cerillo AG, Chiappino D. The levoatriocardinal vein. Pediatr Cardiol 2005;26:494–495
8. Friedman AH, Fogel MA, Stephens P Jr, et al. Identification, imaging, functional assessment and management of congenital coronary arterial abnormalities in children. Cardiol Young 2007;17(Suppl 2): 56–67
9. Van Praagh S, O'Sullivan J, Brili S, Van Praagh R. Juxtaposition of the morphologically left atrial appendage in solitus and inversus atria: a study of 18 postmortem cases. Am Heart J 1996;132(2 Pt 1):391–402
10. Lai WW, Ravishankar C, Gross RP, et al. Juxtaposition of the atrial appendages: a clinical series of 22 patients. Pediatr Cardiol 2001;22: 121–127
11. Carsky EW, Mauceri RA, Azimi F. The epicardial fat pad sign: analysis of frontal and lateral chest radiographs in patients with pericardial effusion. Radiology 1980;137:303–308
12. Eisenberg MJ, Dunn MM, Kanth N, Gamsu G, Schiller NB. Diagnostic value of chest radiography for pericardial effusion. J Am Coll Cardiol 1993;22:588–593

9 Pulmonary Vascularity

The fourth step in chest radiographic interpretation is to assess the pulmonary vascular patterns. The pulmonary vascular patterns can be classified into six categories[1]:

1. Normal vascularity
2. Increased vascularity or plethora
3. Decreased vascularity or oligemia
4. Pulmonary venous hypertension pattern
5. Pulmonary arterial hypertension pattern
6. Uneven, unequal, or asymmetric vascularity

For example, this part of the report in a patient with unilateral absence of the right pulmonary artery can read as follows: *"The pulmonary vascularity is asymmetric with the vascularity of the right lung markedly reduced and that of the left lung increased. The right lung hilum is not only overlain by the displaced heart but also inconspicuous. The right lung is diffusely reticular, which suggests systemic-to-pulmonary arterial collaterals. These findings in conjunction with a reduced volume of the right lung are highly suggestive of unilateral absence of the right pulmonary artery."*

■ Normal Vascularity

The normal pulmonary vascular markings show gradual tapering toward the periphery of the lungs (**Fig. 9.1**). Vascular markings are more prominent in the lower lungs than in the upper lungs, especially when the chest radiograph is obtained in an upright position. The apical parts of the lungs are devoid of sizable vascular markings in most normal individuals. Although the pulmonary vessels show some asymmetric anatomy in the lung hila, the pulmonary vascularity in the lungs is normally symmetric. The symmetry of the peripheral pulmonary vascularity should be assessed region by region. It is common to perceive the vascularity of the left lower lung as being slightly less prominent than that of the right lower lung. This is often a visual illusion. As a significant part of the left lower lung is overlain by the cardiac silhouette, the pulmonary vascularity of this area is perceived as less obvious than the vascularity of the opposite right lower lung. When the left hilum is uncovered on a chest radiograph obtained in a slight left anterior or right posterior oblique view, the vascularity of the left

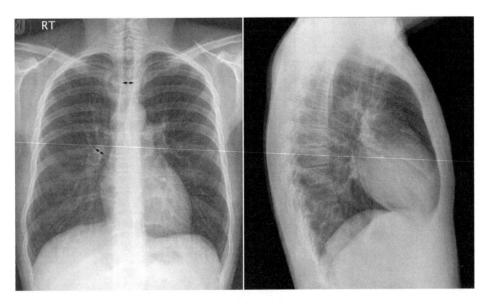

Fig. 9.1 Normal chest frontal and lateral views. The pulmonary vessels show gradual tapering toward the periphery. The descending branch of the right pulmonary artery has a diameter similar to that of the trachea in the thorax (*double-headed arrows*). RT, right.

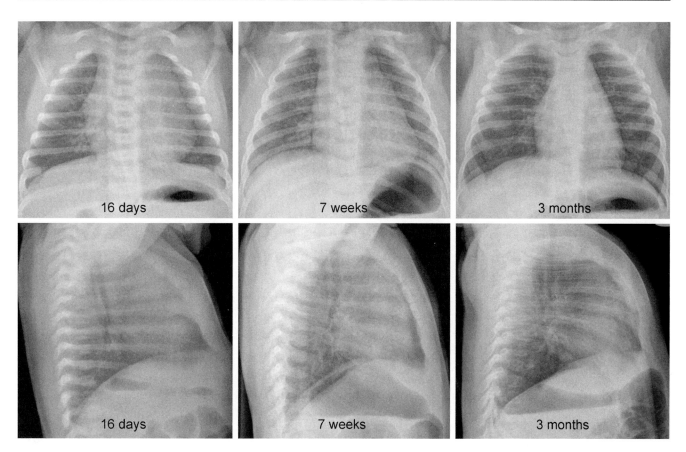

Fig. 9.2 Normal frontal and lateral radiographs in a series of young infants. Pulmonary vascularity appears diminished in the early neonatal period and becomes more prominent with age. A large thymus overlies the cardiac silhouette and central pulmonary vessels. The changing pattern of pulmonary vascularity is more obvious on the lateral images.

lung appears mistakenly increased. When the vascularity is symmetric, the descending branch of the right pulmonary artery can be used as a reference vessel for determination of pulmonary vascular prominence. Normally, the diameter of the descending branch of the right pulmonary artery is equal to the diameter of the trachea in the thorax (**Fig. 9.1**).[2] In the peripheral lungs, the pulmonary vessels and adjacent bronchial lumina are equally sized.

Pulmonary vascularity appears less prominent in newborns and younger infants than in older children (**Fig. 9.2**). This is partly due to the small vessel size in normal newborns. It is also considered to be due to a difference in shape of the thoracic cage. Normally newborns and young infants have a deeper thoracic cage and therefore an increased ratio between the air-filled lung and soft tissue. Consequently, the lungs appear hyperlucent and the pulmonary vascularity less prominent. In addition, a large thymus overlies the larger vessels in the medial lung areas.

Normal pulmonary vascularity can be seen in patients with a milder form of right- and left-sided lesions that is not complicated by an intracardiac or extracardiac shunt or heart failure (**Table 9.1**).

Isolated right-sided lesions including pulmonary valve stenosis, pulmonary regurgitation, and tricuspid regurgitation usually show normal pulmonary vascularity. Decreased pulmonary vascularity in these lesions means that there is right-side heart failure or a right-to-left shunt through the patent foramen ovale. In isolated pulmonary valve stenosis, the pulmonary arterial segment of the left heart border shows a round bulge due to poststenotic dilatation (**Fig. 9.3**). The pulmonary vascularity within the lungs is usually normal. Occasionally the pulmonary

Table 9.1 Cardiac Lesions with Normal Pulmonary Vascularity

Right-sided lesions	Pulmonary stenosis with intact ventricular septum
	Pulmonary regurgitation
	Mild tricuspid regurgitation
Mild forms of left-sided lesions	Aortic valve stenosis
	Supravalvar aortic stenosis
	Aortic regurgitation
	Coarctation of aorta

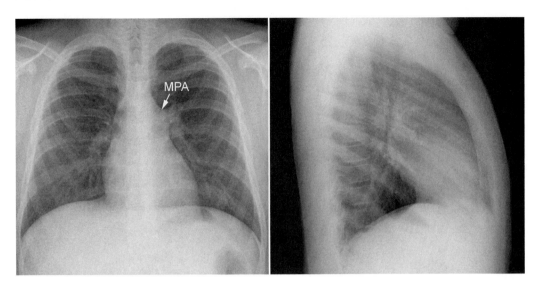

Fig. 9.3 Isolated pulmonary valvar stenosis. The main pulmonary arterial (MPA) segment of the left heart border shows a convex bulge due to poststenotic dilatation. Peripheral pulmonary vascularity is normal. A similar finding can also be seen as a normal variation.

vascularity may be mildly asymmetric because of a preferential pulmonary blood flow to the left lung. Isolated pulmonary regurgitation is also associated with normal peripheral pulmonary vascularity but with cardiomegaly and prominence of the main pulmonary arterial segment of the left heart border (**Fig. 8.37**, right upper panel). Mild to moderate forms of isolated tricuspid regurgitation are associated with normal pulmonary vascularity.

Mild forms of left-sided lesions involving the aortic valve and aorta show normal pulmonary vascularity. However, mitral valve pathology is usually associated with a pulmonary venous hypertension pattern.

■ Increased Vascularity (Plethora)

Increased pulmonary vascularity is typically seen in acyanotic congenital heart diseases causing a left-to-right shunt (**Table 9.2**). It is also seen in cyanotic congenital heart diseases that are not associated with major obstruction to pulmonary arterial blood flow. In these conditions, interatrial or interventricular mixing of the systemic and pulmonary venous returns is necessary with the exchange in favor of the lower pressure pulmonary circulation, resulting in increased pulmonary vascularity. Finally, increased vascularity may also be due to high cardiac output status, which may be secondary to a large vascular malformation or hemangioma in the liver, brain, or extremities; severe anemia; and thyrotoxicosis.

Increased vascularity is characterized by uniformly enlarged vessels at the hila and within the lungs (**Figs. 9.4, 9.5**). The enlarged main pulmonary artery causes a convex bulge of the pulmonary arterial segment of the left heart border. The diameter of the descending branch of the right pulmonary artery exceeds the diameter of the trachea. The peripheral vessels within the lungs are bigger than the adjacent end-on shadows of bronchi. The peripheral pulmonary arteries can be tortuous. The margins of the enlarged vessels are sharp and clean unless there is associated pulmonary edema, atelectasis, or consolidation. Both increased and decreased vascularity can be perceived much more reliably on lateral radiographs than on frontal radiographs. Increased pulmonary vascularity is often not perceived when the pulmonary to systemic blood flow ratio (Qp/Qs) is under 2:1 (**Fig. 9.6**). Although the degree of increased pulmonary vascularity and heart size tend to correlate with the Qp/Qs, chest radiographs cannot be used as a quantitative measurement tool for the shunt lesions as both the pulmonary vascular prominence and heart size at a given amount of left-to-right shunt may vary according to the heart rate and contractility (**Fig. 9.7**). When the left-to-right shunt lesion is complicated by congestive heart failure, the margins of the prominent pulmonary vessels become indistinct (**Fig. 9.8**).

The magnitude of the left-to-right shunt through the atrial septal defect, ventricular septal defect, aortopulmonary window, and patent ductus arteriosus is dependent not only on the size of the defect but also on the differences in vascular resistance between the pulmonary and the systemic circulations.[3] Low pulmonary vascular resistance causes a large shunt, whereas high pulmonary vascular resistance restricts the left-to-right shunt and may result in a reversed shunt. The pulmonary vascular resistance is high in fetal life because the small muscular pulmonary arteries have a thick muscular wall

Table 9.2   Causes of Increased Pulmonary Vascularity or Plethora

Lesions with left-to-right shunt	Partial anomalous pulmonary venous connection
	Atrial septal defect
	Atrioventricular septal defect
	Ventricular septal defect
	Left ventricle-to-right atrial shunt
	Aorto-cameral fistula
	Coronary-cameral fistula
	Aortopulmonary window
	Patent ductus arteriosus
Cyanotic heart diseases with bidirectional shunt	Fenestrated or unroofed coronary sinus
	Common atrium
	Total anomalous pulmonary venous connection
	Double outlet right ventricle without pulmonary stenosis
	Double inlet ventricles without pulmonary stenosis or atresia
	Tricuspid atresia without pulmonary stenosis or atresia
	Complete transposition of the great arteries without pulmonary stenosis or atresia
	Pulmonary atresia with ventricular septal defect and unobstructed major aortopulmonary arterial collateral arteries
	Truncus arteriosus
Hyperkinetic circulatory or high output states	Systemic arteriovenous malformation and hemangiomas, such as vein of Galen aneurysm, hepatic hemangioendothelioma and Klippel-Trenaunay-Weber syndrome
	Severe anemia
	Thyrotoxicosis

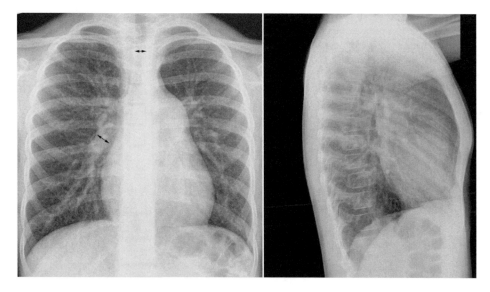

Fig. 9.4 Increased pulmonary vascularity in a 7-year-old patient with a secundum atrial septal defect. The diameter of the descending branch of the right pulmonary artery is greater than the diameter of the trachea (*double-headed arrows*). The main pulmonary arterial segment of the left heart border is convex. There was mild pulmonary hypertension with the systolic pulmonary arterial pressure of 28 mm Hg. The heart is moderately enlarged.

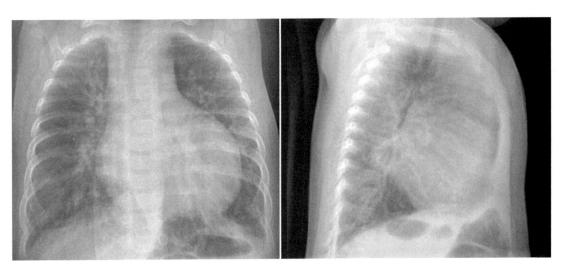

Fig. 9.5 Markedly increased pulmonary vascularity in a 5-month-old patient with a ventricular septal defect. The heart is markedly enlarged. Both lungs show air-trapping.

and small lumen.[4] With initiation of pulmonary ventilation at birth, pulmonary vascular resistance declines rapidly. After the initial rapid decrease in pulmonary vascular resistance and pulmonary arterial pressure, there is a slow, progressive decrease, with adult levels reached after 2 to 6 weeks.[5] This process can be delayed when there is a large shunt. Therefore, the left-to-right shunt lesions do not cause an overt increase in pulmonary vascularity and significant cardiomegaly in the first week of life. As the pulmonary vascular resistance gradually declines in the first few weeks or months of life, the pulmonary blood flow increases with larger amounts of shunt, and

the cardiac chambers enlarge. If the lesion is left untreated, the lungs gradually develop obstructive vascular changes, which result in pulmonary hypertension (discussed later in this chapter).

In certain conditions, the magnitude of the left-to-right shunt is relatively unaffected by the changes in pulmonary vascular resistance. In contrast to the conditions in which the magnitude of the shunt is dependent on pulmonary vascular resistance (dependent shunt lesions), these conditions are called obligatory shunt lesions.[3] An obligatory shunt occurs when the shunt is between chambers having a large pressure difference,

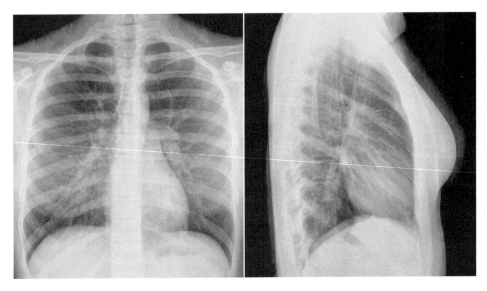

Fig. 9.6 Sinus venosus type atrial sepal defect with the right upper and middle pulmonary veins connecting to the superior vena cava in a 15-year-old girl. The ratio between the pulmonary and systemic blood flow (Qp/Qs) was 2.2 and right ventricular volume index was 151 mL/m² of body surface area, which is moderately increased. The heart is normal in size and the pulmonary vascularity only mildly increased.

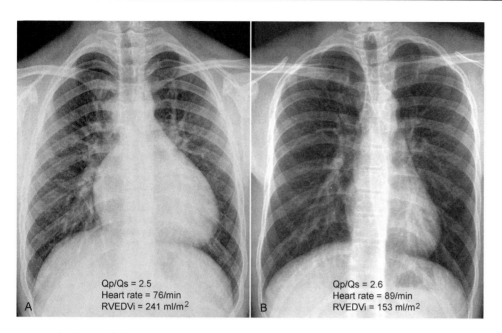

Qp/Qs = 2.5
Heart rate = 76/min
RVEDVi = 241 ml/m^2

Qp/Qs = 2.6
Heart rate = 89/min
RVEDVi = 153 ml/m^2

A

B

Fig. 9.7 (A,B) Frontal chest radiographs from two different 17-year-old patients with an atrial septal defect. The two patients had similar ratios between the pulmonary and systemic blood flow (Qp/Qs) but significantly different heart sizes and prominence of pulmonary vascularity. **(B)** Note that the patient with a normal heart size had a higher heart rate than the patient with a large heart **(A)**. Pulmonary vascularity is moderately increased in **A** and mildly increased in **B**. RVEDVi, right ventricular end diastolic volume index.

such as a left ventricle-to-right atrial shunt, which commonly occurs in an atrioventricular septal defect (**Fig. 9.9**). It also occurs when the shunt lesion is associated with a severe obstructive lesion downstream. For instance, a ventricular septal defect causes a larger amount of left-to-right shunt when it is associated with left ventricular outflow tract obstruction than when it is an isolated lesion (**Fig. 9.10**). Other obligatory shunt lesions include large arteriovenous malformations and aorto–right atrial or coronary artery to right atrial fistula. Increased pulmonary vascularity with overt cardiomegaly in the first few days of life is highly suggestive of an obligatory shunt lesion.

As the bronchi are compressed by the accompanying dilated pulmonary arterial branches, generalized or multifocal obstructive emphysema or segmental or less commonly lobar collapse are often seen even without significant respiratory symptoms (**Fig. 9.5**).

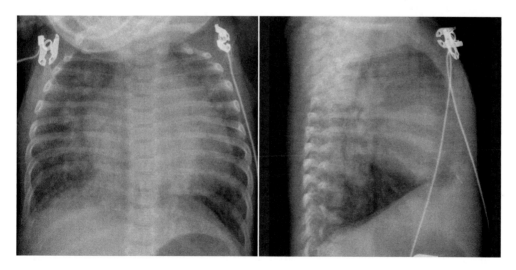

Fig. 9.8 Ventricular and atrial septal defects complicated by congestive heart failure in an 8-week-old infant. The pulmonary vascularity is markedly increased. The vessel margins are blurred because of interstitial edema. The heart is markedly enlarged. The lungs are hyperinflated with posterior atelectasis.

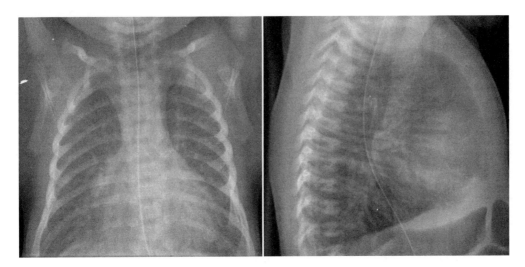

Fig. 9.9 Markedly increased pulmonary vascularity in an 11-day-old newborn with complete atrioventricular septal defect.

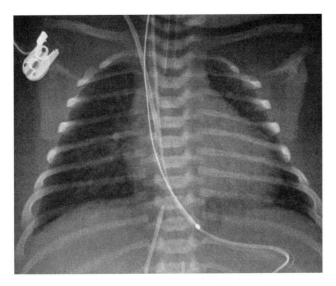

Fig. 9.10 Markedly increased pulmonary vascularity in a 4-day-old newborn with interrupted aortic arch and ventricular septal defect. There are signs of interstitial pulmonary edema and small bilateral effusions, suggesting congestive heart failure.

■ Decreased Vascularity (Oligemia)

Decreased vascularity is seen with a right-to-left shunt, right-sided heart failure, pericardial effusion or constrictive pericarditis, and pulmonary embolism (**Table 9.3**).

Decreased vascularity is characterized by uniformly small size of the pulmonary vessels at the hila and within the lungs (**Fig. 9.11, 9.12, 9.13**). As mentioned, determination of decreased as well as increased vascularity is often easier and perhaps more accurate on lateral radiographs than on frontal radiographs. As the main pulmonary artery and underlying ventricular outflow tract is

also small, the pulmonary arterial segment of the heart border is less prominent than normal. The lungs may appear hyperlucent.

The heart size is normal or small when the right-to-left shunt is primarily associated with an obstructive lesion to the pulmonary blood flow but without valvular regurgitation as in tetralogy of Fallot and other complex congenital heart disease (**Figs. 9.11, 9.12**). However, tetralogy of Fallot may show normal or even increased vascularity and cardiomegaly when the pulmonary outflow tract obstruction is only mild in the initial few weeks to months of life (**Fig. 9.14**). The patient is typically acyanotic in this period and the condition is called "pink" tetralogy of Fallot. With time the right ventricle further hypertrophies due to increased pressure and volume overload. As the right ventricular outflow obstruction worsens with myocardial hypertrophy, right-to-left shunting eventually ensues, and the patient becomes cyanotic. Similar changes over time can also be seen in other cyanotic heart diseases with mild pulmonary outflow tract obstruction and a septal defect.

Decreased pulmonary vascularity is associated with cardiomegaly when there is severe valvular regurgitation or right-sided heart failure. Pulmonary atresia with intact ventricular septum is a good example showing both decreased pulmonary blood flow and an enlarged heart. Cardiomegaly in this condition is mainly due to tricuspid regurgitation causing severe right atrial dilatation, although left ventricular dilatation and right ventricular hypertrophy are additional contributing factors (**Fig. 9.13**).

Pulmonary vascularity is usually reduced when there is a moderate amount of pericardial effusion (**Fig. 9.15A**). In both cardiac tamponade and constrictive pericarditis, reduced pulmonary vascularity is associated with pulmonary venous hypertension (**Fig. 9.15B**).

Table 9.3 Causes of Decreased Pulmonary Vascularity or Oligemia

Lesions with right-to-left shunt	Tetralogy of Fallot
	Pulmonary atresia with ventricular septal defect
	Pulmonary stenosis or atresia with intact ventricular septum, with right-to-left shunt at atrial level
	Ebstein's malformation of tricuspid valve with right-to-left shunt at atrial level
	Complex congenital heart disease with pulmonary stenosis or atresia causing right-to-left shunt
Right-sided heart failure	Right-sided heart failure
	Uhl's anomaly
Pericardial disease	Pericardial effusion
	Constrictive pericarditis
Others	Widespread peripheral pulmonary artery stenosis
	Pulmonary embolism
	Extrinsic compression of the pulmonary artery or right ventricular outflow tract due to tumor, aortic aneurysm, or mediastinal pathology

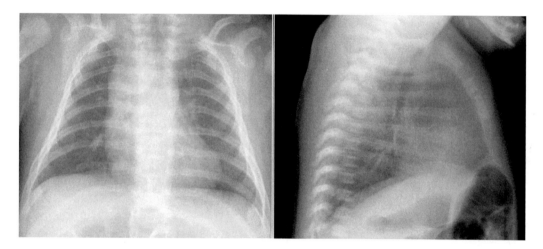

Fig. 9.11 Markedly decreased pulmonary vascularity in a newborn with a severe form of tetralogy of Fallot. The reduced vascularity is more obvious on the lateral view with better visualization of the small hilar pulmonary arteries. There is a right aortic arch.

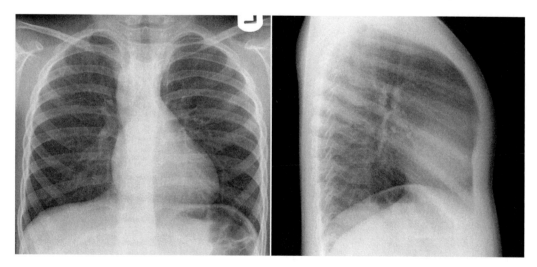

Fig. 9.12 Mildly decreased pulmonary vascularity in a 5-year-old patient with a mild form of tetralogy of Fallot. The pulmonary vascularity looks almost normal on the frontal view. The lateral view clearly shows that the vascularity is decreased as compared with normal vascularity shown in **Fig. 9.1**. There is a right aortic arch.

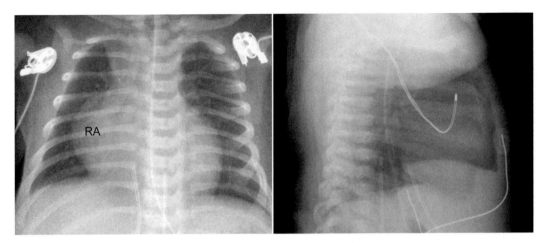

Fig. 9.13 Decreased pulmonary vascularity in a 4-day-old patient with pulmonary atresia with intact ventricular septum. There is moderate cardiomegaly with markedly enlarged right atrium (RA) due to severe tricuspid regurgitation.

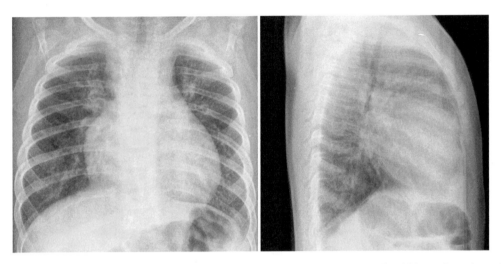

Fig. 9.14 Pink tetralogy of Fallot. Chest radiographs from a 5-month-old patient with mild form of tetralogy of Fallot show moderate cardiomegaly and increased pulmonary vascularity. The arterial oxygen saturation at room air was 98%.

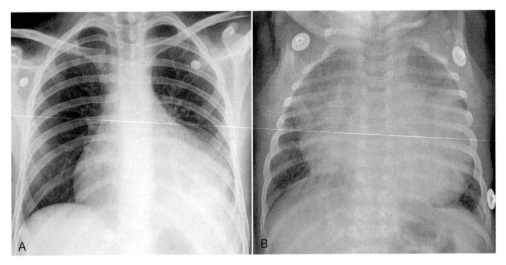

Fig. 9.15 Different manifestations of pericardial effusion. **(A)** This 15-year-old patient with underlying aortic stenosis was supposed to have a rather gradual accumulation of pericardial effusion. The enlarged cardiac silhouette shows a smooth contour. The pulmonary vascularity is reduced. The left lower lobe is collapsed. **(B)** This 11-week-old infant developed pericardial tamponade due to acute pericarditis. The cardiac silhouette is hugely enlarged and both lungs are edematous.

■ Pulmonary Venous Hypertension

Pulmonary venous hypertension is related to increased resistance to flow within the pulmonary veins. As the pulmonary venous pressure is not directly measurable, pulmonary capillary wedge pressure (PCWP) is used as an indirect measure of the pulmonary venous pressure. It is measured by inserting a balloon-tipped catheter into a peripheral vein. Once the catheter tip is advanced into a pulmonary arterial branch, the balloon is inflated and the pressure is measured. The normal mean PCWP is 6 to 12 mm Hg. Pulmonary venous hypertension is defined as a mean PCWP above 12 mm Hg.[6] Pulmonary venous hypertension is caused by obstructive lesions of the pulmonary venous drainage route, mitral regurgitation, and left ventricular dysfunction (**Table 9.4**). The obstruction in the pathway of the pulmonary venous return may be caused

Table 9.4 Causes of Pulmonary Venous Hypertension

Obstruction to pulmonary venous drainage	Pulmonary veins	Obstructive types of total anomalous pulmonary venous connection
		Pulmonary veno-occlusive disease (PVOD)
		Individual pulmonary vein stenosis
		Pulmonary vein atresia
	Left atrium	Cor triatriatum
		Tumor (myxoma)
		Thrombus
Obstruction to left atrial drainage	Left atrial outlet	Supravalvar mitral ring
		Mitral stenosis
		Hypoplastic left heart syndrome with restrictive atrial communication
	Left ventricular inlet	Mitral arcade
		Parachute mitral valve
Mitral regurgitation	Primary pathology of the mitral valve or its tension apparatus	Cleft mitral valve
		Myxomatous mitral valve
		Mitral valve prolapse
		Rheumatic mitral valve diseases
		Ruptured tension apparatus of the mitral valve
	Functional	Left ventricular dilatation
		Localized myocardial dysfunction
Left ventricular failure or dysfunction	With left ventricular dilatation	Aortic regurgitation
		Aorto-left ventricular tunnel
		Myocarditis
		Dilated cardiomyopathy
		Anomalous origin of a coronary artery from the pulmonary artery
		Myocardial ischemia or dysfunction
	With left ventricular diastolic dysfunction	Aortic stenosis
		Supravalvar aortic stenosis
		Severe coarctation of the aorta
		Systemic hypertension
		Hypertrophic cardiomyopathy
		Restrictive cardiomyopathy (amyloidosis, sarcoidosis, hemochromatosis, etc.)
		Storage diseases
	Abnormal rhythm	Complete heart block
		Tachycardia
Pericardial disease		Constrictive pericarditis
		Pericardial tamponade

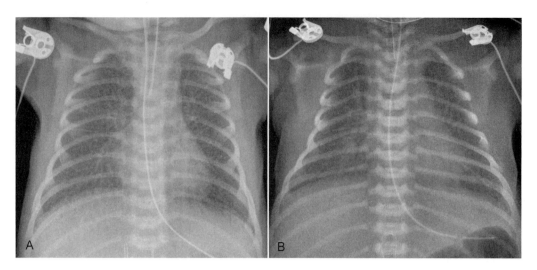

Fig. 9.16 Pulmonary venous hypertension in two newborns with obstructive type of total anomalous pulmonary venous connection. Both lungs show diffusely increased interstitial markings and mild hyperinflation. This radiographic finding is typically seen when the anomalous pulmonary venous drainage is to the portal vein **(A)**. The hepatic parenchyma causes functional obstruction to pulmonary venous drainage with closure of the ductus venosus. A similar finding is also seen when there is severe stenosis of the channel draining the pulmonary veins to an anomalous site **(B)**. This patient had severe stenosis of the draining vein to the right superior vena cava.

by obstruction of the pulmonary veins, but can also be due to an obstructive lesion within the left atrium or left atrial outlet. Mitral regurgitation causes increased left atrial pressure that leads to pulmonary venous hypertension. Left ventricular dysfunction or failure causes elevation of the left ventricular diastolic pressure that leads to impaired diastolic flow into the left ventricle and thus to impaired pulmonary venous drainage (**Table 9.4**). Significant hypertrophy of the left ventricle from any etiology causes impaired relaxation or reduced compliance and therefore impaired filling of the left ventricle and ultimately results in pulmonary venous hypertension. Acute accumulation of pericardial effusion or constrictive pericarditis also may result in pulmonary venous hypertension because of impaired left ventricular filling.

Pulmonary venous hypertension caused by pulmonary venous obstruction is characterized by generalized increase in interstitial markings (**Figs. 9.16, 9.17, 9.18**).

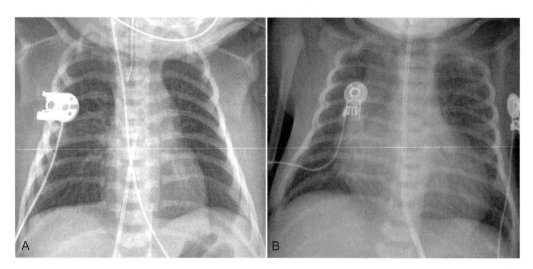

Fig. 9.17 Two different radiographic manifestations of hypoplastic left heart syndrome. **(A)** When the atrial septum is intact or the interatrial defect is restrictive, the heart is normal in size or only mildly enlarged, and the lungs show signs of pulmonary venous hypertension. The finding is very similar to that of the obstructive type of total anomalous pulmonary venous connection as shown in **Fig. 9.16**. **(B)** When the interatrial communication is not restrictive, the pulmonary venous hypertension is not pronounced. The heart tends to be larger and the pulmonary vascularity is increased instead of showing pulmonary venous hypertension.

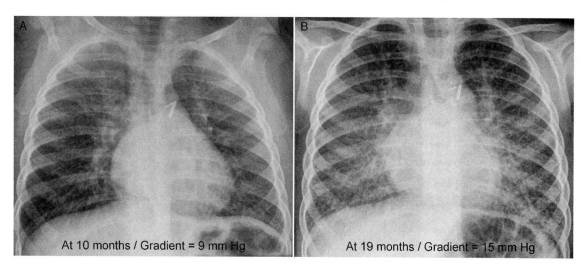

Fig. 9.18 Obstruction of the confluent pulmonary vein at its anastomosis to the left atrium after repair of total anomalous pulmonary venous connection. Chest radiographs show obvious progression of interstitial edema from 10 months to 19 months of age. The pressure gradient across the stenosis rose from 9 to 15 mm Hg during the interval.

Increased interstitial markings are characterized by a reticular pattern and blurred margins of the pulmonary vessels. Pulmonary veno-occlusive disease (PVOD) is a rare fatal condition in which there is gradual obliteration of the pulmonary venules and small veins (**Fig. 9.19**).[7] The importance of suspicion or diagnosis of this rare condition is discussed later in this chapter. Blurring of the hilar pulmonary arteries is called hilar haze (**Fig. 9.19**). Interstitial edema thickens the bronchial walls, which is called peribronchial cuffing. The lungs usually show variable degrees of emphysema. When pulmonary venous obstruction is not associated with intracardiac shunting, the heart size is usually normal. When a newborn with tachypnea shows generalized increase in interstitial markings and mild hyperinflation of the lungs without cardiomegaly, an obstructed type of total anomalous pulmonary venous connection should be considered (**Fig. 9.16**). Total anomalous pulmonary venous connection to the portal vein is the most common type of anomalous connection that causes pulmonary venous obstruction (**Fig. 9.16A**). As the pulmonary venous return needs to pass through the hepatic capillary bed, pulmonary venous drainage is severely impaired unless the ductus venosus is persistently patent after birth. Similar hemodynamic changes and radiographic findings can be seen in any type of total anomalous pulmonary venous connection with the draining vein severely stenosed (**Fig. 9.16B**). In addition, the hypoplastic left heart syndrome and the lesions causing left atrial outlet obstruction that include cor triatriatum and severe mitral stenosis may show a similar feature when the atrial septum is intact or interatrial communication is severely restrictive (**Fig. 9.17A**). When these lesions are associated with a widely patent interatrial communication, the heart is enlarged and the pulmonary vascularity is increased with less severe findings of pulmonary venous hypertension (**Fig. 9.17B**). The radiographic findings of interstitial edema in the newborn are similar to those seen with interstitial pneumonia (**Fig. 9.20**) or congenital lymphangiectasia.

The interstitial edema in older children and adults is characterized by reticular opacities from thickened interlobular septa in the peripheral and central lungs. The peripheral opacities are arranged perpendicular to the nearest pleural surface with a stepladder pattern.[8] They are called Kerley's B lines and are seen best in the costophrenic angle areas. Reticular opacities in more central zones represent either thickened interlobular septa or dilated lymphatics. Interstitial edema associated with mitral regurgitation may predominate in the right upper lobe as a result of regurgitant jet flowing directly into the right upper pulmonary vein.[9] As mentioned previously, interstitial edema causes blurring of the margins of the central and peripheral vessels and bronchi.

Pulmonary venous hypertension caused by mitral regurgitation or left ventricular dysfunction or failure shows pulmonary vascular redistribution as well as increased interstitial markings (**Fig. 9.21**).[1,6,8] Pulmonary vascular redistribution denotes dilatation of the upper lung vessels and relative vasoconstriction of the lower lung vessels. The exact pathogenetic mechanism for vascular redistribution is not clearly understood. Pulmonary vascular redistribution is more obvious with the patient in the upright position than in the supine position. Therefore, infants with pulmonary venous hypertension rarely

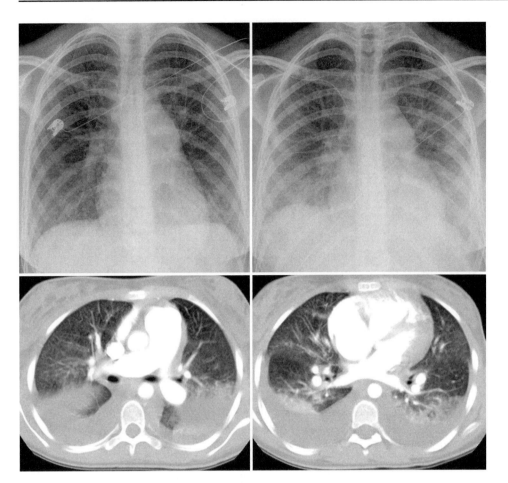

Fig. 9.19 Pulmonary veno-occlusive disease in a 15-year-old patient. The initial chest radiograph (*left upper panel*) shows findings of pulmonary hypertension with dilatation of the main pulmonary arterial segment of the left heart border and central pulmonary arteries. There is generalized increase in interstitial markings. Chest radiograph obtained after administration of a vasodilator (*right upper panel*) shows worsened pulmonary venous hypertension and bilateral pleural effusions. Computed tomography (CT) images show dilated central pulmonary arteries, hypertrophied right ventricle, and patent pulmonary veins. There is generalized increase in interstitial markings. Dependent parts of both lungs show alveolar edema and collapse. Moderate amounts of bilateral pleural effusions are seen.

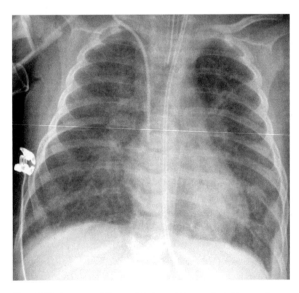

Fig. 9.20 Increased interstitial markings mimicking pulmonary venous hypertension pattern in a young infant with respiratory syncytial viral pneumonia. Both lungs are hyperinflated.

show pulmonary vascular redistribution. Pulmonary vascular redistribution is considered an earlier sign of pulmonary venous hypertension compared with interstitial edema.[6,8] As fluid begins to leak from the vessels into the interstitium when pulmonary vascular pressure exceeds plasma oncotic pressure, interstitial edema seen in radiographs suggests a PCWP above 25 mm Hg.[1] When the combination of cardiomegaly and pulmonary venous hypertension is seen in young infants, an anomalous origin of the left coronary artery from the pulmonary artery (ALCAPA) should be included in the differential diagnosis (**Fig. 9.22**). As the diagnosis of ALCAPA can be missed at routine echocardiography, a high index of suspicion is important in the early detection of this rare but serious anomaly.[10]

Severe pulmonary venous hypertension may be accompanied by alveolar pulmonary edema.[1,6,8] It causes ill-defined central haziness with air-bronchograms and loss

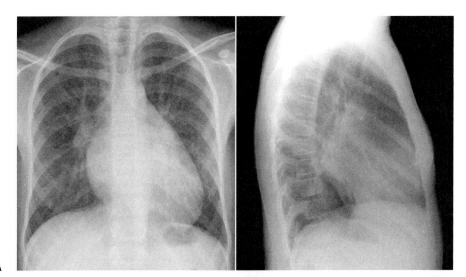

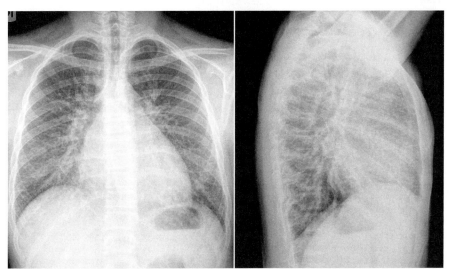

Fig. 9.21 **(A)** Pulmonary venous hypertension in an 11-year-old patient with rheumatic mitral regurgitation and **(B)** a 13-year-old patient with dilated cardiomyopathy. In both patients, the pulmonary vessels in the lower lung zones are smaller compared with the vessels in the upper lung zones. Interstitial markings are mildly increased in **A** and markedly increased in **B**. The overall heart configuration is triangular. The left atrium and left ventricle are dilated.

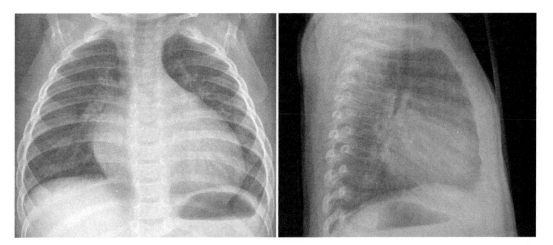

Fig. 9.22 Pulmonary venous hypertension with cardiomegaly in a 7-month-old infant with anomalous left coronary artery arising from the pulmonary artery (ALCAPA). There is moderate cardiomegaly with predominant enlargement of the left atrium and left ventricle. Pulmonary vascularity shows a pulmonary venous hypertension pattern with increased interstitial markings and redistribution. This combination can also be seen in dilated cardiomyopathy and severe mitral regurgitation.

of vessels margins. Long-standing pulmonary venous hypertension may cause hemosiderosis and ossification in the pulmonary interstitium. Pleural effusion is occasionally seen in pulmonary venous hypertension.

Pulmonary venous hypertension can be complicated by elevation of the pulmonary arterial pressure, causing engorged central pulmonary arteries (**Figs. 9.19, 9.21**).

Although the chest radiograph is useful in detecting the presence of pulmonary venous hypertension and in distinguishing severe from mild pulmonary hypertension, precise grading of the severity of pulmonary venous hypertension is difficult.[6,8]

■ Pulmonary Arterial Hypertension

The normal mean pulmonary arterial pressure is 18 to 22 mm Hg. Pulmonary hypertension is defined as a mean pulmonary arterial pressure greater than 25 mm Hg at rest

and greater than 30 mm Hg during exercise.[11] When no etiology is found, pulmonary arterial hypertension is termed idiopathic pulmonary arterial hypertension (formerly primary pulmonary hypertension). Pulmonary arterial hypertension is more commonly secondary to other conditions, such as chronic heart disease, pulmonary thromboembolism, and chronic lung disease (**Table 9.5**).

Pulmonary hypertension is characterized radiographically by discrepancy in central and peripheral pulmonary vascular dimensions with dilatation of the central elastic pulmonary arteries and constriction of the peripheral muscular branches (**Fig. 9.23**).[8,12] The transition varies in level but is usually in the segmental level. The transition can be abrupt or gradual. The peripheral vessels appear reduced in number and size and may appear tortuous. Peripheral vascular paucity gives rise to the so-called pruned-tree appearance. In adults, pulmonary hypertension can be suspected when the descending branch of the right pulmonary artery measures greater than 16 mm or a

Table 9.5   Revised World Health Organization Classification of Pulmonary Arterial Hypertension[12]

1. Pulmonary arterial hypertension	1.1. Idiopathic
	1.2. Familial
	1.3. Associated with:
	1.3.1. Connective tissue disease
	1.3.2. Congenital systemic pulmonary shunts
	1.3.3. Portal hypertension
	1.3.4. Human immunodeficiency virus (HIV) infection
	1.3.5. Drugs and toxins
	1.3.6. Others (thyroid disorders, glycogen storage disease, Gaucher's disease, hereditary hemorrhagic telangiectasia, hemoglobinopathies, myeloproliferative disorders, splenectomy)
	1.4. Associated with significant venous or capillary involvement
	1.4.1. Pulmonary veno-occlusive disease
	1.4.2. Pulmonary capillary hemangiomatosis
	1.5. Persistent pulmonary hypertension of the newborn
2. Pulmonary hypertension associated with left heart diseases	2.1. Left-sided atrial or ventricular heart disease
	2.2. Left-sided valvular heart disease
3. Pulmonary hypertension associated with lung respiratory diseases and/or hypoxemia	3.1. Chronic obstructive pulmonary disease
	3.2. Interstitial lung disease
	3.3. Sleep-disordered breathing
	3.4. Alveolar hypoventilation disorders
	3.5. Chronic exposure to high altitudes
	3.6 Developmental abnormalities
4. Pulmonary hypertension due to chronic thrombotic and/or embolic disease	4.1. Thromboembolic obstruction of proximal pulmonary arteries
	4.2. Thromboembolic obstruction of distal pulmonary arteries
	4.3. Nonthromboembolic pulmonary embolism (tumor, parasites, foreign material)
5. Miscellaneous	Sarcoidosis, histocytosis X, lymphangiomatosis, compression of pulmonary vessels (adenopathy, tumor, fibrosing mediastinitis)

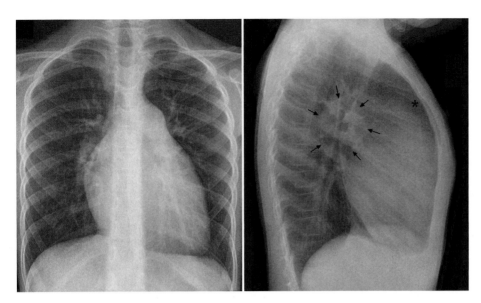

Fig. 9.23 Idiopathic pulmonary hypertension in a 7-year-old patient. The central pulmonary arteries are markedly dilated, whereas the peripheral branches are small. Note the prominence of the branch pulmonary arteries at the hilum evident both on frontal and lateral views. The right and left pulmonary arteries together form a mass-like shadow (*arrows*) in the hilum on the lateral view. The pulmonary arterial segment of the left heart border shows a round bulge. The hypertrophied right ventricle and dilated main pulmonary artery obliterate the retrosternal clear space (*asterisk*) on the lateral view. The sternum is bowed forward.

hilar-to-thoracic ratio is greater than 0.44 in the absence of any shunt lesion (**Fig. 9.24**).[8] Although this radiographic sign is specific, it is not sensitive for the diagnosis of pulmonary hypertension.[13] Redistribution of pulmonary vascularity can also be seen in pulmonary arterial hypertension.[14] The peripheral lungs may show a mosaic pattern of oligemia. The chest radiograph plays a limited role in the assessment of pulmonary hypertension, but may show evidence of underlying lung pathology. Nonetheless, it should be emphasized that any suspicion of this potentially fatal disease from the chest radiographic findings can prompt the diagnosis of pulmonary hypertension that has been mistaken for other commoner diseases.

Pulmonary hypertension may complicate chronic left-to-right shunts (**Fig. 9.25A**). With increased pulmonary arterial pressure secondary to a left-to-right shunt, the peripheral muscular arteries develop medial hypertrophy and vasoconstriction, which results in fast and turbulent blood flow. The intima of the constricted vessels is damaged, which induces intimal proliferation and thrombus formation. As a result, the effective peripheral vascular cross-sectional area is reduced, further elevating the pulmonary arterial pressure. Pulmonary hypertension secondary to a left-to-right shunt shows some different findings depending on the underlying pathology and severity of hypertension. In general, central-peripheral discrepancy of the pulmonary vascularity in shunt lesions is less obvious than in idiopathic pulmonary hypertension, and the degree of discrepancy

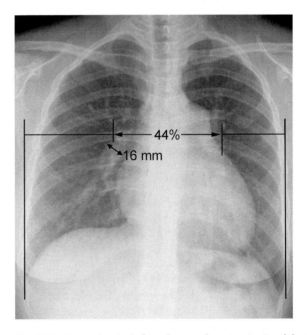

Fig. 9.24 Diagnostic criteria for pulmonary hypertension in adults. The hilar-to-thoracic ratio is measured by dividing the distance between the lateral margins of the pulmonary arteries at the hilum by the transverse diameter of the thorax. Pulmonary hypertension is suspected when the hilar-to-thoracic ratio is over 0.44 or the descending branch of the right pulmonary artery measures 16 mm or more.

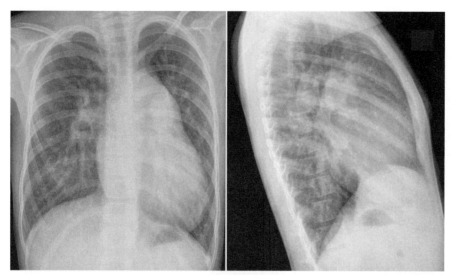

A

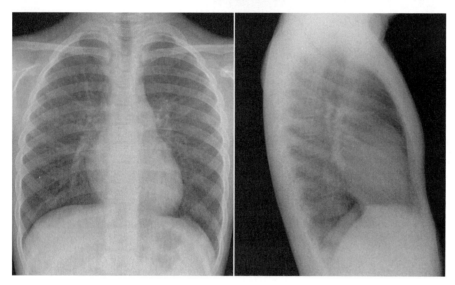

B

Fig. 9.25 **(A)** Patent ductus arteriosus complicated by pulmonary arterial hypertension in a 6-year-old patient. The central parts of the pulmonary arteries are markedly enlarged, whereas the peripheral branches are small compared with the central vessels. The main pulmonary arterial segment of the left heart border is markedly convex. The pulmonary arterial pressure was three quarters of the systemic arterial pressure. **(B)** Eisenmenger syndrome in a 7-year-old patient with a large perimembranous ventricular septal defect. The heart is not enlarged and the pulmonary arterial segment of the left heart border is slightly convex. The pulmonary vascularity appears otherwise normal.

does not correlate well with the pulmonary arterial pressures. Disproportionately prominent pulmonary vascular markings relative to the size of the heart in a patient with a shunt lesion are suggestive of pulmonary hypertension (**Fig. 9.25A;** also see **Fig. 8.37,** lower middle panel). Uncommonly, the findings of pulmonary hypertension, especially when it occurs with a ventricular septal defect, is hardly perceivable (**Fig. 9.25B**).

As discussed, pulmonary venous hypertension is associated with various degree of pulmonary arterial hypertension. PVOD is a rare fatal disease with progressive obliteration of the pulmonary venules and veins resulting in severe pulmonary hypertension. Radiologic suspicion of PVOD is of paramount importance because inadvertent administration of vasodilator in PVOD may cause catastrophic effect (**Fig. 9.19**). When the chest radiographs of the patient with

pulmonary hypertension of unknown origin show increased interstitial markings in addition to general features of pulmonary hypertension, computed tomography (CT) scan is indicated. The classic CT features of PVOD include mosaic distribution of centrilobular ground-glass appearance, generalized thickening of septal interstitial markings that extend to the pleural surfaces, and mediastinal edema in the presence of patent central pulmonary veins and features of pulmonary hypertension.[6]

Markedly dilated central pulmonary arteries with small peripheral branches can also be seen without pulmonary hypertension. When tetralogy of Fallot is associated with absent pulmonary valve syndrome, the branch pulmonary arteries and proximal segmental arteries are markedly dilated as a result of severe pulmonary regurgitation from in utero (**Fig. 9.26**).[15]

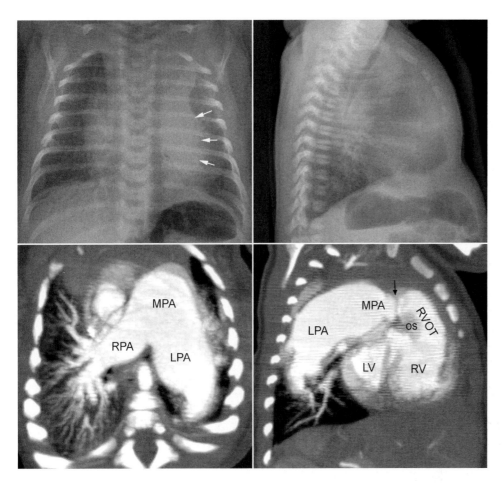

Fig. 9.26 Marked dilatation of the central pulmonary arteries in tetralogy of Fallot with absent pulmonary valve syndrome. The central pulmonary arteries are markedly dilated. There is abrupt transition to small peripheral branches. Frontal chest radiograph shows a large descending branch (*arrows*) of the left pulmonary artery through the cardiac silhouette. Central-peripheral discrepancy in pulmonary vascularity is also obvious on the lateral view. CT angiograms in the *lower panels* show a huge main and branch pulmonary arteries. The right ventricular outflow tract (RVOT) is mildly narrowed by the anteriorly deviated outlet septum (os). The pulmonary valve annulus (*arrow*) forms a ridge-like defect between the RVOT and main pulmonary artery (MPA). LPA, left pulmonary artery; RPA, right pulmonary artery.

■ Uneven, Unequal, or Asymmetric Vascularity

Uneven, unequal, or asymmetric vascularity indicates abnormal distribution of pulmonary perfusion (**Table 9.6**). This abnormal perfusion pattern is more commonly due to the pathology on the pulmonary arterial side. Less frequently the abnormal perfusion is secondary to the abnormal venous drainage. In addition, pulmonary vascular malformations and primary pathology of the lung may cause abnormal distribution of pulmonary vascular markings.

Stenosis of a branch pulmonary artery causes reduced pulmonary vascular markings in the affected lung and increased vascularity in the other lung regions (**Figs. 9.27,** **9.28, 9.29**). It is most commonly seen as a complication of a surgical procedure that involves the pulmonary outflow tract augmentation or enlargement of a branch pulmonary artery, which is performed in patients with tetralogy of Fallot, tetralogy of Fallot with pulmonary atresia, truncus arteriosus, and other diseases with pulmonary outflow tract obstruction (**Fig. 9.27**). The stenosis of a branch pulmonary artery can be due to intrinsic narrowing, kinking, or extrinsic compression from an aneurysmal pulmonary outflow tract. Narrowing of one or both branch pulmonary arteries is not an uncommon complication of the arterial switch operation with a LeCompte procedure, in which the transected main pulmonary artery and its branches are brought forward to encircle the newly made ascending aorta. As the branch pulmonary arteries have longer courses around the ascending aorta

Table 9.6   Causes of Uneven, Unequal, or Asymmetric Pulmonary Vascularity

Pulmonary arterial obstruction	Stenosis of a branch pulmonary artery
	Unilateral absence of a pulmonary artery
	Pulmonary artery sling
	Peripheral pulmonary artery stenosis
	Isolated
	Williams-Beuren syndrome
	Takayasu's arteritis
	Alagille syndrome
	Congenital rubella syndrome
	Cutis laxa
	Ehlers-Danlos syndrome
	Holt-Oram syndrome
	Keutel syndrome
	Noonan syndrome
	Postrubella syndrome
	After unifocalization surgery
	With other congenital heart disease
	Pulmonary thromboembolism
Preferential pulmonary blood flow to a lung	Pulmonary valvar stenosis (to the left lung)
	Tetralogy of Fallot (to the right lung)
	Complete transposition of the great arteries (to the right lung)
	After bidirectional cavopulmonary connection, Fontan operation, or Blalock-Taussig shunt
Systemic arterial supply to the lung	Pulmonary atresia with ventricular septal defect
	Truncus arteriosus with stenosis or hypoplasia of a pulmonary artery
	Origin of a pulmonary artery from the aorta (so-called hemitruncus arteriosus)
	Aberrant systemic arterial supply to a normal lung
	Systemic arterial to pulmonary arterial fistulas
Pulmonary venous obstruction	Individual pulmonary vein stenosis
	Unilateral pulmonary vein atresia
	Postoperative pulmonary vein obstruction
	Pulmonary venous infarction
Pulmonary arteriovenous fistula or malformation	Congenital
	Isolated
	Osler-Weber-Rendu disease
	Acquired
	After Glenn operation
	After bidirectional cavopulmonary connection
	Hepatic failure (hepatopulmonary syndrome)
	Pulmonary infection (actinomycosis, schistosomiasis)
	Chest trauma/surgery
	Amyloidosis
	Mitral stenosis
Pathology of a lung	Scimitar syndrome
	Horseshoe lung
	Congenital lobar emphysema
	Primary hypoplasia of a lung
	Swyer-James syndrome

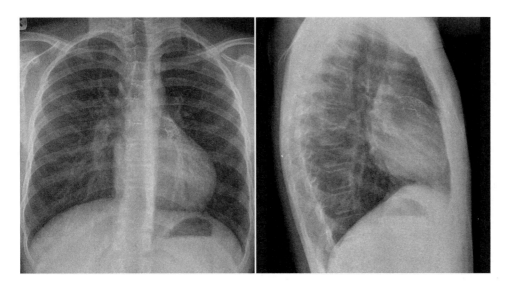

Fig. 9.27 Stenosis of the left pulmonary artery in a 15-year-old patient with repaired tetralogy of Fallot. The pulmonary vessels in the left lung are smaller than those in the right lung. The difference can be recog- nized by comparing the vascularity region by region. Opaque stents are seen in the right ventricular outflow tract and main pulmonary artery.

to reach the pulmonary hila, they tend to be stretched, causing variable degrees of stenosis of one or both branches (**Fig. 9.28**).[16] Primary stenosis of a branch pulmonary artery as an isolated lesion is not common. Stenosis of the left pul- monary arterial origin is occasionally seen in tetralogy of Fallot with pulmonary atresia and in severe forms of tetral- ogy of Fallot (**Fig. 9.29**). This condition is known as juxta- ductal stenosis because it is at the ductal insertion site and it is related to the closure of the ductus arteriosus.[17] The left pulmonary artery may show hypoplasia or stenosis in a

pulmonary artery sling where the left pulmonary artery arises from the proximal right pulmonary artery and courses to the left hilum through the space between the lower trachea and esophagus. Pulmonary artery sling is dis- cussed in detail in Chapter 11 (**Fig. 11.11**).

Unilateral absence of a pulmonary artery is a rare dis- ease causing asymmetric pulmonary vascularity. Invari- ably the absent segment is the mediastinal segment of the branch pulmonary artery and the distal pulmonary artery is connected to the closing or closed ductus arteriosus.

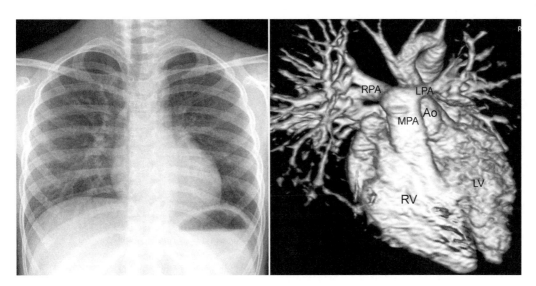

Fig. 9.28 Stenosis of the left pulmonary artery in a 7-year-old patient who underwent arterial switch operation for complete transposition of the great arteries. Chest radiograph shows reduced vascularity in the left lung and increased vascularity in the right lung. Volume-rendered magnetic resonance angiogram seen from the front and above shows the small size of the left pulmonary artery (LPA) as it courses around the ascending aorta (Ao). The blood flow ratio between the right and left pulmonary arteries was 72/28%. LV, left ventricle; RPA, right pul- monary artery; RV, right ventricle; MPA, main pulmonary artery.

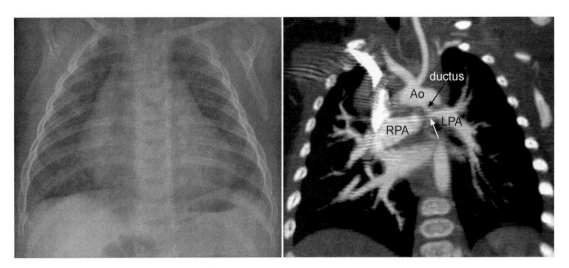

Fig. 9.29 Juxtaductal stenosis of the left pulmonary artery (LPA) in a 3-month-old patient with tetralogy of Fallot. Chest radiograph shows asymmetric pulmonary vascularity. The vascularity of the left lung is less prominent than that of the right lung. CT angiogram reformat in coronal plane shows severe narrowing (*white arrow*) of the left pulmonary artery where the ductus arteriosus is inserted. Ao, aorta; RPA, right pulmonary artery.

Typically, the absent pulmonary artery is on the side opposite the aortic arch and arises from the ductus arteriosus coming from the innominate or subclavian artery on the same side.[18] This ductus arteriosus that gives rise to the pulmonary artery is completely occluded in most cases but can rarely be patent or severely narrowed. Almost always, the affected lung shows variable degree of hypoplasia with the heart and mediastinal structures displaced to the affected side (**Figs. 9.30, 9.31**). The vascularity is typically reduced in the affected lung and increased in the unaffected lung. Systemic arterial collateral vessels are the sole source of pulmonary blood flow to the affected lung. Initially the systemic collateral circulation is through existing vessels including the bronchial arteries. As the patient grows, the affected lung recruits additional collateral arteries, with many developing across the pleura. These vessels produce a reticular pattern in the peripheral part of the lung. Radiographic recognition of this condition is important because a small lung volume and reticular lung densities in a child with or without repeated pulmonary infections may lead to an incorrect diagnosis of chronic lung disease. The diagnosis is often delayed until the

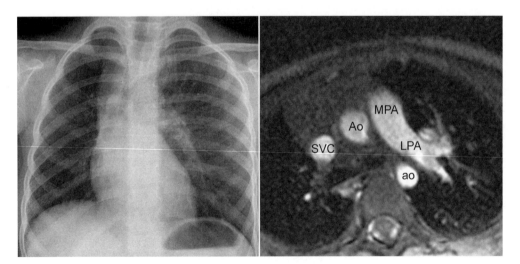

Fig. 9.30 Congenital absence of the right pulmonary artery in a 12-month-old child. The right lung volume is reduced. The mediastinal structures and heart are displaced to the right, and the right hemidiaphragm is elevated. The right hilar vessels are hardly visible. The vascularity of the left lung is increased. The left pulmonary artery (LPA) looks prominent not only because it is large but also because it is uncovered. Axial magnetic resonance image shows no right pulmonary artery arising from the main pulmonary artery. The aortic arch is left-sided. Ao, ascending aorta; ao, descending aorta; MPA, main pulmonary artery; SVC, superior vena cava.

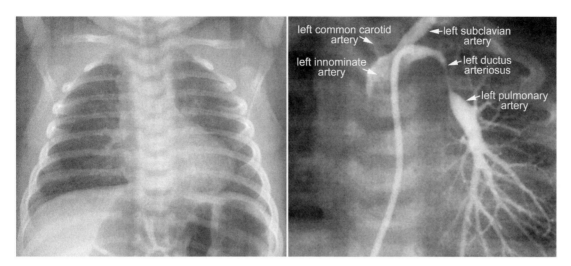

Fig. 9.31 Congenital absence of the left pulmonary artery in a 6-week-old patient. The left lung volume is mildly reduced. The left lung shows reduced pulmonary vascularity. The small left hilar vessels are visible through the cardiac silhouette. The vascularity of the right lung is increased. Conventional angiogram shows that the left pulmonary artery arises from the obliterated left ductus arteriosus. The aortic arch was right sided and had a mirror-image branching pattern.

patient develops hemoptysis caused by the rupture of systemic collateral arteries. A high index of suspicion of this rare entity can lead to the correct diagnosis.

Asymmetric distribution of pulmonary vascularity may also be due to preferential flow to either lung without anatomic stenosis. Tetralogy of Fallot is often associated with preferential flow to the right lung because the right ventricular outflow tract is inclined to the right by the deviated infundibular septum (**Fig. 9.32**). In pulmonary valve stenosis, the poststenotic jet is directed preferentially to the left pulmonary artery (**Fig. 9.33**). Complete transposition of the great arteries is also known to have preferential flow to the right lung because of a geometric distortion of the left pulmonary arterial origin. Asymmetric distribution of pulmonary blood flow is not uncommonly seen after the Blalock-Taussig (**Fig. 9.34**) shunt, bidirectional cavopulmonary connection, and Fontan-type of operation.

Pulmonary thromboembolism may cause increased radiolucency and oligemia distal to the obstruction (**Fig. 9.35**).[8] Atelectasis of the involved lung is common.

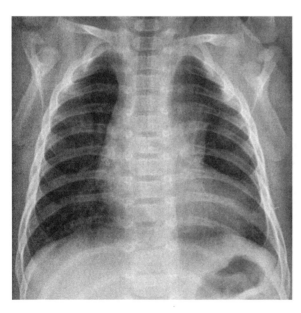

Fig. 9.32 Asymmetric vascularity with mild preferential flow to the right lung in an 11-week-old patient with tetralogy of Fallot.

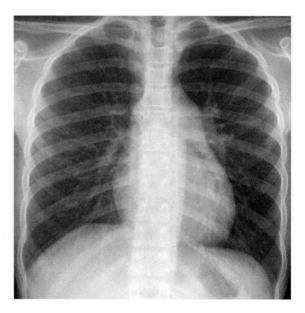

Fig. 9.33 Asymmetric vascularity with mild preferential flow to the left lung in a 12-year-old patient with isolated pulmonary valve stenosis.

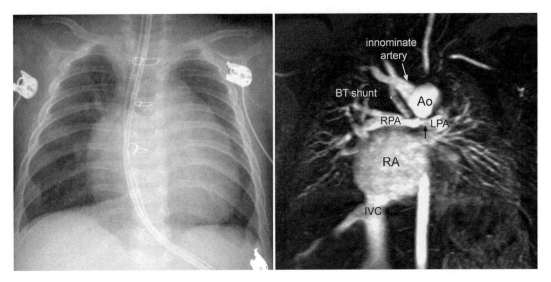

Fig. 9.34 Asymmetric vascularity in a 4-month-old patient with hypoplastic left heart syndrome who underwent Norwood operation and right-side modified Blalock-Taussig (BT) shunt. The vascularity of the right lung is more prominent than that of the left lung. There was preferential flow to the right pulmonary artery (RPA). The left pulmonary artery (LPA) was small and slightly narrowed. Ao, aorta; IVC, inferior vena cava; RA, right atrium.

The hilar pulmonary artery of the affected lung may be enlarged. Depending on the extent of disease, the radiographic findings vary. With development of infarct, the lung shows wedge-shaped patch consolidation along the pleura, pleural effusion, and elevation of the diaphragm.

Peripheral pulmonary arterial stenosis involves the pulmonary arterial tree at any level.[19] Various etiologies of peripheral pulmonary arterial stenosis are listed in **Table 9.6**. Although it may occur at a single level, multifocal stenosis is more common. It causes uneven distribution of pulmonary vascular markings between the lungs and within a lung (**Fig. 9.36**).

Uneven pulmonary vascularity between the lungs and within a lung is also seen in tetralogy of Fallot with pulmonary atresia when the pulmonary arterial supply is from multiple major aortopulmonary collateral arteries (MAPCAs) (**Fig. 9.37**). When a lung gets blood flow through the collateral circulation, it is almost always supplied by multiple MAPCAs. The vascularity varies

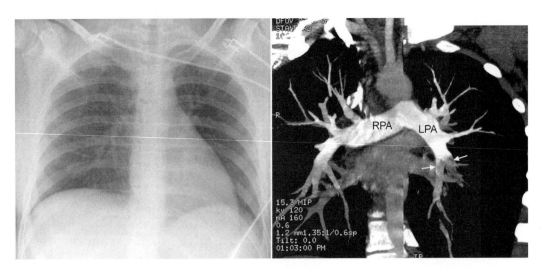

Fig. 9.35 Uneven pulmonary vascularity in a 15-year-old patient with pulmonary emboli in the pulmonary arterial branches to the left lower lobe. Left lower lobe is hyperlucent and has smaller vascular markings as compared with the corresponding area in the right lung. Composite CT angiogram shows thrombi (*arrows*) in the pulmonary arterial branches in the left lower lobe. LPA, left pulmonary artery; RPA, right pulmonary artery.

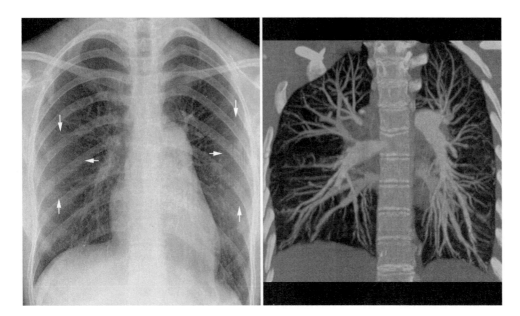

Fig. 9.36 Uneven vascularity due to disseminated peripheral pulmonary arterial vasculopathy and stenosis. Chest radiograph shows reduced vascularity in the right middle lung zone and the lateral aspect of the left middle lung (marked by *arrows*). CT angiogram reformated from one zone to the other according to the size of the in coronal plane correlate very well with the chest radiographic finding. There was secondary pulmonary hypertension causing dilatation of the main and branch pulmonary arteries.

from one zone to the other according to the size of the supplying collateral arteries. Rarely, one lung is supplied by the patent ductus arteriosus and the other lung by multiple MAPCAs. The pulmonary vascularity may also be asymmetric in truncus arteriosus when one pulmonary artery is smaller than the other or the origin of a pulmonary artery is stenotic. Asymmetric vascularity is obvious when one branch of the pulmonary artery arises

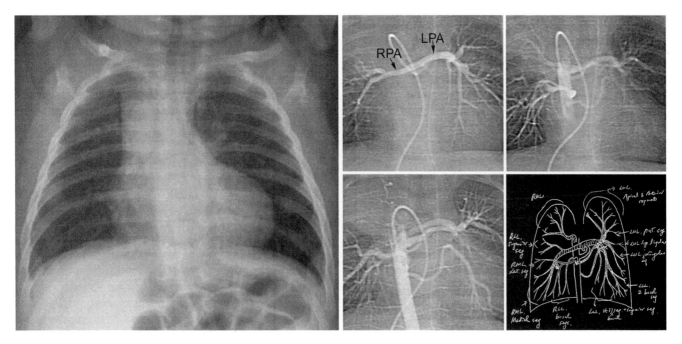

Fig. 9.37 Uneven pulmonary vascularity in a 9-week-old patient with tetralogy of Fallot, pulmonary atresia, and major aortopulmonary collateral arteries. Conventional angiograms show multiple collateral arteries of different sizes supplying the lungs. Note that the pulmonary vascularity of the left lower lung is significantly diminished as compared with the other areas. RPA, right pulmonary artery; LPA, left pulmonary artery.

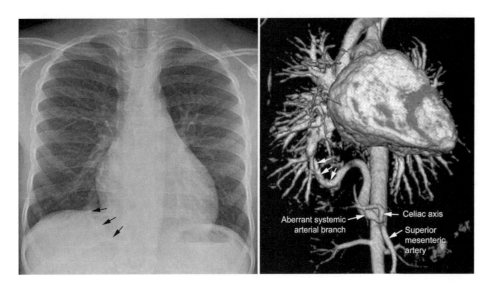

Fig. 9.38 Aberrant systemic arterial supply to a normal lung. Chest radiograph shows an oblique vascular shadow (*arrows*) in the medial aspect of the right lower lung. Magnetic resonance angiogram demonstrates an aberrant arterial branch arising from the celiac axis and supplies the right lower lung. White arrows indicate the segment of the aberrant branch shown on the chest radiograph.

from the aorta and the other from the main pulmonary artery.

Rarely, an area of an otherwise normal lung, most commonly the basal part of the left lower lobe, has an aberrant systemic arterial supply from the lower thoracic or upper abdominal aorta.[20] This condition is different from the classic bronchopulmonary sequestration in that the involved lung tissue retains a normal connection to the bronchial tree. This rare condition is called aberrant systemic arterial supply to a normal lung. The involved area of the lung may show increased vascularity, abnormal orientation of the vessels, or nodular opacities.

The lungs recruit systemic arterial collateral arteries (**Fig. 9.38**) when the pulmonary blood flow is reduced or maintained without pumping action of a ventricle, as may occur after a bidirectional cavopulmonary anastomosis or Fontan-type of operation. The systemic collateral arteries produce a reticular pattern in the involved lung areas, which are commonly the upper lung areas (**Fig. 9.39**).

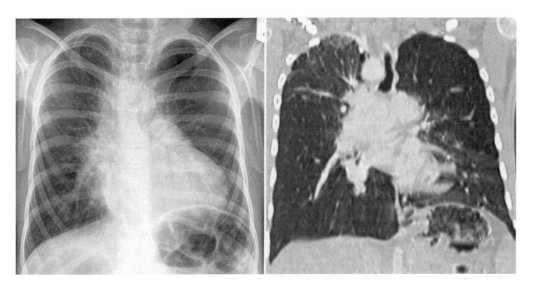

Fig. 9.39 Localized increased vascularity in the right upper lobe in a 5-year-old patient who underwent surgical repair of tetralogy of Fallot and absent pulmonary valve syndrome. Increased reticular markings in the right upper lung extend to the pleural surface. The findings correlate very well with the CT image in which transpleural systemic-to-pulmonary arterial collateral channels are shown in the same region of the lung.

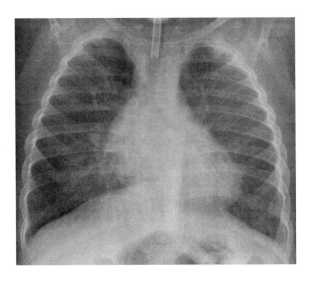

Fig. 9.40 Asymmetric pulmonary vascularity in an 18-month-old patient with severe stenosis of the left pulmonary veins. The left lung shows increased interstitial markings and diminished vascularity, whereas the right lung shows increased vascularity.

Stenosis or atresia of an individual pulmonary vein causes interstitial edema in the involved region. The pulmonary arterial blood flow is redistributed to the lung areas that have normal venous drainage, and therefore the affected area also shows reduced vascularity. The lung volume may also be reduced. The unaffected lung areas show increased vascularity (**Fig. 9.40**).[21] Unilateral pulmonary vein atresia is an extreme example showing a small volume with a reticular pattern of pulmonary vascularity of the evolved lung (see Chapter 11, **Fig. 11.25**).[22] The findings are often difficult to differentiate from those of unilateral absence of a branch pulmonary artery.

Congenital pulmonary arteriovenous fistulas or malformations may occur as an isolated pathology, but more commonly are seen in hereditary hemorrhagic telangiectasia (Osler-Weber-Rendu).[23] The malformations are seen as round or oval opacities or masses (**Figs. 9.41, 9.42**). On close observation, the feeding artery or arteries and draining vein or veins can be identified. The arteriovenous malformations occur as a known complication of a Glenn operation or bidirectional cavopulmonary anastomosis.[24] They are also seen in patients with chronic hepatic failure, such as liver cirrhosis; this condition is called hepatopulmonary syndrome.[25] They are considered to develop because the lungs are deprived of the hepatic humoral factor that has an inhibitory effect in the development of pulmonary arteriovenous malformations (**Fig. 9.43**). These malformations are hardly discernible on a chest radiograph. Other causes of pulmonary arteriovenous malformation are listed in **Table 9.6**.

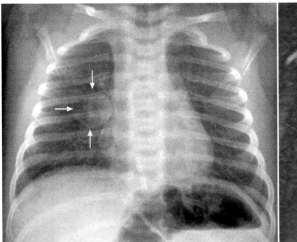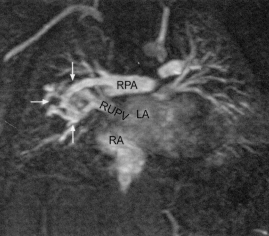

Fig. 9.41 Pulmonary arteriovenous malformation in a 20-day-old neonate. There is a round mass-like lesion (*arrows*) in the right middle lung. Magnetic resonance angiogram (*right panel*) shows that the mass consists of entangled vessels of an arteriovenous malformation supplied by branches of the right pulmonary artery (RPA) and drained by the right upper pulmonary vein (RUPV). LA, left atrium; RA, right atrium.

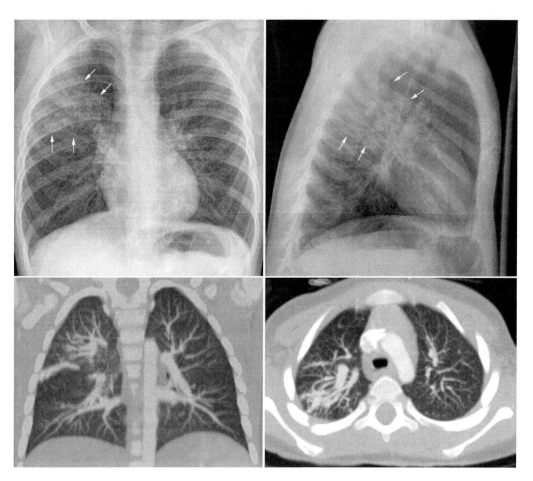

Fig. 9.42 Pulmonary arteriovenous malformations in a 2-year-old child with Osler-Weber-Rendu syndrome. Chest radiographs show mottled, granular, and tubular densities in the posterior aspect of the right upper lobe (*arrows*). The plain radiographic findings correlate very well with CT findings (*lower panels*). Note the entangled vessels in the posterior segment of the right upper lung.

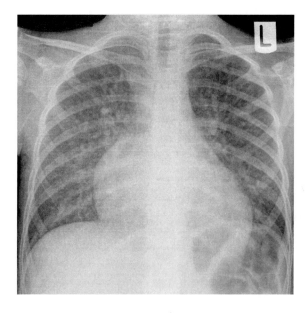

Fig. 9.43 Pulmonary arteriovenous malformations in a 6-year-old patient with hepatic failure. Both lungs show increased vascularity with disseminated short tubular and small nodular opacities. There is cardiomegaly. Contrast echocardiography with agitated normal saline, so-called bubble study, demonstrated the appearance of bubbles in the left atrium.

Asymmetric pulmonary vascularity is also seen in unilateral lung diseases, including primary pulmonary hypoplasia, scimitar syndrome, horseshoe lung, congenital lobar emphysema, and Swyer-James syndrome. These conditions will be discussed in further detail in Chapter 11.

Pearls

- Pulmonary vascular pattern can be classified into six categories: (1) normal; (2) increased; (3) decreased; (4) pulmonary venous hypertension pattern; (5) pulmonary arterial hypertension pattern; and (6) uneven, unequal, or asymmetric distribution.

- The diameter of the descending branch of the right pulmonary artery is a good indicator of increased or decreased pulmonary vascularity. Normally it is equal to the diameter of the trachea in the thorax.

- Increased pulmonary vascularity is characterized by enlarged size of the central and peripheral pulmonary vessels with sharp margins.

- Pulmonary venous hypertension is characterized by increased interstitial markings with blurred vascular margins and peribronchial cuffing. Pulmonary vascular redistribution is rather an early radiographic sign of pulmonary venous hypertension but can also be seen in pulmonary arterial hypertension. Overt alveolar edema suggests severe pulmonary venous hypertension.

- Pulmonary arterial hypertension is characterized by dilatation of the central vessels and reduced size and number of peripheral branches.

- Uneven, unequal, or asymmetric pulmonary vascularity should be assessed by carefully comparing the right and left lungs, region by region.

References

1. Ravin CE. Pulmonary vascularity: radiographic considerations. J Thorac Imaging 1988;3:1–13
2. Coussement AM, Gooding CA. Objective radiographic assessment of pulmonary vascularity in children. Radiology 1973;109:649–654
3. Rudolph AM. The changes in the circulation after birth. Their importance in congenital heart disease. Circulation 1970;41:343–359
4. Haworth SG. The pulmonary circulation. In: Anderson RH, Baker EJ, Macartney FJ, et al, eds. Paediatric Cardiology, 2nd ed. Edinburgh: Churchill Livingstone; 2002:57–93
5. Fineman JR, Heymann MA, Morin FC III. Fetal and postnatal circulations: pulmonary and persistent pulmonary hypertension of the newborn. In: Allen HD, Gutgesell HP, Clark EB, Driscoll DJ, eds. Moss and Adams' Heart Disease in Infants, Children, and Adolescents Including the Fetus and Young Adult, 6th ed. Philadelphia: Lippincott Williams & Wilkins; 2001:41–52
6. Sharma S, Bhargava A, Krishnakumar R, Rajani M. Can pulmonary venous hypertension be graded by the chest radiograph? Clin Radiol 1998;53:899–902
7. Resten A, Maitre S, Humbert M, et al. Pulmonary hypertension: CT of the chest in pulmonary venoocclusive disease. AJR Am J Roentgenol 2004;183:65–70
8. Levin DL, Goodman ET. Radiology of pulmonary vascular disease. Cardiol Clin 2004;22:375–382, vi vi.
9. Gurney JW, Goodman LR. Pulmonary edema localized in the right upper lobe accompanying mitral regurgitation. Radiology 1989;171:397–399
10. Yang YL, Nanda NC, Wang XF, et al. Echocardiographic diagnosis of anomalous origin of the left coronary artery from the pulmonary artery. Echocardiography 2007;24:405–411
11. Widlitz A, Barst RJ. Pulmonary arterial hypertension in children. Eur Respir J 2003;21:155–176
12. Simonneau G, Galiè N, Rubin LJ, et al. Clinical classification of pulmonary hypertension. J Am Coll Cardiol 2004;43(12, Suppl S):5S–12S
13. Widimsky J. Noninvasive diagnosis of pulmonary hypertension in chronic lung diseases. Prog Respir Res 1985;20:69–75
14. Ravin CE, Greenspan RH, McLoud TC, Lange RC, Langou RA, Putman CE. Redistribution of pulmonary blood flow secondary to pulmonary arterial hypertension. Invest Radiol 1980;15:29–33
15. Taragin BH, Berdon WE, Printz B. MRI assessment of bronchial compression in absent pulmonary valve syndrome and review of the syndrome. Pediatr Radiol 2006;36:71–75
16. Freedom RM, Yoo SJ, Williams WG. Transposition of the great arteries: arterial repair. In: Freedom RM, Yoo SJ, Mikailina H, Williams WG, eds. The Natural and Modified History of Congenital Heart Disease. New York: Futura; 2004:323–347
17. Momma K, Takao A, Ando M, et al. Juxtaductal left pulmonary artery obstruction in pulmonary atresia. Br Heart J 1986;55:39–44
18. Presbitero P, Bull C, Haworth SG, de Leval MR. Absent or occult pulmonary artery. Br Heart J 1984;52:178–185
19. Kreutzer J, Landzberg MJ, Preminger TJ, et al. Isolated peripheral pulmonary artery stenoses in the adult. Circulation 1996;93:1417–1423
20. Do KH, Goo JM, Im JG, Kim KW, Chung JW, Park JH. Systemic arterial supply to the lungs in adults: spiral CT findings. Radiographics 2001;21:387–402
21. Roman KS, Kellenberger CJ, Macgowan CK, et al. How is pulmonary arterial blood flow affected by pulmonary venous obstruction in children? A phase-contrast magnetic resonance study. Pediatr Radiol 2005;35:580–586
22. Heyneman LE, Nolan RL, Harrison JK, McAdams HP. Congenital unilateral pulmonary vein atresia: radiologic findings in three adult patients. AJR Am J Roentgenol 2001;177:681–685
23. Carette MF, Nedelcu C, Tassart M, Grange JD, Wislez M, Khalil A. Imaging of hereditary hemorrhagic telangiectasia. Cardiovasc Intervent Radiol 2009;32:745–747
24. Srivastava D, Preminger T, Lock JE, et al. Hepatic venous blood and the development of pulmonary arteriovenous malformations in congenital heart disease. Circulation 1995;92:1217–1222
25. Lenci I, Alvior A, Manzia TM, Toti L, Neuberger J, Steeds R. Saline contrast echocardiography in patients with hepatopulmonary syndrome awaiting liver transplantation. J Am Soc Echocardiogr 2009; 22:89–94

10 Aorta and Systemic Veins

The fifth step of the chest radiographic interpretation is to assess the size and configuration of the ascending aorta, aortic arch, descending aorta, superior and inferior venae cavae, and azygos-hemiazygos veins. For example, this part of the report in a patient with known bicuspid aortic valve may read: *"The right upper mediastinal border is mildly convex outward, suggesting a dilated ascending aorta in association with aortic stenosis."*

■ Ascending Aorta and Aortic Sinus

The ascending aorta is not normally seen as a border-forming structure on a frontal chest radiograph in children and young adults. When it is dilated, the ascending aorta can bulge to the right beyond the superior vena caval border (**Fig. 10.1**). Dilatation of the ascending aorta can be caused by diseases affecting the aortic wall, increased blood flow volumes through the ascending aorta, or deformation of the aortic wall by the fast blood flow across a stenotic aortic valve (**Table 10.1**).

Dilatation of the aortic root and ascending aorta is seen in various connective tissue diseases, particularly in Marfan syndrome (**Figs. 10.2, 10.3**). Aortic dilatation and mitral valve prolapse are the two most common cardiovascular manifestations of Marfan syndrome.[1,2] Both manifestations usually develop later in childhood and progress gradually. Rarely, aortic dilatation is seen in early infancy, with very poor prognosis.[3] The prevalence of both aortic dilatation and mitral valve prolapse in pediatric cohorts is approximately 80%.[1] Aortic regurgitation develops as a complication of aortic dilatation during childhood and adolescence in 25% of Marfan patients, whereas mitral valve prolapse results in mitral regurgitation in 50%. Loeys-Dietz syndrome is a much more aggressive and lethal disease characterized by aortic and arterial tortuosity, aneurysm formation, and a propensity for early dissection.[3] Aortic dilatation is also common in other connective tissue diseases, such as Ehlers-Danlos syndrome and pseudoxanthoma elasticum.[4,5] Aortic dilatation, however, can occur without definable underlying disease and can cause aortic regurgitation.[6] Familial dilatation of the aorta has also been reported. Aneurysm of the aortic sinus of Valsalva may cause a localized bulge of the lower part of the right upper heart border.

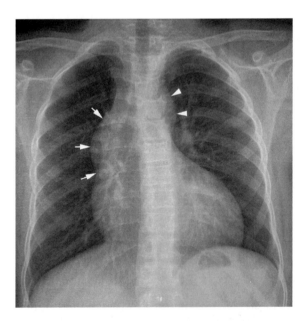

Fig. 10.1 Dilated ascending aorta in an 11-year-old patient with aortic stenosis and insufficiency. The dilated ascending aorta results in a rounded bulging contour of the right upper mediastinum (*arrows*). This dilatation is caused by a poststenotic jet and increased blood flow volume from aortic regurgitation. The aortic knob (*arrowheads*) is also prominent when there is significant aortic insufficiency.

Table 10.1 Conditions that Cause Dilatation of the Ascending Aorta

Diseases affecting the aortic wall	Marfan syndrome
	Loeys-Dietz syndrome
	Ehlers-Danlos syndrome
	Pseudoxanthoma elasticum
	Familial
	Idiopathic
Increased blood flow volumes	Aortic regurgitation
	Aortopulmonary window
	Patent ductus arteriosus
	Congenital heart diseases with right-to-left shunt, for instance tetralogy of Fallot
	Truncus arteriosus
Poststenotic dilatation	Aortic valve stenosis

132

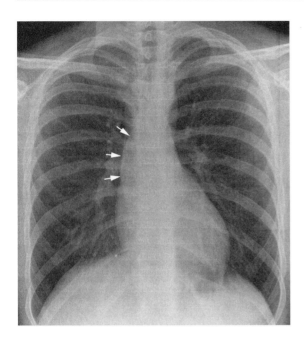

Fig. 10.2 Dilated ascending aorta in a 15-year-old patient with Marfan syndrome. The ascending aorta has a mildly convex contour (*arrows*) in the right upper mediastinum. The aortic knob and descending aorta appear normal

Aortic regurgitation results in aortic and left ventricular dilatation because of volume overload (**Fig. 10.1**). Aortic regurgitation can be due not only to aortic valvular abnormalities but also to aortic root dilatation, as

discussed in the previous paragraph. Bicuspid aortic valve is often complicated by later development of aortic stenosis and regurgitation due to chronic mechanical injury and inflammation. Among patients with aortic valve stenosis or regurgitation, dilatation of the ascending aorta develops earlier and is more severe in patients with bicuspid aortic valve than in those with tricuspid aortic valve.[7] Aortic regurgitation is typically related to shrunken valvular tissue in rheumatic or rheumatoid disease and ankylosing spondylitis and to perforated valvular cusps in infective endocarditis. Aortic valve prolapse is not an uncommon complication of a ventricular septal defect that is located below the aortic valve and may result in aortic regurgitation (**Fig. 10.4**).[8] Congenital aortic regurgitation is rare. Congenital regurgitation presenting in the neonatal period occurs more commonly through a route in the paravalvular space, which is called an aorto–left ventricular tunnel.[9]

Left-to-right shunt lesions at the great arterial level also cause dilatation of the ascending aorta. They include patent ductus arteriosus and aortopulmonary window. However, we rarely see obvious radiographic findings of dilatation of the ascending aorta in these conditions in children. Congenital heart diseases with an intracardiac right-to-left shunt are also characterized by a dilated ascending aorta (**Fig. 10.5**). There is a reciprocal relationship in size between the two great arteries in most cases. The ascending aorta becomes smaller after surgery, but residual dilatation is common. Common

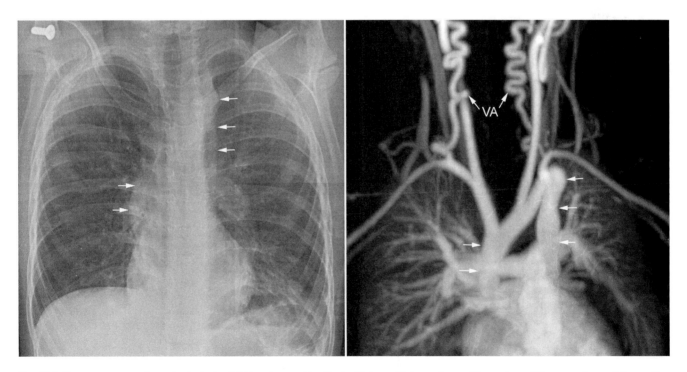

Fig. 10.3 Tortuous aorta and vertebral arteries (VA) in a 4-year-old patient with Loeys-Dietz syndrome. The contour of the ascending and descending aorta (*arrows*) seen on a frontal chest radiograph is well correlated with that seen on a contrast-enhanced magnetic resonance angiogram.

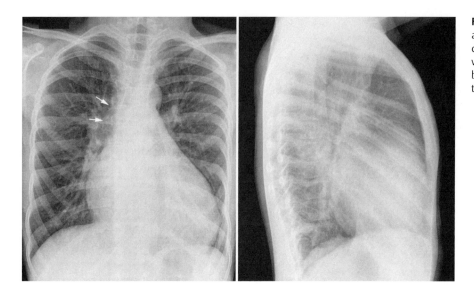

Fig. 10.4 Prominent ascending aorta (*arrows*) and aortic knob and cardiomegaly with a dilated left ventricle in an 11-year-old patient with a ventricular septal defect complicated by aortic valve prolapse and aortic regurgitation. The pulmonary vascularity is increased.

arterial trunk in truncus arteriosus can also be seen as a round bulge of the right upper mediastinum. Dilated ascending aorta is more obvious when the thymus is shrunken after birth or is congenitally hypoplastic or aplastic in association with chromosome 22q11 deletion that is common in truncus arteriosus and tetralogy of Fallot.

Significant aortic valve stenosis results in acceleration of the blood flow. The accelerated flow usually streams toward the right anterior wall of the ascending aorta,

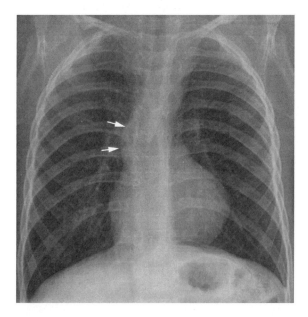

Fig. 10.5 Dilated ascending aorta in a 26-month-old patient with tetralogy of Fallot. The dilated ascending aorta (*arrows*) is clearly seen when there is involution of the thymus, which when present often hides the enlarged aorta.

causing a rounded outward bulge of the right upper mediastinal margin (**Fig. 10.1**). The degree of post-stenotic dilatation of the ascending aorta varies according to the severity of aortic stenosis. Newborns with severe aortic stenosis show a hypoplastic ascending aorta because of reduced blood flow volume through the aortic valve. Bicuspid aortic valve is the most common underlying substrate for later development of aortic valve stenosis. The bicuspid leaflets are prone to develop thickening and calcification later in life, causing stenosis, regurgitation, or both.[7] Rheumatic fever, which was the leading cause of aortic stenosis up through the early 20th century, has become rare in developed countries. Recurrent inflammation from rheumatic fever causes fibrous thickening and contracture of the cardiac valve leaflets, resulting in stenosis and regurgitation. Rheumatic fever affects most commonly the mitral valve, less commonly the aortic valve, and rarely the tricuspid valve. Aortic stenosis is associated with left ventricular hypertrophy, although the left ventricle may dilate when it fails.

The ascending aorta may have an abnormal left-sided position in congenitally corrected transposition of the great arteries and double inlet left ventricle with the transposed aorta arising from the left-sided rudimentary right ventricle (**Figs. 10.6, 10.7**). The left-sided ascending aorta causes an unusual prominence of the left upper mediastinum, often with a rounded bulge. When this configuration is seen in the presence of dextrocardia, the diagnosis of congenitally corrected transposition or double-inlet left ventricle with discordant ventriculoarterial connection can be entertained. However, asymmetric prominence of the left lobe of the thymus may mimic this configuration (**Fig. 10.8**).

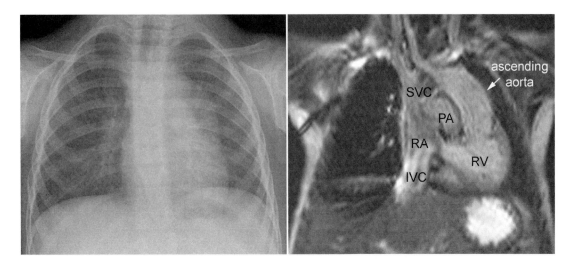

Fig. 10.6 Left-sided ascending aorta in a patient with congenitally corrected transposition of the great arteries. The left upper mediastinum shows a large rounded contour, which is characteristic of the left-sided ascending aorta, which is typically seen in congenitally corrected transposition. The finding is well correlated with the magnetic resonance findings. IVC, inferior vena cava; PA, pulmonary artery; RA, right atrium; RV, right ventricle; SVC, superior vena cava.

■ Aortic Knob and Descending Aorta

The aortic knob is the rounded protuberance of the distal part of the aortic arch seen on a frontal chest radiograph. It is seen on the left side of the distal trachea and continues to the shadow of the descending aorta. A prominent aortic knob is seen when there is dilatation of the aortic arch as in Marfan syndrome and other causes of aortic dilatation (**Figs. 10.1, 10.3**). It can be prominent also with a patent ductus arteriosus, aortopulmonary window, truncus arteriosus, and tetralogy of Fallot. A significant left-to-right intracardiac shunt is associated with a small aortic knob.

The aortic knob and proximal descending aorta together may show a figure-of-3 configuration (**Figs. 10.9, 10.10**). The focal indentation represents a discrete coarctation lesion. The rounded contour below the indentation is the descending aorta that usually shows some poststenotic dilatation. This sign is characteristic of coarctation of the aorta but is not always seen or recognizable. This sign is usually seen after a few years of age and may be associated with rib changes related to dilatation of the intercostal arteries.

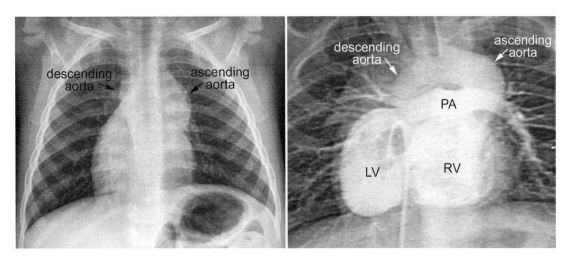

Fig. 10.7 Left-sided ascending aorta in a patient with dextrocardia and congenitally corrected transposition of the great arteries. The left upper mediastinum shows a large rounded bulge due to a dilated left-sided ascending aorta. The left-sided ascending aorta connects to the right-sided descending aorta through a very elongated aortic arch. LV, left ventricle; PA, pulmonary artery; RV, right ventricle.

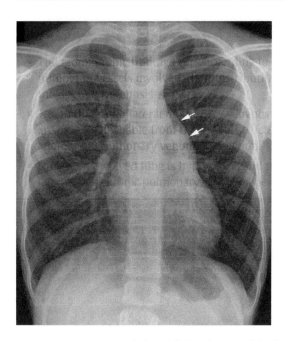

Fig. 10.8 An asymmetrically large left lobe (*arrows*) of the thymus in a 7-year-old patient with a small patent ductus arteriosus simulates a left-sided ascending aorta seen with congenitally corrected transposition of the great arteries.

The aortic knob and descending aorta may show an irregular undulated margin with or without calcification, which is highly suggestive of aortitis, most commonly Takayasu arteritis (**Fig. 10.11**). Extensive calcification of the entire aorta and its branches is seen in idiopathic calcifying arteritis in the newborn.

The right aortic arch indents the right side of the trachea and continues as a right-sided descending aortic contour (**Fig. 10.7;** also see **Fig. 7.13,** middle panel). Double aortic arch may cause bilateral indentation of the tracheal lumen with concentric narrowing (**Fig. 7.13**, right panel), but unilateral indentation of the right side of the trachea is a more common finding.[10] When the tracheal indentation by the aortic arch and the vertical stripe of the proximal descending aorta are seen on opposite sides, the diagnosis of a circumflex retroesophageal aortic arch or double aortic arch should be considered (**Fig. 7.14**).[10,11]

A cervical aortic arch is a condition in which the apex of the aortic arch is located unusually high above the level of the clavicles (**Fig. 7.15**). It occurs slightly more commonly with a right aortic arch, often taking a circumflex retroesophageal course to form a vascular ring. It is often associated with tracheal obstruction because of crowding of vascular structures and airway in a confined small space. It is commonly associated with tortuosity, aneurysmal dilatation, and narrowing of the aortic arch itself or its branches.[10,12]

■ Systemic Veins

On frontal chest radiographs, the superior vena cava occupies the upper half of the right mediastinal border in adults and older children. On lateral chest radiographs, the superior vena cava can be seen as a band of haziness in front of the tracheal air column. The azygos venous arch can be seen as a round structure at the right tracheobronchial angle where the trachea continues to the right

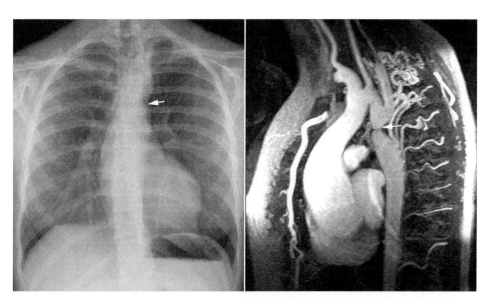

Fig. 10.9 Figure-of-3 configuration of the proximal descending aorta in a 16-year-old patient with coarctation of the aorta. A focal indentation (*arrow*) is seen at the junction of the aortic knob and the prominent descending aorta, causing a figure-of-3 configuration.

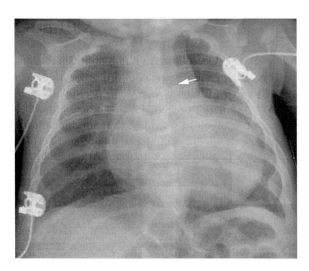

Fig. 10.10 Figure-of-3 configuration of the proximal descending aorta in a 12-week-old infant with coarctation of the aorta. A mild indentation (*arrow*) is seen in the proximal descending aorta. The descending aorta shows a mild outward convexity because of poststenotic dilatation.

Table 10.2   Conditions that Cause Dilatation of the Superior Vena Cava

Right-sided heart failure	Severe tricuspid regurgitation
	Right ventricular dysfunction/failure
	Pulmonary hypertension
	Chronic lung diseases
	Airway diseases
	Left-sided heart failure
Increased blood flow volumes	Supracardiac type of anomalous pulmonary venous connection
	Vascular malformation in the upper compartment of the body
	Inferior vena caval obstruction
	Interruption of the inferior vena cava with azygos-hemiazygos continuation
Obstruction to superior vena caval drainage	Obstruction of lower superior vena cava
	Tumor or thrombus within the right atrium

main bronchus on frontal radiographs (**Fig. 10.12**, upper panel). The superior vena cava and azygos venous arch are usually overlain by a large thymus and not identifiable in young children. They are visible only when the thymus is shrunken or underdeveloped, or when they are dilated. The inferior vena cava is only occasionally visible in the angle between the right atrium and right diaphragm on frontal chest radiographs. It is nearly always seen on the lateral chest radiograph as a small but distinct web-like shadow, filling the angle formed by the lower posterior margin of the left ventricle and the right diaphragm (**Fig. 10.12**, lower panel).

A dilated superior vena cava should be suspected when there is right upper mediastinal widening, although this may be due to other mediastinal lesions including postsurgical hematomas or seromas, enlarged lymph nodes and mediastinal tumors, or a collapsed right upper lobe. The superior mediastinal widening in children is difficult to assess because of a large thymus overlying the mediastinal vessels and heart. The causes of dilatation of the superior vena cava include right-sided heart failure, increased blood flow returning through the superior vena cava, and obstruction to the superior vena caval drainage (**Table 10.2**).

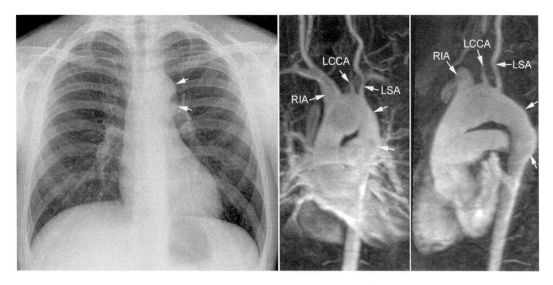

Fig. 10.11 Prominent round bulge of the aortic knob and proximal descending aorta (*arrows*) in a 15-year-old patient with Takayasu arteritis. The bulge is well correlated with contrast-enhanced magnetic resonance angiography. The right innominate artery (RIA) is also dilated. The left common carotid artery (LCCA) is completely occluded and the left subclavian artery (LSA) is mildly stenotic.

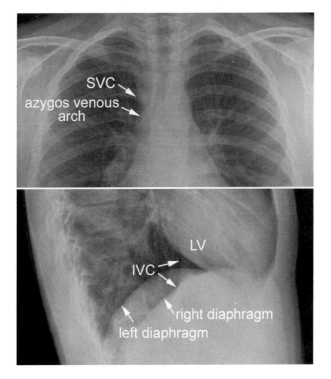

Fig. 10.12 Systemic veins shown on the frontal and lateral chest radiographs. The azygos vein is seen at the corner of the right tracheobronchial angle on the frontal view. The superior vena cava (SVC) forms the right upper mediastinal border. The inferior vena cava (IVC) is seen as a web-like structure filling the angle formed by the left ventricular (LV) margin and the right diaphragm on the lateral view.

Right-sided heart failure is caused by a variety of conditions that are listed in **Table 10.2**. Right-sided heart failure is characterized by engorgement of the systemic veins with generalized edema, enlarged liver, and ascites (**Fig. 10.13**).

The pulmonary vascularity may be decreased especially when there is a right-to-left shunt at the atrial level. When right-sided heart failure is secondary to a left-sided lesion, the findings of pulmonary venous hypertension are also seen.

The superior vena cava is dilated when there is a supracardiac type of partial or total anomalous pulmonary venous connection (**Figs. 10.14, 10.15**). The dilated superior vena cava produces an outward convexity of the right upper mediastinal border (**Fig. 10.14**). The dilated vein may cast a vertical band of haziness in front of the tracheal air column when a large thymus does not occupy the anterior upper mediastinum. When the connection is to the innominate vein through a left-sided vertical vein, the dilated superior vena cava and vertical vein are responsible for a so-called snowman or figure-of-8 appearance (**Fig. 10.15**). However, this finding is not clearly seen in the first one or two years when the thymus overlies the mediastinal great vessels. The superior vena cava is also dilated when there is a large vascular malformation in the upper compartment of the body, such as vein of Galen malformation in the brain and large hemangioma in the upper extremity.

The superior vena cava may show an unusual outward convexity when there is left juxtaposition of the atrial appendages, in which the right atrial appendage is displaced to the left and lies above the left atrial appendage (**Fig. 10.16**).[13] The displacement is through the space behind the great arterial trunks in the transverse sinus of the pericardial cavity. The rounded course of the superior vena cava can be explained by the medial displacement of the lower part of the superior vena cava accompanying the displaced right atrium.

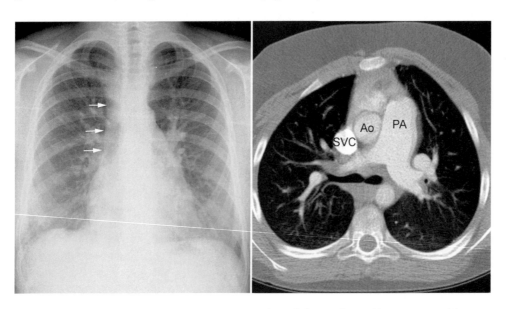

Fig. 10.13 Dilated right superior vena cava (*arrows* on frontal chest radiograph) in a 12-year-old patient with restrictive cardiomyopathy. Ao, ascending aorta; PA, pulmonary artery; SVC, superior vena cava.

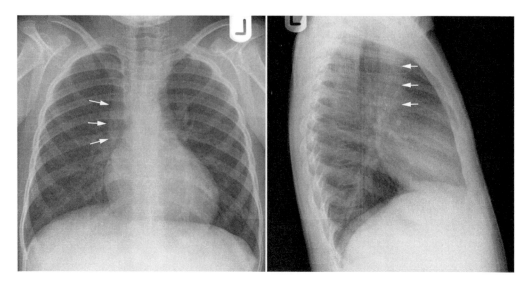

Fig. 10.14 Dilated superior vena cava in a 6-year-old patient with unilateral total anomalous pulmonary venous connection of the left lung to the innominate vein. The dilated superior vena cava results in a convex contour of the right upper mediastinal border (*arrows*) on the frontal view. It is also seen as a vertical band-like haziness (*arrows*) in front of the tracheal air-column on the lateral view.

The superior vena cava may become dilated when there is an obstruction of its lower part (**Figs. 10.17, 10.18**). When the inferior vena cava is obstructed or interrupted, the veins of the lower part of the body drain to the superior vena cava causing dilatation (**Fig. 10.19**).

The collateral channels between the inferior and superior vena caval systems are mainly the azygos-hemiazygos veins, although other mediastinal and chest wall veins may contribute. As the azygos and hemiazygos veins and their tributaries are located along both sides of the vertebral

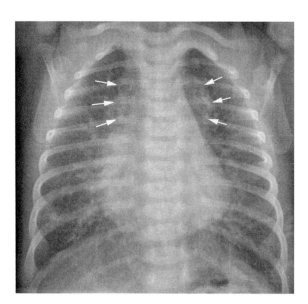

Fig. 10.15 Figure-of-8 configuration of the cardiovascular silhouette in a 5-week-old infant with total anomalous pulmonary venous connection to the innominate vein. The superior mediastinum is wide and convex. The convexity of the left upper mediastinum (*arrows*) is formed by the dilated vertical vein that connects the confluent pulmonary vein to the innominate vein. The convexity of the right upper mediastinum (*arrows*) is formed by the dilated superior vena cava. This finding is not usually apparent in infants. The heart is enlarged and the pulmonary vascularity is increased.

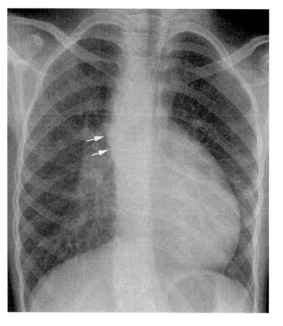

Fig. 10.16 Convex superior vena caval contour in a 10-year-old patient with left juxtaposition of the atrial appendages. The lower aspect of the superior vena cava (*arrows*) is inclined medially as a result of the leftward displacement of the upper part of the right atrium. The patient had double-inlet left ventricle and transposition of the great arteries.

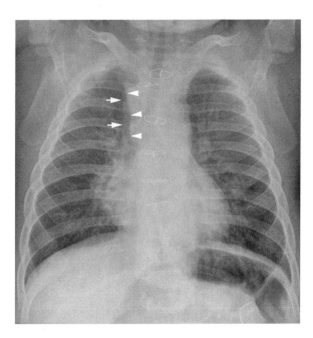

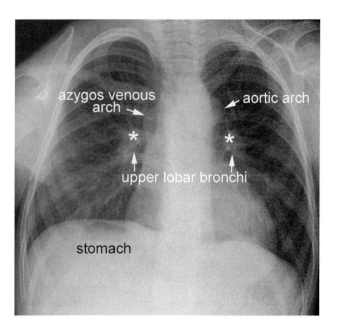

Fig. 10.17 Widening of the right upper mediastinum related to a dilated azygos vein and superior vena cava due to obstruction of the superior vena cava in an 8-month-old child with repaired complete transposition of the great arteries. The right upper mediastinal border is double contoured. The outer margin (*arrows*) is the dilated superior vena cava. The inner contour (*arrowheads*) is the dilated azygos vein.

Fig. 10.19 Dilated azygos venous arch in a patient with left isomerism and interrupted inferior vena cava. The azygos vein is dilated as the interrupted inferior vena cava connects to the dilated azygos vein on the right. Note that the stomach is on the right and that the pulmonary arteries and bronchi show symmetric branching patterns. The pulmonary arteries (*asterisks*) are seen above the upper lobar bronchi in the hila.

column, the engorged veins can be seen as unilateral or bilateral paravertebral stripes on frontal chest radiographs (**Fig. 10.18**). The stripes usually show an undulating contour when the vena caval obstruction is an acquired lesion. When the azygos venous arch is dilated and is in direct contact with the right lung, it can be seen as a distinct structure. A dilated azygos venous arch can be a telltale sign for an interrupted inferior vena cava that occurs in over 80% of patients with left isomerism (**Fig. 10.19**).[14]

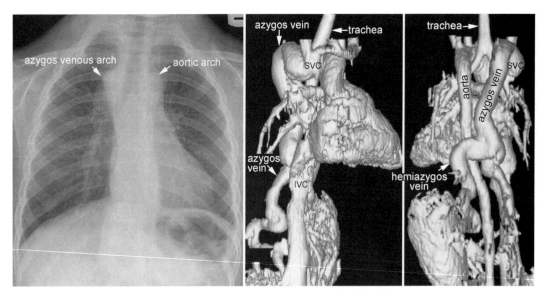

Fig. 10.18 Dilated azygos and hemiazygos veins in a patient with obstruction of the lower part of the superior vena cava (SVC). The dilated veins cast undulating paraspinal stripes in the thorax. Note that the stripes extend to the lower extent of the thorax where they lose their interfaces with the aerated lungs. The plain radiographic findings are well correlated with three-dimensional computed tomography (CT) images. IVC, inferior vena cava.

Dilatation of the inferior vena cava is hard to identify because its conspicuity changes significantly with subtle obliquity of the lateral view and cardiomegaly. In the old literature, absence of the inferior vena caval web was introduced as a sign of interruption of the inferior vena cava. However, this sign is of little value because the common hepatic vein, which is in fact the hepatic and posthepatic segment of the inferior vena cava, is present in this location in most cases with an interrupted inferior vena cava.

Pearls

- Dilated ascending aorta may bulge to the right beyond the superior vena caval border on the frontal radiograph.
- Left-sided ascending aorta in situs solitus is highly suggestive of congenitally corrected transposition of the great arteries or double inlet left ventricle with discordant ventriculoarterial connection arising from the left-sided rudimentary right ventricle.
- Focal indentation of the proximal descending aorta with a figure-of-3 configuration is a reliable sign of coarctation of the aorta.

- Irregularly undulated margin of the descending aorta suggests aortitis, such as Takayasu arteritis.
- Dilatation of the superior vena cava is seen in conditions having a large amount of venous drainage through the superior vena cava, such as anomalous pulmonary venous connection and vein of Galen aneurysm. Dilated superior vena cava and azygos/hemiazygos vein suggests lower superior vena caval obstruction or interruption or occlusion of the inferior vena cava.

References

1. Hwa J, Richards JG, Huang H, et al. The natural history of aortic dilatation in Marfan syndrome. Med J Aust 1993;158:558–562
2. van Karnebeek CD, Naeff MS, Mulder BJ, Hennekam RC, Offringa M. Natural history of cardiovascular manifestations in Marfan syndrome. Arch Dis Child 2001;84:129–137
3. Pearson, GD, Devereux, R, Loeys, B. Report of the national heart, lung, and blood institute and national Marfan foundation working group on research in Marfan syndrome and related disorders. Circulation 2008;118; 785–791
4. Wenstrup RJ, Meyer RA, Lyle JS, et al. Prevalence of aortic root dilation in the Ehlers-Danlos syndrome. Genet Med 2002;4:112–117
5. Farmakis D, Vesleme V, Papadogianni A, Tsaftaridis P, Kapralos P, Aessopos A. Aneurysmatic dilatation of ascending aorta in a patient with beta-thalassemia and a pseudoxanthoma elasticum-like syndrome. Ann Hematol 2004;83:596–599
6. Roman MJ, Devereux RB, Niles NW, et al. Aortic root dilatation as a cause of isolated, severe aortic regurgitation. Prevalence, clinical and echocardiographic patterns, and relation to left ventricular hypertrophy and function. Ann Intern Med 1987;106:800–807
7. Bauer M, Bauer U, Siniawski H, Hetzer R. Differences in clinical manifestations in patients with bicuspid and tricuspid aortic valves undergoing surgery of the aortic valve and/or ascending aorta. Thorac Cardiovasc Surg 2007;55:485–490
8. Saleeb SF, Solowiejczyk DE, Glickstein JS, Korsin R, Gersony WM, Hsu DT. Frequency of development of aortic cuspal prolapse and aortic regurgitation in patients with subaortic ventricular septal defect diagnosed at <1 year of age. Am J Cardiol 2007;99:1588–1592
9. Sousa-Uva M, Touchot A, Fermont L, et al. Aortico-left ventricular tunnel in fetuses and infants. Ann Thorac Surg 1996;61:1805–1810
10. Yoo SJ. Bradley TJ. Vascular rings, pulmonary artery sling and related conditions. In: Anderson RH, Edward JB, Penny D, Redington AN, Rigby ML, Wernovsky G, eds. Pediatric Cardiology, 3rd ed. Philadelphia: Elsevier, 2009, in press
11. Philip S, Chen SY, Wu MH, Wang JK, Lue HC. Retroesophageal aortic arch: diagnostic and therapeutic implications of a rare vascular ring. Int J Cardiol 2001;79:133–141
12. Baravelli M, Borghi A, Rogiani S, et al. Clinical, anatomopathological and genetic pattern of 10 patients with cervical aortic arch. Int J Cardiol 2007;114:236–240
13. Lai WW, Ravishankar C, Gross RP, et al. Juxtaposition of the atrial appendages: a clinical series of 22 patients. Pediatr Cardiol 2001;22:121–127
14. Lim JS, McCrindle BW, Smallhorn JF, et al. Clinical features, management, and outcome of children with fetal and postnatal diagnoses of isomerism syndromes. Circulation 2005;112:2454–2461

11 Airways, Lungs, Pleurae, Mediastinum, Diaphragm, and Chest Wall

The final step of the chest radiographic interpretation is to assess the abnormalities in the airways, lung parenchyma, pleurae, mediastinum, diaphragm, and bones and soft tissue of the chest wall. For example, this part of the report may read: *"The left lower lobe is collapsed, which may result from compression of the left lower lobar bronchus by an enlarged left atrium or direct compression of this part of the lung by the enlarged and displaced left ventricle. The collapsed left lower lobe obliterates the left diaphragmatic contour. There are small amounts of pleural effusion in both thoraces. The sternum is mildly bowed forward by the enlarged heart."*

■ Airways and Lungs

Abnormalities of the airways and lungs are common in patients with cardiovascular disease (**Table 11.1**). These abnormalities may be due to a mechanical effect by enlarged or abnormally positioned cardiovascular structures on adjacent airways or lung parenchyma. Less commonly, the abnormalities of the airway or lungs may be associated with congenital heart disease without any obvious causal relationship.

Table 11.1 Abnormalities of the Airways and Lungs Associated with or Related to Heart Diseases

Airway compression	Aorta or its branches - Dilated aortic arch - Posterior displacement of the ascending aorta and aortic arch - Long transverse aortic arch - Low lying aortic arch - Innominate artery compression syndrome - Vascular ring or sling - Aortic diverticulum of Kommerell
	Pulmonary arteries - Dilated pulmonary arteries with left-to-right shunt - Dilated branch pulmonary arteries in pulmonary hypertension - Absent pulmonary valve syndrome - Displacement of a pulmonary artery
	Cardiac chambers - Dilated left atrium
	Secondary to small thoracic cage
Intrinsic airway abnormality	Abnormal branching pattern - Tracheal bronchus - So-called bridging bronchus
	Intrinsic stenosis of the trachea or a bronchus
	Tracheomalacia and bronchomalacia
Tracheal and bronchial calcifications	Idiopathic calcification in children
	Warfarin sodium administration
	Adrenogenital syndrome
	Skeletal dysplasias - Chondrodysplasia punctata – Diastrophic dysplasia – Hydrops ectopic calcification, moth-eaten skeletal dysplasia

Table 11.1 *(Continued)* **Abnormalities of the Airways and Lungs Associated with or Related to Heart Diseases**

Lung collapse	Extrinsic airway compression
	Endobronchial mucous plug or retention of secretions
	Direct compression of the lung
Emphysema	Extrinsic airway compression
	Endobronchial mucous plug or retention of secretions
	Diffuse interstitial edema
	Compensatory emphysema
	Small airway disease
Consolidation	Pneumonia complicating already compromised ventilation
	Pneumonia secondary to frequent aspiration
	Pulmonary hemorrhage
	Pulmonary infarction
Lung hypoplasia	Scimitar syndrome
	Unilateral absence of a pulmonary artery
	Unilateral stenosis of a pulmonary artery
	Unilateral pulmonary vein atresia/stenosis
	Isolated
Horseshoe lung	Associated with scimitar syndrome
	Isolated

Airway Compression

The major airways are neighbored by the aortic arch, branch pulmonary arteries, and left atrium. Abnormal positions and dilatation of any of these structures may compress the trachea or main bronchi. A classic airway compression is due to vascular rings and slings.[1] Infrequently, the airway may be compressed by a normally formed but abnormally positioned vascular structure.[2,3] The severity of airway compression by cardiovascular structures depends not only on the vascular anatomy but also on the size and shape of the thoracic cage.

Tracheal compression is typically seen in aortic arch anomalies causing a vascular ring.[1,4] The tracheal and esophageal compression is most obvious and consistent when there is a double aortic arch (**Fig. 11.1**). A right or left aortic arch with an aberrant subclavian or innominate artery characteristically causes compression of the esophagus due to its retroesophageal course in front of the spine. A posterior indentation of the trachea can be obvious when the aberrant artery arises from the descending aorta through a large diverticulum of Kommerell (**Fig. 11.2**). A similar but more severe indentation can be seen with so-called circumflex retroesophageal aortic

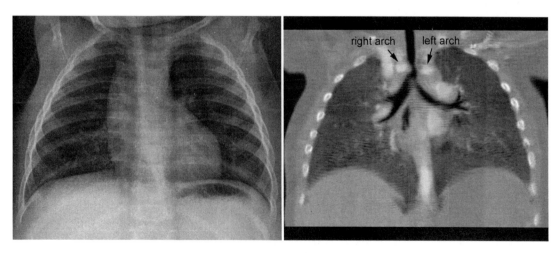

Fig. 11.1 Double aortic arch causing narrowing of the distal trachea. The right aortic arch is larger than the left arch and makes a sharp indentation of the trachea on the right side. Airway narrowing is obvious on the frontal chest radiograph but this finding is not specific for double aortic arch.

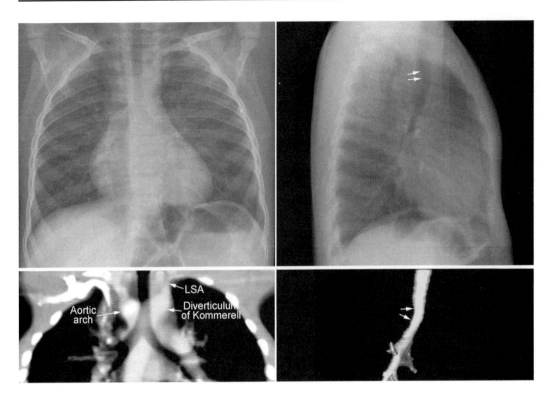

Fig. 11.2 Right aortic arch with aberrant origin of the left subclavian artery (LSA) from the descending aorta through the diverticulum of Kommerell. The distal trachea shows mild narrowing. The trachea is not significantly deviated to the left but it is bent forward by the distal aortic arch and diverticulum (*arrows* on the lateral views).

arch (**Fig. 11.3**).[5] Tracheal narrowing can be minimal or absent when the diverticulum is small or absent. The trachea may be compressed by the ascending aorta and aortic arch that have a more posterior position or by the aortic arch that has a long transverse course in front of the trachea (**Fig. 11.4**).[2,3] The innominate artery as well may compress the distal trachea when it arises more distally from the aortic arch on the left side and crosses the midline in front of the trachea.[6] This condition has been described as innominate artery compression syndrome. Nonetheless, the pretracheal location of the innominate artery is often seen but rarely symptomatic.[7]

Tracheal compression and narrowing may be identified on the frontal and lateral chest radiographs. Severe tracheal narrowing may be associated with emphysema of both lungs, especially with tracheomalacia. As air trapping develops, the hyperinflated lungs displace the ascending aorta and aortic arch further backward, causing a vicious cycle of airway obstruction and emphysema.

As the left main bronchus is normally crossed over by the aortic arch and left pulmonary artery, dilatation of those vessels may cause left bronchial compression from above (**Figs. 11.5, 11.6**). The left main bronchus is more vulnerable to compression when the aortic arch has an unusually low position. The most proximal part of the left main bronchus is also close to the proximal right

pulmonary artery. Therefore, the left main bronchus may be compressed by the dilated right pulmonary artery. The right main bronchus is transversely positioned in the mediastinum behind the right pulmonary artery and in front of the spine. A dilated right pulmonary artery may therefore compress both main-stem bronchi (**Fig. 11.6**). As the ascending aorta is immediately in front of the right pulmonary artery, dilatation or an abnormal posterior position of the ascending aorta may cause or contribute to right main bronchial compression. A proximal descending aorta on the right side seen with a right or double aortic arch may also compress the right main bronchus. Significant compression of the main-stem bronchi is almost always seen when there is severe dilatation of the branch pulmonary arteries with absent pulmonary valve syndrome (**Fig. 11.6**) and less commonly with more modest dilatation in pulmonary arterial hypertension.

The left main bronchus or left lower lobar bronchus may also be obstructed by a markedly dilated left atrium (**Figs. 11.7, 11.8**). A dilated left atrium typically displaces and compresses the left main bronchus and its lower lobar bronchus backward and upward, causing left lung or left lower lobe collapse (**Fig. 11.7**).

Patients with congenital heart disease with large left-to-right shunts often develop wheezing with obstructive

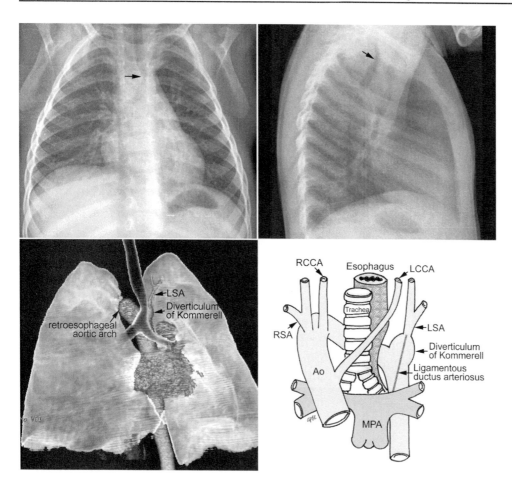

Fig. 11.3 Circumflex retroesophageal right aortic arch. The proximal part of the aortic arch is on the right side, indenting the right tracheal wall (*arrow* on the frontal chest radiograph). The aortic arch then takes a long oblique downward course behind the trachea and esophagus to connect to the descending aorta on the left. The trachea shows forward bending by the retroesophageal part of the aortic arch (*arrow* on the lateral chest radiograph). In the majority of cases, the left subclavian artery (LSA) arises from the top of the descending aorta through the diverticulum of Kommerell. Ao, ascending aorta; LCCA, left common carotid artery; MPA, main pulmonary artery; RCCA, right common carotid artery; RSA, right subclavian artery.

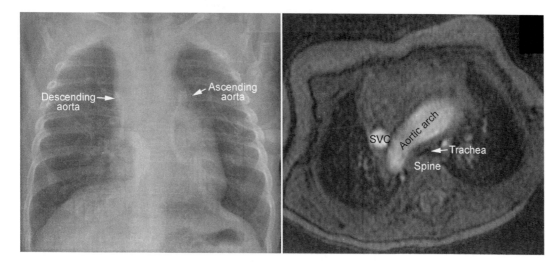

Fig. 11.4 Right aortic arch in corrected transposition of the great arteries. The aorta ascends on the left side, forming a convex bulge of the left upper mediastinal border. As the ascending aorta and descending aorta are on the opposite sides of the mediastinum, the aortic arch has a long transverse course in front of the trachea, causing compression of the trachea against the spine. SVC, superior vena cava.

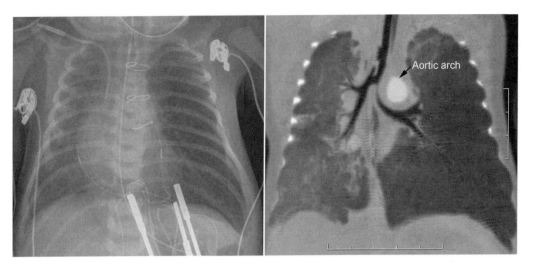

Fig. 11.5 Left main bronchial compression by an augmented aortic arch and surrounding edema in a newborn with complete transposition of the aorta and aortic arch narrowing. The left lung is hyperinflated.

emphysema or atelectasis (**Figs. 11.9, 11.10**). As the bronchi and pulmonary arteries course together in the lungs, dilatation of the pulmonary arteries causes some degree of bronchial compression. This may be further complicated by any insult to the respiratory system, causing significant symptoms and signs of airway obstruction.

Patients with frequent episodes of aspiration may show patchy lung parenchymal consolidation or atelectasis in the lower lobes. Patients who aspirate in the supine position may show lung opacities in the upper lobes and superior segments of the lower lobes.

Intrinsic Abnormalities of the Airway

Airway narrowing can also be due to inadequate rigidity of the tracheal or bronchial wall causing tracheomalacia

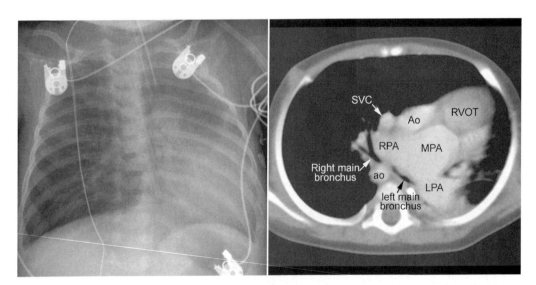

Fig. 11.6 Severe hyperinflation of the right lung with compression of the proximal right main bronchus between the dilated right pulmonary artery (RPA) and right-sided descending aorta (ao) in a patient with tetralogy of Fallot, absent pulmonary valve syndrome, and right aortic arch. The hyperinflated right lung herniates into the left thorax and displaces the heart and mediastinal structures leftward and backward. Most of the left lung is collapsed. Airway compression and hyperinfla-

tion can result in a vicious cycle and rapid deterioration. As hyperinflation secondary to airway compression pushes the heart and mediastinal structures backward, the main bronchi are further compressed against the spine and descending aorta. Ao, ascending aorta; LPA, left pulmonary artery; MPA, main pulmonary artery; RVOT, right ventricular outflow tract; SVC, superior vena cava.

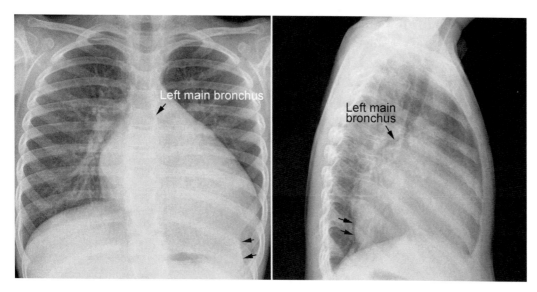

Fig. 11.7 Left lower lobe collapse in a 3-year-old child with dilated cardiomyopathy. The heart is markedly enlarged with a dilated left atrium and left ventricle. The left main bronchus is displaced upward and backward. The left lower lobe is collapsed (*arrows*). The left diaphragmatic silhouette is obliterated. There is compensatory hyperinflation of the left upper lobe.

or bronchomalacia, which can develop in utero or anytime after birth (**Fig. 11.8**).[8] Tracheomalacia may be due to primary intrinsic weakness of the tracheal cartilage but more commonly is a result of chronic extrinsic compression by an abnormal vessel such as a vascular rings or pulmonary artery sling. In addition, narrowing of the airway may be due to an intrinsic stenosis from complete cartilaginous rings, typically seen with pulmonary artery sling (**Fig. 11.11**).[9,10]

An abnormal branching pattern of the airway can be recognized on well-taken chest radiographs. Abnormal bronchial branching patterns in situs inversus and visceral heterotaxy with right or left thoracic and atrial isomerism are discussed in Chapter 7. A tracheal bronchus is the most common form of abnormal branching of the airway in which an abnormal bronchus arises from the lateral wall of the trachea and supplies the entire or a part of the upper lobe, more commonly on the right than the left.[11] Bilateral

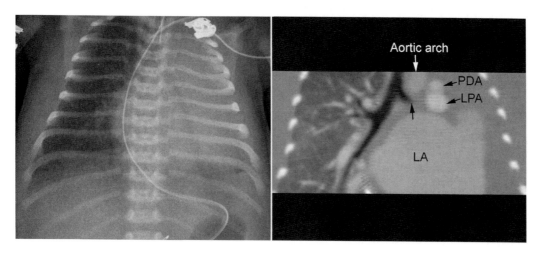

Fig. 11.8 Left lung collapse due to complete obstruction of the left main bronchus in a 6-day-old patient with critical aortic stenosis and severe mitral regurgitation. Computed tomography (CT) angiogram shows complete obstruction of the left main bronchus (*arrow*). Although the left atrium is hugely dilated and certainly compresses the left main bronchus, the level of proximal obstruction is at some distance from the site of left atrial compression. The patient was considered to have bronchomalacia. LA, left atrium; LPA, left pulmonary artery; PDA, patent ductus arteriosus.

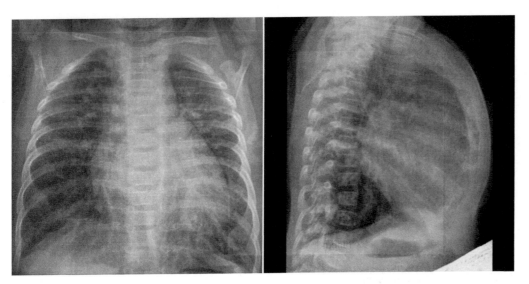

Fig. 11.9 Hyperinflation of both lungs in an infant with ventricular septal defect. The heart is moderately enlarged and the pulmonary vascularity is markedly increased. The diaphragm does not form a clear contour on the frontal view because it is flattened by the hyperinflated lungs. The sternum is bowed forward due to both cardiomegaly and hyperinflation.

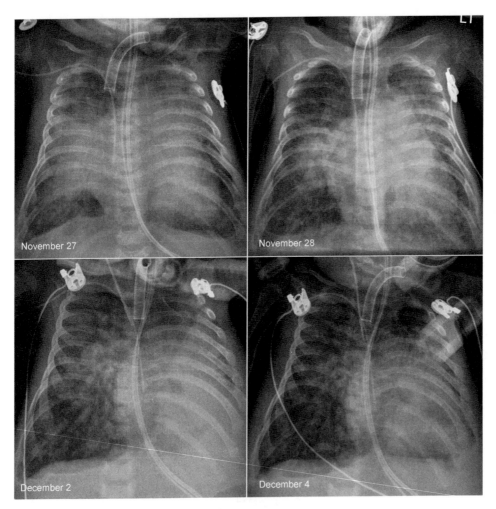

Fig. 11.10 Rapidly changing lung ventilation in a 3-month-old neonate with atrioventricular septal defect. The heart is moderately enlarged and the pulmonary vascularity is markedly increased. On the first radiograph on November 27, the right middle lobe and the upper part of the left upper lobe were collapsed. On the following day, the right middle and left upper lobes showed better aeration. Five days later, the left lower lobe and the lingular segment of the left upper lobe are collapsed and the right lung is hyperinflated. On the final radiograph, the left lower lobe showed improved aeration, whereas the right lung showed persistent hyperaeration. There was poor correlation between the patient's clinical findings and radiographic changes.

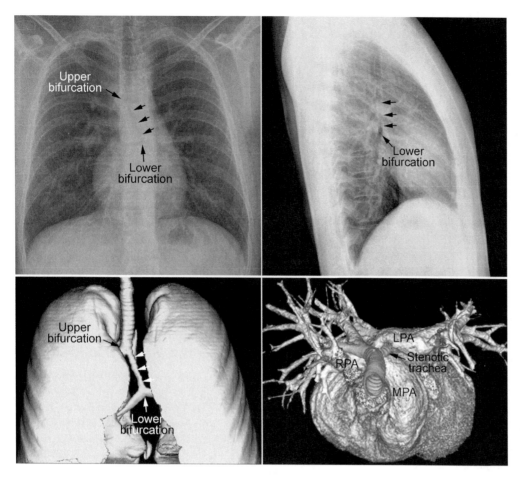

Fig. 11.11 Abnormal bronchial branching and congenital tracheal stenosis in pulmonary artery sling. There are two bifurcations of the airway in the mediastinum. The upper bifurcation gives rise to a bronchus to the right upper lobe. The lower bifurcation is into the left main bronchus and the bronchus to the right middle and lower lobes. The airway between the two bifurcations is diffusely narrowed due to complete cartilaginous rings (*arrows*). The three-dimensional CT angiogram as seen from above and front shows that the left pulmonary artery (LPA) arises far distally from the right pulmonary artery (RPA), encircling the right side of the stenotic trachea and then coursing leftward behind the trachea to reach the left hilum. MPA, main pulmonary artery.

tracheal bronchi have rarely been described. Tracheal bronchus is usually asymptomatic and found as an incidental finding on an imaging study or bronchoscopy but can be associated with chronic atelectasis, recurrent infection, or bronchiectasis. The main clinical implication of tracheal bronchus is during endotracheal intubation (**Fig. 11.12**).[12,13] The tracheal bronchus can be occluded by an endotracheal or tracheostomy tube, resulting in persistent atelectasis of the affected upper lobe. Inadvertent intubation of the tracheal bronchus results in regional variation in ventilation and may be complicated by pneumothorax with mechanical ventilation. There is an apparent increased incidence of tracheal bronchus in Down syndrome. An abnormal branching pattern of the tracheobronchial tree is seen in 40 to 80% of cases with pulmonary artery sling (**Fig. 11.11**).[9,10] Typically the trachea bifurcates into the

main-stem bronchi at a lower level than normal, with a wide angle between the right and left bronchi, producing an inverted-T appearance. In approximately one third of the cases with a low inverted-T bifurcation of the airway, the right upper lobar bronchus arises from the trachea slightly above the level of normal tracheal bifurcation. The left pulmonary artery forms a sling on the right side of the airway immediately above the lower bifurcation. The low inverted-T pattern of airway bifurcation has previously been described as a bridging bronchus.[9] Almost all cases with a low inverted-T bifurcation of the airway, with or without a separate origin of the right upper lobe bronchus, are associated with long segment narrowing of the lower airway above the bifurcation. The narrowing is due to complete cartilaginous rings with absence of the membranous part of the trachea posteriorly.

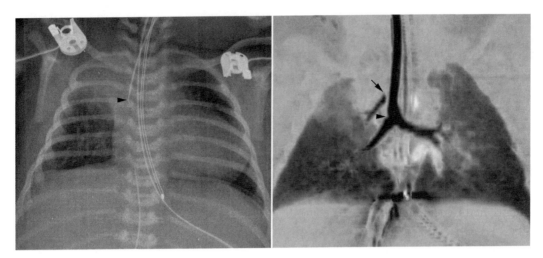

Fig. 11.12 Right upper lobe collapse in a newborn with truncus arteriosus. The endotracheal tube tip (*arrowhead*) is close to the carina. The right upper lobe is collapsed. Subsequent CT scan showed a tracheal bronchus supplying the collapsed right upper lobe. The orifice of the tracheal bronchus was occluded (*arrow*) by the endotracheal tube.

Warfarin Sodium-Induced Calcification of Tracheal and Bronchial Cartilaginous Rings

Progressive calcification of the cartilaginous rings of the trachea and bronchi has been observed in up to 50% of the patients undergoing prolonged anticoagulant therapy with warfarin sodium.[14] The calcification appears linear or beaded along the wall of the trachea and major bronchi on chest radiographs (**Fig. 11.13**). Other causes of airway calcifications are listed in **Table 11.1**.

Collapse, Emphysema and Consolidation

Segmental or lobar collapse involving lower lobes is common when the heart is enlarged. Collapse can be due to mechanical compression of a main, lobar, or segmental bronchus by the enlarged heart or dilated vessel (**Figs. 11.7, 11.8, 11.14**). The left lower lobe is most commonly affected especially when the left atrium is dilated (**Fig. 11.7**). A completely collapsed lobe or segment is seen as a triangular hazy area without visible vascular or

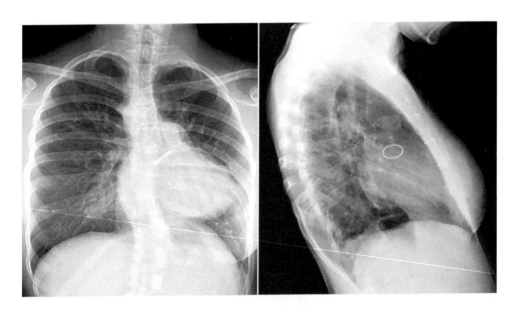

Fig. 11.13 Warfarin sodium-induced calcification of the trachea and bronchi in a 16-year-old girl. The patient underwent repair of truncus arteriosus followed by replacement of the regurgitant truncal valve in the aortic position with a mechanical valve. She was on prolonged administration of warfarin sodium for her mechanical aortic valve. The walls of the trachea and major bronchi are lined with beaded calcification.

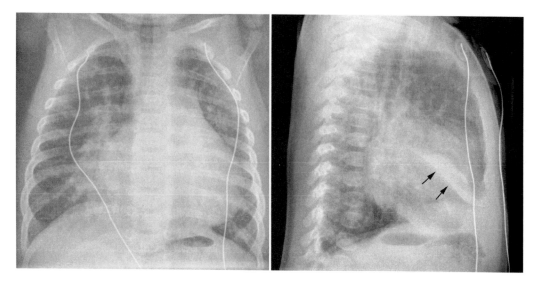

Fig. 11.14 Right middle lobe collapse in a 5-week-old infant with ventricular septal defect. The pulmonary vascularity is moderately increased. The medial segment of the right middle lobe is collapsed. On the frontal view, ill-defined haziness is seen in the medial aspect of the right lower lung partially obliterating the right lower cardiac border. On the lateral view, a fusiform dense haziness is seen in the lower aspect of the right middle lobe area. The inferior margin of the haziness is sharply demarcated by the major fissure (*arrows*). Loculated pleural effusion in the major fissure may show a similar finding.

bronchial markings. The base of the triangular haziness is on the pleural surface, whereas its apex is directed toward the lung hilum. A poorly ventilated lung area is characterized by crowded vascular markings. Collapse can also be due to retention of secretions or a mucus plug in an already narrowed bronchus or bronchi. In addition the enlarged heart may directly compress the lung parenchyma. A poorly ventilated lung area due to direct compression may show air-bronchograms as well as crowded vascular markings. In contrast, a pneumonic consolidation typically does not show significant loss of lung volume.

The lungs are hyperinflated when the airways are partially obstructed by extrinsic vascular compression, as discussed earlier (**Figs. 11.5, 11.6, 11.9, 11.10**). Hyperinflation is common when heart disease is complicated by pulmonary edema. Hyperinflation is primarily due to increased resistance to gas flow through the edematous small airway, but reflex bronchoconstriction is also considered to play a role.[15] The most typical combination of interstitial edema and hyperinflation is seen in newborns with an obstructive type of total anomalous pulmonary venous connection (**Fig. 11.15**). Hyperinflation can also be due to

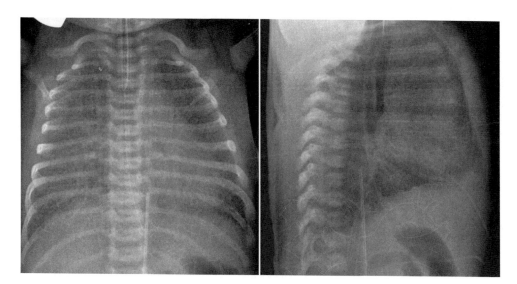

Fig. 11.15 Hyperinflation and interstitial edema of both lungs in a 2-day-old newborn with total anomalous pulmonary venous connection to the portal vein. Both lungs show generalized increase in interstitial markings. Both lung volumes are increased with flattening of the diaphragm.

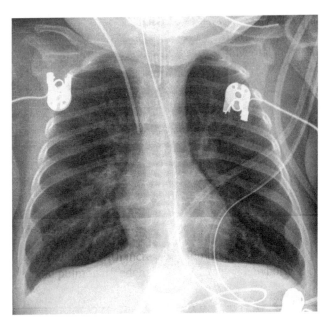

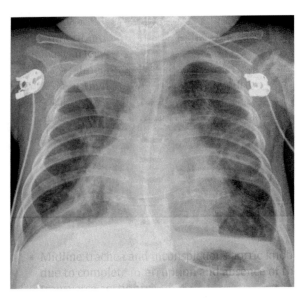

Fig. 11.16 Hyperinflation of both lungs in a 3-month-old infant with bronchiolitis. Both lungs show increased interstitial markings and are hyperinflated. The findings are similar to those seen in obstructive type of total anomalous pulmonary venous connection as in **Fig. 11.15.**

Fig. 11.17 Respiratory syncytial viral pneumonia complicating atrial sepal defect in a 5-month-old infant. The right upper lobe, the right middle lobe, and parts of both lower lobes are collapsed and reticular-streaky lesions are seen in the remaining aerated lung.

associated small airway disease such as bronchiolitis or asthma (**Fig. 11.16**). On a frontal chest radiograph, the lung volumes are increased with downward displacement of the diaphragms. When the displaced diaphragm is flat or convex downward, the diaphragmatic contour on the frontal view is blurred (**Figs. 11.9, 11.14**). In addition, the cardiac silhouette appears to be floating above the diaphragm, which is pushed downward by the hyperinflated lower lobes. The flattened or inverted diaphragm can also be

readily appreciated on lateral radiographs. Severe hyperinflation of the lungs results in increased anteroposterior diameter of the thorax (**Fig. 11.9**). Hyperinflation of the lungs is often associated with scattered areas of subsegmental, segmental, or lobar atelectasis (**Fig. 11.10**). Not uncommonly, the collapsed lung areas become hyperinflated and the hyperinflated areas become collapsed in a short interval, and therefore the radiographs may appear quite different from day to day without any significant change in clinical findings. Finally, severely cyanotic patients can develop

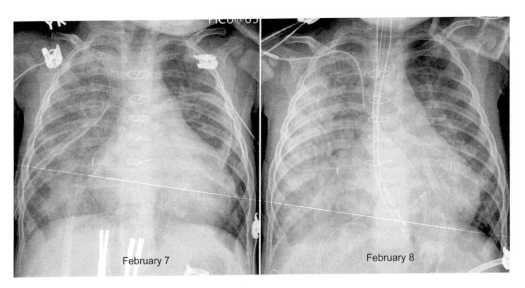

February 7   February 8

Fig. 11.18 Postoperative pulmonary hemorrhage in a child who underwent a Ross-Konno operation for aortic stenosis. The patient developed bleeding from the nose after chest tube removal. Frontal chest

radiograph obtained on the day of nasal bleeding shows a wide area of confluent haziness in the right lung, which is consistent with pulmonary hemorrhage.

compensatory hyperinflation of the lungs due to reflex hyperventilation.

Pneumonia is particularly common in patients with congenital heart disease because of impaired ventilation of the lungs related to airway compression, vascular congestion, and interstitial and alveolar pulmonary edema (**Fig. 11.17**). Frequent aspiration pneumonia can be seen when the esophagus is atretic or compressed by an abnormal cardiovascular structure. When a lobar or segmental type of pulmonary consolidation is seen in a cardiac patient, pulmonary hemorrhage and pulmonary infarction as

well as pneumonia should be included in the differential diagnoses. Pulmonary hemorrhage in cardiac patients can be a complication of administration of anticoagulant agents for a surgical or interventional procedure or a manifestation of disseminated intravascular coagulation. The patient usually has a sudden onset of overt hemoptysis, and the chest radiograph shows new development of bilateral or unilateral dense confluent opacity (**Fig. 11.18**). Pulmonary infarct with a pulmonary arterial embolus or thrombus typically produces a pleura-based triangular or lobular haziness and is commonly associated with pleural effusion (**Fig. 11.19**).[16] Although rare, pulmonary infarction can be due to pulmonary venous occlusion (**Fig. 11.20**).[17]

Patients with frequent episodes of aspiration may show evidence of lung parenchymal consolidation or atelectasis in the lower lobes. Patients who aspirate in the supine position may show lung lesions in the upper lobes and superior segments of the lower lobes.

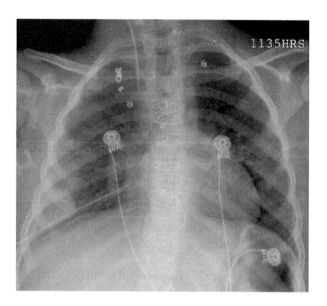

Fig. 11.19 Pulmonary infarction in a child who underwent a modified Fontan operation and coil embolization of internal mammary arteries. A pleural-based homogeneous haziness in the right lower lung is accompanied by a small amount of pleural effusion.

Unilateral Pulmonary Hypoplasia

Hypoplasia of a lung is seen in scimitar syndrome and its variants (**Figs. 11.21, 11.22**), unilateral absence of a branch pulmonary artery (**Figs. 11.23, 11.24**), and unilateral pulmonary vein atresia or stenosis (**Fig. 11.25**). Rarely does it occur as an isolated primary anomaly (**Table 11.2**). Hypoplasia of a lung is characterized by the small size of the thoracic cage with decreased intercostal spaces; elevation of the ipsilateral hemidiaphragm; and displacement of the mediastinal structures, including the heart and trachea, to the affected side. Diminished volume of a lung in these conditions is often mistakenly regarded as a manifestation or sequela of lung infection or chronic lung disease, and delayed diagnosis is not uncommon.

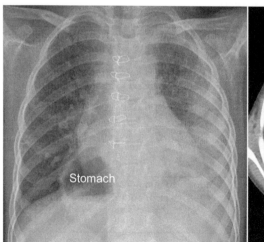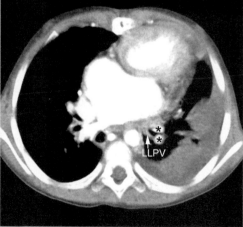

Fig. 11.20 Pulmonary venous infarction in a 5-year-old patient with left pulmonary vein obstruction after repair of total anomalous pulmonary venous connection and bidirectional cavopulmonary anastomosis. A pleural-based homogeneous haziness is seen in the left lower lung. There is pleural effusion surrounding the lung parenchymal lesion. CT shows nonopacification of the left lower pulmonary vein. The adjacent pulmonary arterial branches (*asterisks*) are opacified. The patient has right isomerism, and the right-sided stomach is partly within the thorax.

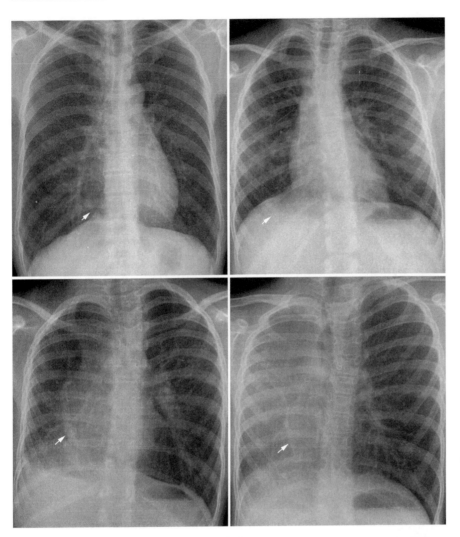

Fig. 11.21 Four different cases of scimitar syndrome showing various degrees of right lung hypoplasia. The two cases in the *lower panels* show severe hypoplasia, which is associated with hypoplasia of the thoracic cage and obliteration of the right heart border. All cases show abnormal branching pattern and arrangement of the pulmonary vessels. Scimitar veins (*arrows*) are visible in all cases.

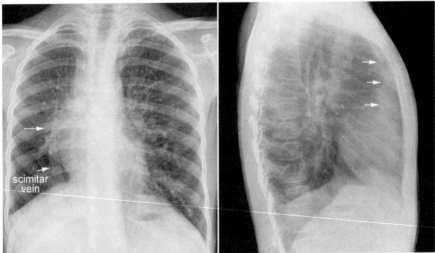

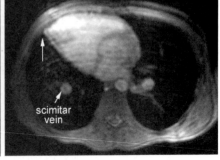

Fig. 11.22 Scimitar syndrome showing obliteration (*arrow*) of the lower right heart border on the frontal chest radiograph, and a retrosternal hazy band (*arrows*) on the lateral view. An axial MR image shows that the heart is displaced and rotated to the right and has wide contact with the anterior chest wall. As the lung does not surround the right margin of the heart, the heart border is obliterated at this level. The part of the heart and mediastinal tissue in front of the right lung produce a band-like haziness behind the sternum on the lateral view. It is demarcated by the anterior extent of the right lung (*arrows* on lateral chest radiograph and *arrow* on MR image).

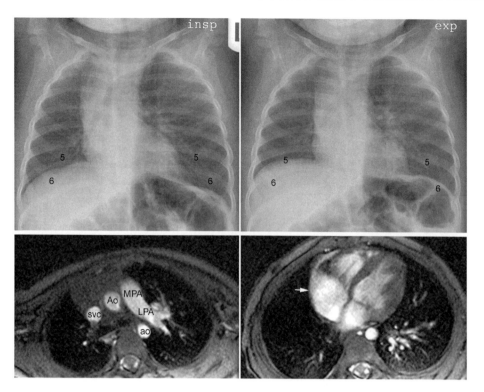

Fig. 11.23 Absence of the right pulmonary artery. As a foreign body was suspected, frontal chest radiographs were obtained in inspiration and expiration. There was no significant difference in mediastinal shift on the two frontal chest radiographs with different levels of inspiration, making the possibility of a foreign body unlikely. The right lung is mildly hypoplastic, with the trachea bent to the right and shows diminished vascularity. The left lung shows increased vascularity. The right heart border is not obliterated. Axial MR image in *lower left panel* shows that the right pulmonary artery is absent in the mediastinum. Axial image in *lower right panel* shows that the right lung surrounds the right heart margin (*arrow*). This finding is in contrast to that seen in most scimitar syndrome cases in which the right lung does not surround the far right margin of the heart as shown in **Fig. 11.22.** Ao, ascending aorta; ao, descending aorta; LPA, left pulmonary artery; MPA, main pulmonary artery; svc, superior vena cava.

Table 11.2 Differential Radiographic Findings in Three Major Causes of Congenital Right Lung Hypoplasia

	Scimitar Syndrome	Absence of the Right Pulmonary Artery	Unilateral Pulmonary Vein Atresia or Stenosis
Severity of right lung hypoplasia	Mild to severe	Usually moderate	Mild to moderate
Right cardiac border	Partly or completely obliterated in most cases	Clear	Visible but can be blurred due to edema in the adjacent lung
Retrosternal hazy band	Usually present	Not present	Not present
Right diaphragm	Elevated and often blurred	Elevated but usually sharp	Can be elevated
Right lung vascularity	Abnormal branching pattern of the pulmonary arteries Scimitar vein can be identified Small branches from aberrant systemic artery arising from the abdominal aorta can be identified	Decreased Collateral arteries may appear reticular	Reticular pattern with indistinct margins of the vessels
Abnormal airway branching	Majority of cases	No	No
Abnormal lung lobation	Majority of cases Often with horseshoe lung	No	No

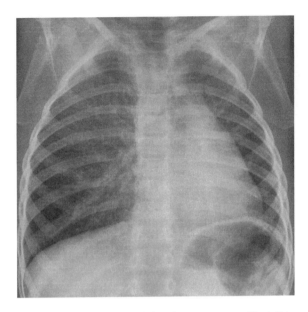

Fig. 11.24 Absence of the left pulmonary artery. The left lung volume is reduced, with the heart and mediastinal structures displaced to the left. The left diaphragm is elevated. The intercostal spaces of the left thorax are mildly narrowed. The pulmonary vascularity is reduced in the left lung and increased in the right lung.

Inclusion of the congenital causes on the list of differential diagnosis for diminished lung volume of a lung is important in the early detection of these rare conditions. The acquired conditions that may cause asymmetric lung volume include recurrent pneumonia, foreign body aspiration (**Fig. 11.26**), viral bronchiolitis (**Fig. 11.27**), and postinfectious obliterative bronchiolitis termed Swyer-James syndrome.

Scimitar syndrome and unilateral absence of a branch pulmonary artery are the most commonly encountered congenital lesions that are associated with lung hypoplasia (**Table 11.2**). Scimitar syndrome almost exclusively affects the right lung, whereas absence of a branch pulmonary artery has a mild predilection for the right side.[18,19] The severity of lung hypoplasia varies widely in scimitar syndrome. It is usually moderate with absence of a branch pulmonary artery. In scimitar syndrome, the right heart border is obliterated when there is severe right lung hypoplasia. In almost all cases with absence of a branch pulmonary artery, the heart border remains clear. The reason for this difference can be well appreciated on axial computed tomography (CT) or magnetic resonance (MR) images (**Figs. 11.22, 11.23**). In scimitar syndrome, the mediastinum contacts a wide part of the right anterior chest wall so that the hypoplastic right lung does not silhouette the cardiac margin. With absence of a branch pulmonary artery, in contrast, the mediastinum contacts the anterior chest wall far medial to the interface between the heart and the hypoplastic lung, and therefore the heart border remains clear. The pulmonary arteries and veins as well as bronchi of the affected lung show variable abnormal branching patterns in scimitar syndrome. Absence of a branch pulmonary artery is characterized by diminished vascularity with or without a reticular pattern, but is not associated with an abnormal branching pattern of the pulmonary arteries and veins and bronchi. Scimitar syndrome is commonly associated

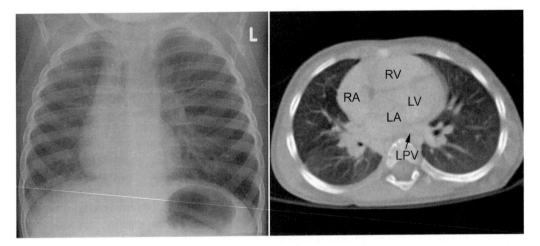

Fig. 11.25 Right pulmonary vein atresia in a 2-year-old child. The right lung volume is reduced and shows diminished vascularity with a reticular pattern. The findings are not unlike those seen in absence of the right pulmonary artery in **Fig. 11.23**. Axial CT image shows a large left pulmonary vein (LPV) connecting to the left atrium (LA). No vein from the right lung was found to connect to the left atrium. The patient had hemoptysis from bronchial varices. LV, left ventricle; RA, right atrium; RV, right ventricle. (Courtesy of L.P. Koopman and N. de Graaf, Erasmus Medical Center, Sophia Children's Hospital, Rotterdam, the Netherlands.)

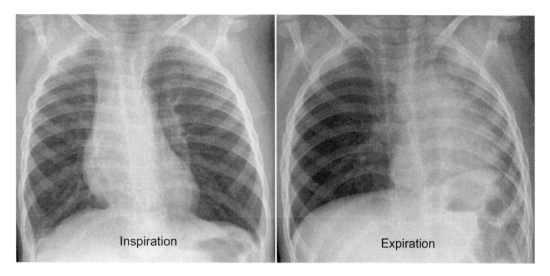

Inspiration

Expiration

Fig. 11.26 Peanut in right main bronchus. On inspiration, the right lung volume is smaller than the left lung volume. The findings are similar to those seen in absence of the right pulmonary artery in **Fig. 11.23** and in right pulmonary vein atresia in **Fig. 11.22.** Chest radiograph obtained during expiration shows air trapping of the right lung. No reticular pattern related to collaterals present.

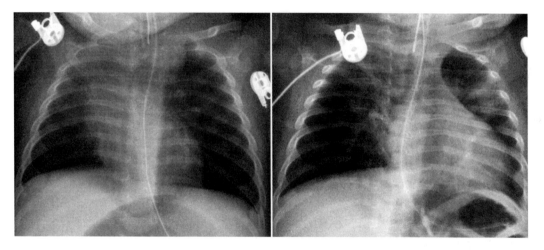

Fig. 11.27 Bronchiolitis mimicking absence of the right pulmonary artery or right pulmonary vein atresia with partial right upper lobe collapse and interstitial thickening. On a follow-up study, the right lung is better aerated, whereas the left lung shows areas of atelectasis.

with abnormal lobation of the right lung. Horseshoe lung is a rare form of abnormal lung lobation that can accompany scimitar syndrome.[20,21] There are a few variations of horseshoe lung. In its most classic form, a tongue of lung tissue arising from the right lower lobe extends to the left thorax through a tunnel between the right and left pleural cavities with or without parenchymal fusion to the left lower lobe. Rarely, a crossover portion of one lung can be without a pleural tunnel. Also reported is a separate midline lobe with its own pleural envelope that straddles the right and left thorax. A horseshoe lung may be suspected when one or a few horizontal vascular markings are seen in the medial aspect of the left lower lung. The pleural fissure separating the herniated right lung and the left lung, when present, can be seen as an oblique linear shadow in the left lower lung region (**Figs. 11.28, 11.29**).

A meandering right pulmonary vein is a condition in which the right pulmonary vein has an unusually meandering course in the right lower lung but retains a connection to the left atrium (**Fig. 11.29**).[21] It is considered a variant of scimitar syndrome, as most cases of meandering right pulmonary vein share the common features of classic

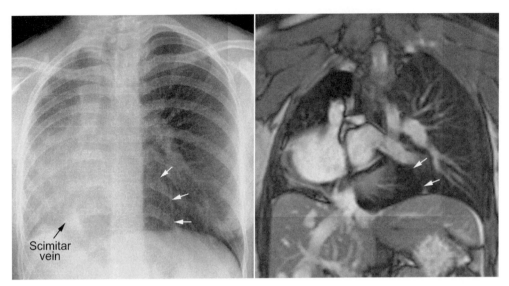

Fig. 11.28 Scimitar syndrome with horseshoe lung in a 17-year-old patient. The right lung is hypoplastic. There is a vertically oriented scimitar vein that drained to the inferior vena cava in the right lower lung. There is an oblique fissure (*arrows*), demarcating the left border of the right lower lung that extended to the left through the retrocardiac space.

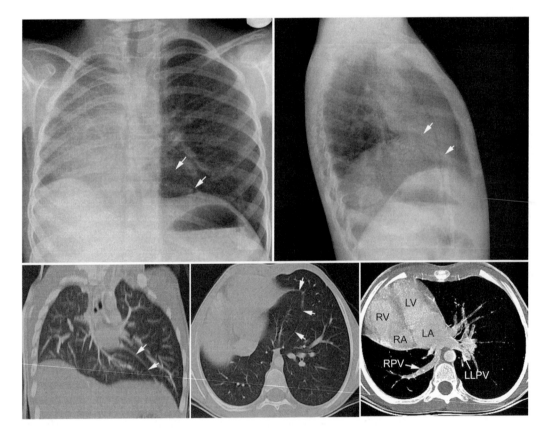

Fig. 11.29 Meandering right pulmonary vein (RPV) with severe hypoplasia of the right lung in a 6-year-old child. The chest radiographic findings are not unlike classic scimitar syndrome with an abnormal branching pattern of the pulmonary vessels in the right lung visible through the cardiac silhouette. There was systemic collateral arterial supply to the right lower lung. A single vein draining the right lung (RPV) has an unusual course but was connected to the left atrium (LA). An oblique fissure (*arrows*) is seen in the medial aspect of the left lung. This fissure demarcates the right lung that extends to the left thorax through the space between the heart and spine, which is characteristic of horseshoe lung. LLPV, left lower pulmonary vein; LV, left ventricle; RA, right atrium; RV, right ventricle.

scimitar syndrome, including right lung hypoplasia, horseshoe lung, and aberrant systemic arterial supply to the right lower lung. Rarely, the scimitar vein can have connections to both the inferior vena cava and left atrium.[22]

Unilateral pulmonary vein atresia is characterized by a reticular pattern of pulmonary vascularity with interlobular septal thickening in a hypoplastic lung (**Fig. 11.25**).[23] The reticular pattern of engorged pulmonary venous tributaries and collateral channels is often difficult to differentiate from the reticular pattern of the systemic collateral arteries associated with unilateral absence of a branch pulmonary artery. In fact, systemic arterial collateral arteries may develop secondary to pulmonary venous obstruction.

■ Pleura

In patients with known heart disease, pleural effusion is a sign of congestive heart failure. Pleural effusion is seen in the majority of patients with congestive heart failure.[24] Pleural effusion in congestive heart failure is usually bilateral and but can be unilateral. Congestive heart failure is by far the most common cause of bilateral pleural effusion (**Fig. 11.30**). Although unilateral left-sided pleural effusion

had been regarded as atypical for congestive heart failure, a large series showed no statistically significant difference in right-left side distribution.[25] Pleural effusion is seen in approximately 50% of patients with pulmonary embolism (**Fig. 11.19**). Pleural effusion can be secondary to pneumonia complicating heart disease.

Pleural effusion typically accumulates in the dependent part of the thorax. In an erect position, pleural effusion accumulates along the diaphragm. Blunting of the costophrenic angles where the diaphragmatic contour meets the chest wall is the earliest sign of a small pleural effusion. Larger amounts of pleural effusion cast a homogeneous haziness in the lower thorax that obliterates the diaphragmatic silhouette and forms a meniscus that is concave upward (**Fig. 11.31**). In contrast to atelectasis, pneumonia, or other forms of lung consolidation, vascular markings are seen through the haziness of a pleural effusion. On an erect radiograph, pleural effusion often accumulates between the undersurface of the lung and the diaphragm (**Fig. 11.31**, left panels). This subpulmonic pleural effusion is often misinterpreted as an elevated diaphragm. In contrast to an elevated diaphragm, the crest of the shadow of the subpulmonic effusion tends to lie more lateral than that of an elevated diaphragm. Pleural effusion within the interlobar fissures is seen as a linear, band-like, or ovoid shadow when the fissure is aligned with the radiographic beam.

In the supine position, pleural effusion layers along the posterior chest wall, causing a diffuse increased haziness of the affected thorax with the vascular and bronchial markings remaining visible. Unilateral diffuse haziness of the lung density on a supine chest radiograph is an important telltale sign of fluid collection in the pleural cavity (**Fig. 11.32**). Differential diagnosis of unilateral haziness includes an abnormality of the lung or asymmetric chest wall or breast tissues. In addition, there are technical pitfalls that may result in asymmetric blackness of a frontal chest radiograph. The pitfalls are an oblique projection and less commonly an asymmetric radiographic exposure. When pleural effusion is suspected, a lateral decubitus view can be obtained to visualize shift of pleural effusion to the dependent part of the thorax.

Pneumothorax can develop as a complication of positive pressure ventilation (**Fig. 11.33**). Increased transalveolar pressure may result in air leak into the pleural cavity, causing a pneumothorax, and into the interstitium and mediastinum, causing pulmonary interstitial emphysema and pneumomediastinum (**Figs. 11.33, 11.34**). A large-tension pneumothorax is characterized by an increase in volume of the hemithorax with displacement of the heart and mediastinum to the contralateral side. In the supine position, pneumothorax accumulates anteriorly and medially first and then laterally along the chest wall (**Fig. 11.35**).

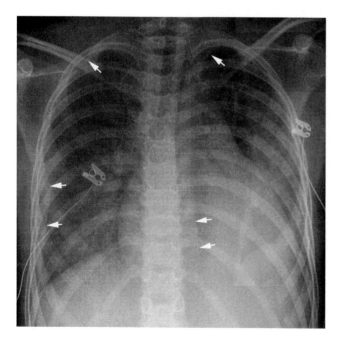

Fig. 11.30 Bilateral pleural effusion in a 10-year-old patient with dilated cardiomyopathy. In this supine frontal chest radiograph, pleural effusion layered in the dependent part of the thorax causes diffuse haziness of the hemithoraces. Some effusion is accumulated laterally within the pleural cavity around the lungs (*arrows*). Left lower lobe is collapsed.

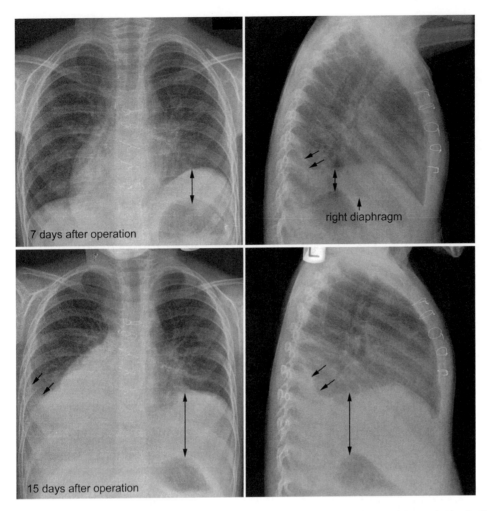

Fig. 11.31 Subpulmonic left pleural effusion in a 4-year-old patient after modified Fontan operation. There is dextrocardia. Upright frontal and lateral chest radiographs obtained 7 days after the operation show that the dome of interface between the left thorax and abdomen is abnormally high and convex more laterally than that of a usual hemidiaphragm. This pseudo-diaphragm contour is higher than the right hemidiaphragm and is some distance from the gastric bubble (*double-headed arrow*). On the lateral view, the posterior costophrenic sulcus is obliterated (*arrows*). The findings are quite characteristic of a subpulmonic pleural effusion. Fifteen days after the operation, a larger amount of subpulmonic pleural effusion is seen in the left thorax, with a wider gap between the pseudo-diaphragm and the gastric bubble. There is new accumulation of a large amount of pleural effusion in the right thorax, which shows a typical meniscus of pleural fluid in the right and posterior costophrenic angles (*arrows*).

Infrequently, pneumothorax can accumulate predominantly along the diaphragm (**Fig. 11.36**), making a differential diagnosis from a loculated pneumomediastinum along the diaphragm difficult (**Fig. 11.37**). Spontaneous pneumothorax is a rare complication of connective tissue disease such as Marfan syndrome (**Fig. 11.38**).[26]

■ Mediastinum

The mediastinal contour varies significantly in infants and young children because of the variable size and appearance of the thymus. The thymus increases in size during childhood and reaches its maximum weight at puberty. The thymus is most prominent between birth and 2 years of age. After 2 years of age, the rate of thymic growth decelerates and the thymus gradually becomes less prominent. At about 5 years of age in most children, the thymus is often no longer recognizable on radiographs. On frontal chest radiographs, the thymus is a well-defined soft tissue density that projects from both sides of the upper mediastinum with the bronchovascular markings remaining visible through it (**Fig. 11.39**). The thymus is usually asymmetric in size and configuration (**Fig. 11.40**). The right lobe of the thymus is more frequently larger than the left lobe. The contour of each lobe varies from triangular, quadrilateral-shaped, or rounded appearance. The

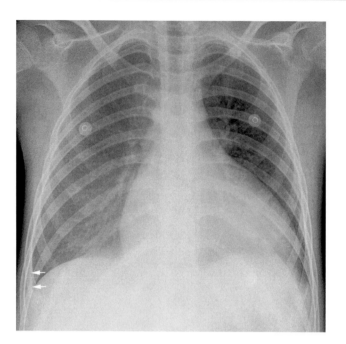

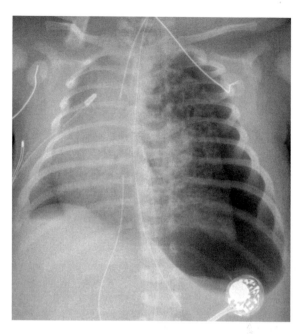

Fig. 11.32 Unilateral layered right pleural effusion in a 7-year-old patient with dilated cardiomyopathy. The right hemithorax is diffusely hazy but the pulmonary vessels are identifiable. A small effusion is profiled along the lateral chest wall (*arrows*).

Fig. 11.33 Tension pneumothorax and interstitial emphysema in a newborn with tetralogy of Fallot and absent pulmonary valve syndrome. There is a large left pneumothorax displacing the heart and mediastinum to the right and the left hemidiaphragm downward. The underlying left lung contains numerous tubular and round air bubbles in the interstitium. Because of splinting effect of interstitial emphysema, the left lung is not completely collapsed in spite of the severe mass effect of the pneumothorax.

right lobe of the thymus often projects over the right middle lung zone with a sharp horizontal inferior margin, called the thymic sail sign. When both lobes of the thymus have a rounded contour, the thymicocardiac silhouette might look like a snowman. The contour of the left lobe of the thymus usually appears less prominent than the right lobe as it merges with the left cardiac silhouette. The normal thymic contour often shows a notch where it

meets the cardiac silhouette as well as showing indentations from the adjacent ribs, causing the thymic wave sign (**Fig. 11.39**). On a lateral view, the thymus appears as homogeneous soft tissue occupying the retrosternal clear

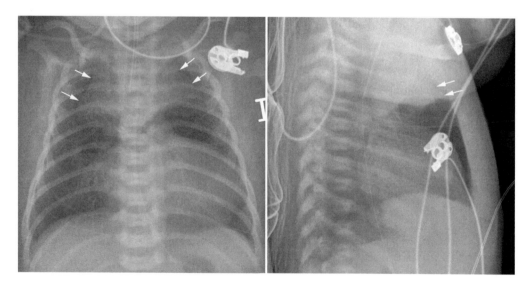

Fig. 11.34 Pneumomediastinum causing elevation of thymic lobes in a newborn with pulmonary atresia and intact ventricular septum. The elevated thymic lobes (*arrows*) are likened to angel wings on the frontal

view. Elevation of the thymus is also noticeable on the lateral view anteriorly. The mediastinal air is faintly outlined from the air in the lungs on the frontal view and more obviously on the lateral view.

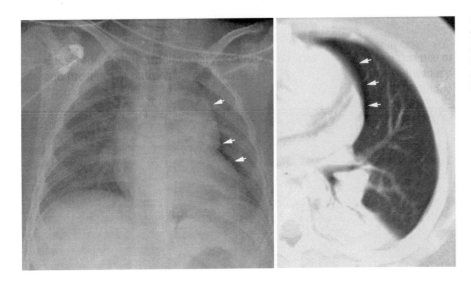

Fig. 11.35 Small medial pneumothorax along the left heart border. Pneumothorax begins to accumulate medially along the heart border because this part of the pleural cavity is highest in the supine position (*arrows*). The left lower lobe is partly collapsed.

space and is frequently demarcated inferiorly by a sharp horizontal interface with the normal lung.

Thymic hypoplasia or aplasia is common in microdeletion 22q11.2 syndrome that encompasses DiGeorge syndrome, velocardiofacial syndrome, and conotruncal face syndrome.[27] When a newborn infant with congenital cardiac defect shows a narrow superior mediastinum, microdeletion 22q11.2 syndrome should be excluded (**Fig. 11.41**). Approximately 75% of patients with microdeletion 22q11.2 have congenital heart disease. The most common types of cardiac defects include tetralogy

of Fallot, interrupted aortic arch type B, ventricular septal defect, persistent truncus arteriosus, and various aortic arch anomalies. A further consideration that mimics an absent thymus is involution of the thymus, which can occur very rapidly when the patient experiences a critical postnatal course (**Fig. 11.42**).[28,29] With recovery of the general condition after treatment, the thymus may show rapid rebound growth.

When the mediastinum is unusually wide or shows a lobulated contour without typical signs of a normally prominent thymus for the patient's age, pathologic lesions

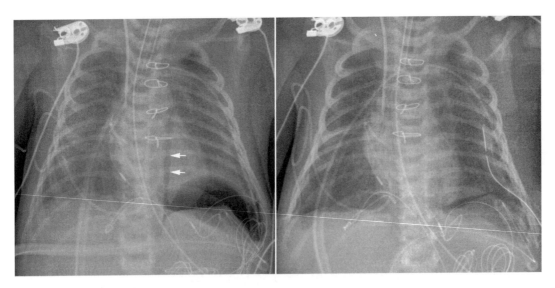

Fig. 11.36 Loculated pneumothorax along the left diaphragm in a newborn after repair of complete transposition of the great arteries and aortic arch obstruction. An oval air pocket is seen along the left hemidiaphragm. The extrapulmonary air extends along the medial border of the left lung (*arrows*), suggesting that the air is in the pleural cavity. After insertion of a new chest tube, the pneumothorax was successfully drained.

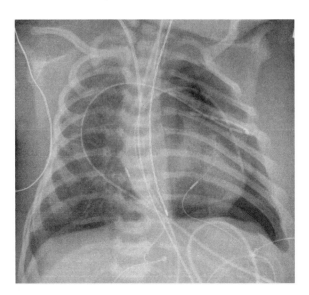

Fig. 11.37 Pneumomediastinum along diaphragm. In this patient with the chest wall kept open after open-heart surgery, air collections are seen along both hemidiaphragms as well as in the mediastinum. These air collections are considered to be extrapleural. It is considered that pneumomediastinum can reach the subpleural space along the diaphragm, where a loculated air pocket or pockets can be made. A differential diagnosis between a loculated pneumothorax and a loculated pneumomediastinum can be difficult.

including thymic masses and mediastinal tumors should be considered. With a recent history of cardiovascular surgery, postoperative hematomas, mediastinal abscesses, or vascular aneurysms within the mediastinum should be

suspected, and cross-sectional imaging, most preferably a contrast-enhanced CT, should be performed (**Fig. 11.43**).

■ Diaphragm

The diaphragm normally forms a sharp dome-shaped silhouette between the lungs and abdomen. Obliteration of part or all of diaphragmatic silhouette suggests an adjacent lung parenchymal lesion or accumulation of pleural effusion. When the diaphragm straightens or makes a downward convexity due to hyperinflation of the lungs, the diaphragmatic contour loses its sharpness on the frontal view (**Fig. 11.9**). An upward bulge of a part of the diaphragmatic contour is seen in congenital diaphragmatic eventration or hernia through a defect (**Fig. 11.44**). A larger defect of the hemidiaphragm with herniation of abdominal contents into the thorax causes contralateral shifting of the heart and mediastinum, hypoplasia and collapse of the ipsilateral lung, and extrinsic compression of the contralateral lung. The abdomen is typically scaphoid.

Unilateral elevation of the hemidiaphragm can be due to ipsilateral phrenic nerve injury at the time of surgery (**Fig. 11.45**). Diaphragmatic paralysis or paresis is characterized by paradoxical or reduced movement of the affected diaphragm on respiration, which can be assessed with ultrasound. It should be noted that a paradoxical movement of the diaphragmatic domes is also seen in

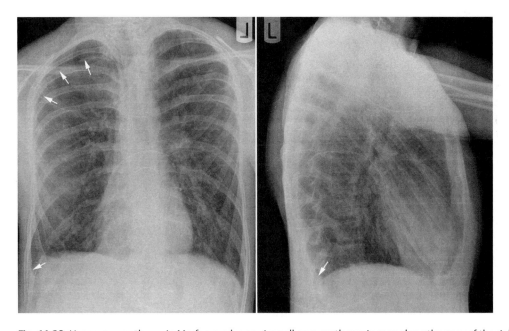

Fig. 11.38 Hemopneumothorax in Marfan syndrome. A small pneumothorax is seen along the apex of the right lung (*arrows*). A small fluid collection is also seen in the right costophrenic angle area (*arrow*).

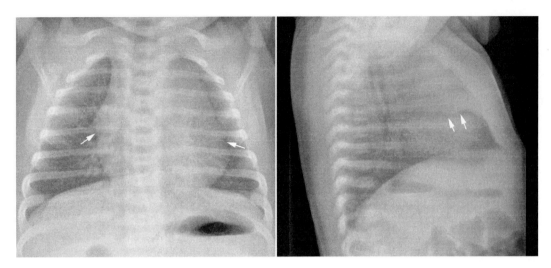

Fig. 11.39 Normal thymus obscuring the cardiac contour on the frontal chest radiograph in a 16-day-old neonate. Wavy appearance of the left margin is characteristic of normal thymus. The lower extent of the thymus is demarcated by distinct notches (*arrows*). The retrosternal clear space is occupied by the thymus. The horizontal lower margin of the thymus (*arrows*) is straight on the lateral view.

unilateral bronchial obstruction such as foreign body aspiration (**Fig. 11.26**). As discussed in this chapter, subpulmonic pleural effusions can simulate diaphragmatic paralysis radiographically (**Fig. 11.31**, upper left panel).

■ Chest Wall

The chest wall consists of the rib cage, spine, adjacent muscles, connective tissue, and overlying skin. Skeletal abnormalities are commonly seen in patients with congenital

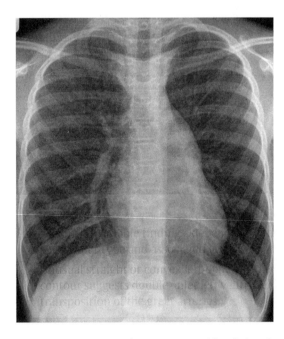

Fig. 11.40 Asymmetric thymus causing a blunt bulge along the left heart border in a 7-year-old patient with patent ductus arteriosus.

heart disease as part of syndromes or associations. Skeletal abnormalities can occur as a consequence of cardiomegaly or vascular engorgement, as an associated lesion without any obvious known causal relationships, and as a shared feature of a generalized connective tissue disease affecting the cardiovascular system (**Table 11.3**).

A large heart may cause forward bowing of the sternum and protrusion of the adjacent thoracic cage, which is termed pectus carinatum (**Fig. 11.10**). Chronic air-trapping secondary to engorgement of the pulmonary vessels may also cause forward bowing of the sternum. As the diaphragms tend to contract rather forcefully in response to air-trapping, the lower ribs may be retracted.

As discussed earlier in this chapter, scimitar syndrome, unilateral absence of a branch pulmonary artery, and unilateral pulmonary vein atresia or severe stenosis are associated with unilateral hypoplasia of a lung (**Figs. 11.21, 11.22, 11.23, 11.24, 11.25**). Unilateral hypoplasia of the lung is characterized by a reduced size of the thoracic cage with narrowed intercostal spaces, upward displacement of the ipsilateral diaphragm, and scoliosis.

Rib notches are well-known skeletal findings of coarctation of the aorta (**Fig. 11.46**). They are erosive changes caused by increased pulsation of the dilated intercostal arteries that deliver collateral flow to the descending aorta. Rib notches are typically seen along the inferior margins of the posterolateral aspects of the ribs where the intercostal arteries are in close proximity to the ribs in these locations. Despite its well-recognized name, obvious rib notching is rare in children. Erosive changes are usually preceded by sclerotic changes, and asymmetric sclerosis of the inferior cortical margins of the ribs is more commonly seen. Sclerosis or erosions in coarctation of the aorta typically affect the third to ninth ribs. The reason

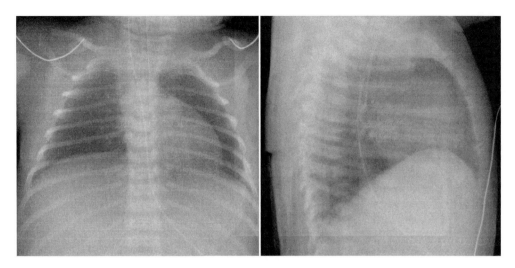

Fig. 11.41 No radiographically visible thymus in a newborn with tetralogy of Fallot and chromosome 22q11.2 microdeletion syndrome.

the first two ribs are not affected is that the first two intercostal arteries arise from the costocervical trunk of the subclavian artery and therefore do not contribute to intercostal collateral circulation supplied by the internal mammary arteries. Acquired stenosis of the aorta such as Takayasu's aortitis may also be associated with sclerosis and erosions of the ribs below the level of obstruction. Other rare causes of rib sclerosis or erosions include superior vena caval obstruction, Blalock-Taussig shunt, systemic arterial collateral circulation to the lung(s) (**Fig. 11.47**), and arteriovenous fistula and intercostal neurofibromas.

Intravenous infusion of prostaglandin E1 is used to maintain ductal patency in infants with ductal-dependent congenital heart disease. Prostaglandin infusion may be complicated by fever, diarrhea, hypotension, apnea, bradycardia, gastric outlet obstruction, and skin edema. Prolonged use of prostaglandin is often associated with skeletal side effects, including periosteal reaction with bone-within-bone appearance in the long bones, ribs, clavicles, and scapulae; pseudowidening of the cranial sutures; and underossification of the calvarial bones (**Fig. 11.48**).[30,31] The bone changes are both dose and duration dependent and associated with increased serum alkaline phosphatase level.

Straight back syndrome is a congenital condition in which cardiac murmurs are associated with unusual straightening of the thoracic spine and vertical orientation

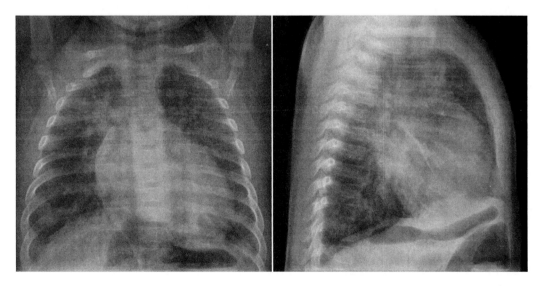

Fig. 11.42 No radiologically visible thymus in a 3-month-old infant with complete transposition of the great arteries. Postnatal thymic hypoplasia uncovers the narrow vascular pedicle. The heart is enlarged and the pulmonary vascularity is increased.

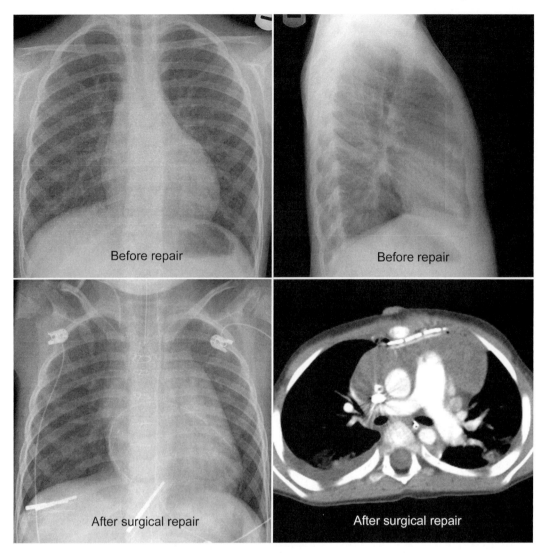

Fig. 11.43 Mediastinal widening due to postoperative hematoma in a 4-year-old patient following surgical repair of atrioventricular septal defect. The superior mediastinum was not prominent prior to surgery (*upper panels*). Postoperatively, there was marked superior mediastinal widening. Axial CT image shows a large hematoma in the anterior mediastinum (*lower panels*).

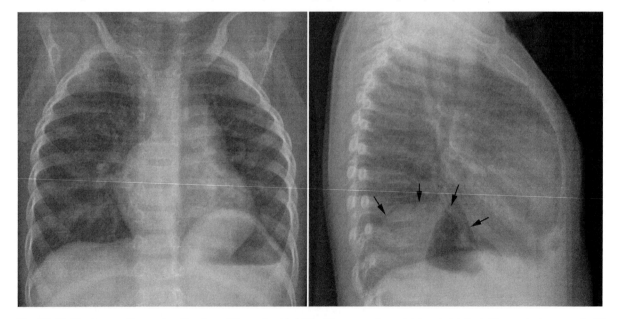

Fig. 11.44 Diaphragmatic eventuration in an 18-month-old child with a secundum atrial septal defect. The posterior aspect of the diaphragm shows a focal upward bulge (*arrows*).

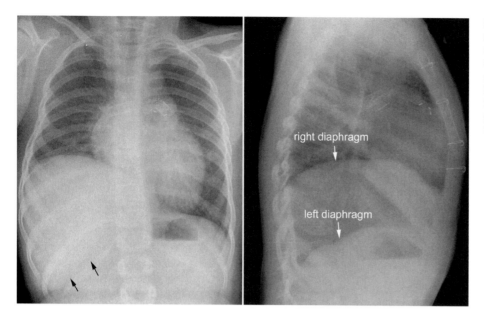

Fig. 11.45 Right diaphragmatic paresis in a patient with tetralogy of Fallot and pulmonary atresia who underwent corrective surgery and stent dilatation of the stenotic right and left pulmonary arteries. The right diaphragm is much higher than the left diaphragm. The lower margin of the hepatic silhouette is displaced upward.

Table 11.3 Skeletal Abnormalities in Pediatric Cardiac Patients

As a consequence of cardiovascular disease	Sternal bowing (pectus carinatum)
	Hypoplasia of the thorax
	Rib notching and sclerosis
	Prostaglandin osteopathy
As an associated abnormality	Straight back syndrome
	Sternal depression (pectus excavatum)
	Deficient sternal ossification
	Scoliosis
As skeletal manifestations of systemic disease	Marfan syndrome
	Loeys Dietz syndrome
	Ehlers-Danlos syndrome
	Pseudoxanthoma elasticum
	Osteogenesis imperfecta
	Turner's syndrome
	Mucopolysaccharidosis
	Trisomies
	Alagille syndrome
	Ellis–van Creveld syndrome
	Holt-Oram syndrome
	Polydactyly-syndactyly syndrome
	VACTERL* association

*Vertebral abnormalities, anal atresia, cardiac abnormalities, tracheoesophageal fistula, esophageal atresia, renal agenesis, and limb defects.

of the sternum.[32] The cardiac murmurs have been attributed to compression of the heart secondary to the reduced anteroposterior dimension of the thoracic cage. On chest radiographs, the thorax is flat anteroposteriorly with diminished distance between the straightened spine and sternum (**Fig. 11.49**). The heart appears squashed between the spine and sternum on the lateral view. The cardiac silhouette on the frontal view is enlarged or displaced leftward. The descending aorta may also be pushed further to the left and backward by the displaced left atrium. It has been reported that the straight back syndrome is inherited as an autosomal dominant condition.[32] Although the heart can be structurally normal, approximately two thirds of the individuals showing a straight back have mitral valve prolapse.

Pectus excavatum or funnel chest is characterized by depression of the lower midline chest caused with backward displacement of the lower part of the sternum (**Fig. 11.50**). As in straight back syndrome, the heart is displaced to the left and an ejection systolic murmur is heard along the left heart border. The lower part of the heart is compressed by the depressed sternum and therefore appears unusually lucent. The anterior parts of the ribs are often abnormally vertical. Pectus excavatum, although not commonly associated with congenital heart disease, has been associated with an increased incidence of an atrial septal defect.

The sternum normally has one ossification center for the manubrium, three to four centers for the body, and one for the xiphoid. The ossification centers for the manubrium and upper sternal body appear in fetal life,

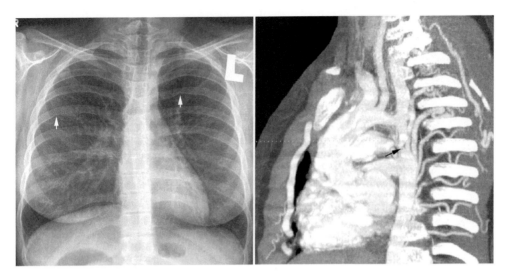

Fig. 11.46 Rib notching in a 13-year-old patient with severe coarctation of the aorta. Rib notches (*arrows*) are seen along the inferior cortex of the posterior parts of the ribs with a sharp one on the left fifth rib and a shallow one on the right sixth rib. In addition, the posterior parts of the ribs show asymmetric sclerosis of the inferior cortex. Most pronounced sclerosis is seen on the third and fourth ribs. CT angiogram shows a severe discrete coarctation (*arrow*) and tubular hypoplasia of the aortic arch, and a well-developed collateral network with large intercostal arteries coursing along the inferior margins of the ribs.

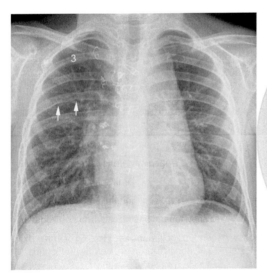
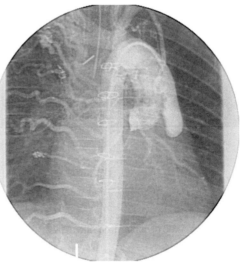

Fig. 11.47 Rib notches in a 4-year-old patient after Fontan operation for double-inlet left ventricle and discordant ventriculoarterial connection. The patient developed florid systemic collateral arterial supply to the right lung. The inferior margins of the posterior parts of the right ribs are irregular. The right fifth rib shows distinct notches (*arrows*) on the inferior cortex. The right third rib appears hyoplastic due to surgical injury at the time of a Blalock-Taussig shunt in the early neonatal period. Aortogram shows that the right intercostal arteries are markedly dilated as compared with the left intercostal arteries. There has been previous coil embolization of collateral arteries.

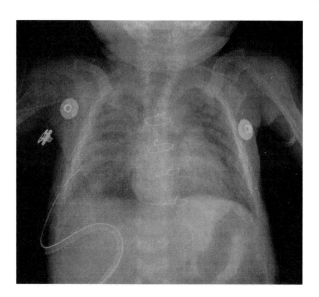

Fig. 11.48 Prostaglandin osteopathy in a neonate. Widespread periosteal reaction is seen in the clavicles, ribs, and left humerus. Note that the intercostal spaces are encroached on by the thickened ribs.

whereas the centers for the lower sternal body appear after birth, and the center for the xiphoid appears still later. Fusion of the ossification centers of the sternal body occurs in childhood and young adulthood, whereas bony union across the manubriosternal joint and sternoxiphoid joints is occasionally seen later in adulthood. Premature fusion of the sternal ossification centers leads to an abnormally short and thick sternum, which may be bowed or angled forward. Deficient sternal segmentation is commonly associated with congenital heart disease, such as ventricular septal defect and atrial septal defect.

Congenital scoliosis is often associated with congenital heart disease.[33] Atrial septal defect, ventricular septal defect, and tetralogy of Fallot with pulmonary atresia are the most common defects seen in patients with scoliosis. Scoliosis can be idiopathic with no abnormality of the individual spines (**Fig. 11.51**). Rarely, scoliosis is due to major abnormalities of spinal segmentation, such as hemivertebrae, butterfly vertebrae, etc. (**Fig. 11.52**). Severe scoliosis may be associated with deficient alveolar growth of the compressed lung and pulmonary hypertension. Children who underwent median sternotomy for congenital

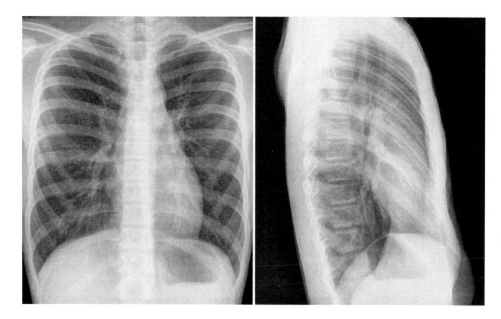

Fig. 11.49 Straight back syndrome in a 14-year-old boy. The thorax is flat with an unusually straight spinal column and vertically oriented sternum. The heart appears squashed between the spine and sternum.

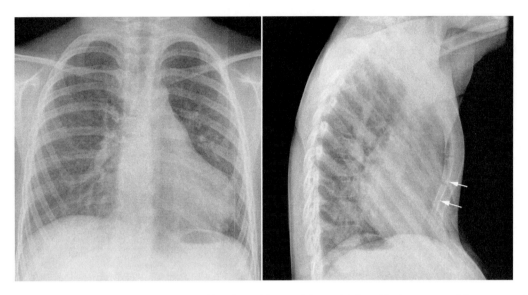

Fig. 11.50 Pectus excavatum in a 5-year-old patient with an atrial septal defect. The lower part of the sternum (*arrows*) is bent backward, compressing the heart. The heart is displaced to the left on the frontal view. The lower part of the heart appears lucent.

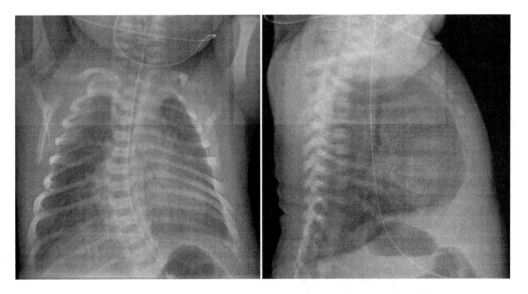

Fig. 11.51 Idiopathic thoracic scoliosis in a newborn infant with total anomalous pulmonary venous connection. The curvature is rather prominent but gentle. The spinal curvature is also abnormal on the lateral view. No vertebral segmentation abnormalities are seen.

heart disease surgery are at a higher risk of developing scoliosis or kyphosis later in life.[34,35]

Finally, skeletal manifestations of systemic diseases can be appreciated on the chest radiographs. Systemic diseases affecting connective tissues, such as Marfan, Loeys Dietz, and Ehlers-Danlos syndromes, frequently show deformity of the thoracic cage with scoliosis, kyphosis, and pectus excavatum (**Fig. 11.53**).

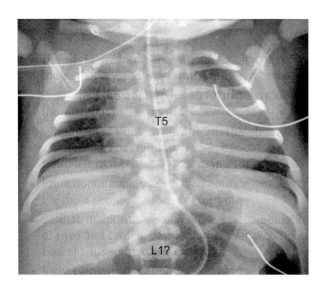

Fig. 11.52 Spinal segmentation abnormalities in a newborn with mitral atresia, transposition of the great arteries, and pulmonary atresia. The lower thoracic spine show multiple segmentation abnormalities including butterfly vertebrae and lateral hemivertebrae. Note the asymmetric development and orientation of the ribs. There is mild scoliosis.

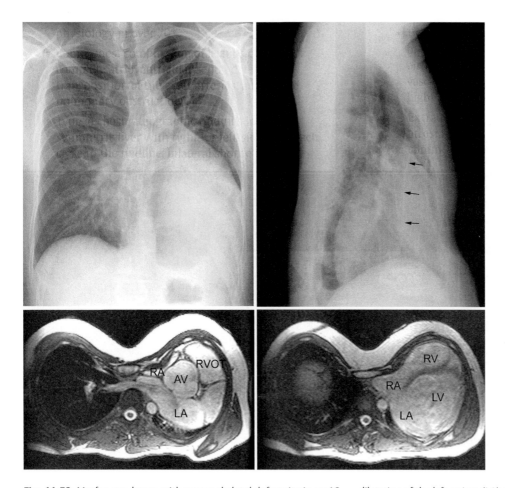

Fig. 11.53 Marfan syndrome with severe skeletal deformity in an 18-year-old patient. The sternum shows severe bowing backward (*arrows*), leaving a small space for the heart as shown on MR images. The heart is displaced into the left thorax. There is moderate cardiomegaly with dilatation of the left atrium (LA) and left ventricle (LV) due to aortic and mitral regurgitation. The aortic valve (AV) sinuses are markedly dilated. The right atrium (RA) and right ventricle (RV) are squashed. RVOT, right ventricular outflow tract.

Pearls

- Airway compression can result from abnormal vascular structures such as vascular rings and aneurysmally dilated vessels. It can also be due to normally formed but abnormally positioned vascular structures. The severity of vascular compression depends not only on vascular pathology but also on the size and shape of the thoracic cage.

- Pulmonary artery sling is commonly associated with an abnormal branching pattern of the airway and congenital tracheal stenosis.

- Collapse of the left lower lobe is common in patients with a large heart especially when the left atrium or left ventricle is enlarged.

- Hypoplasia of a lung is seen in scimitar syndrome, unilateral absence of a branch pulmonary artery,

and unilateral pulmonary vein stenosis or atresia, although it may occur as an isolated anomaly.

- In the supine position, pneumothorax tends to collect anteromedially along the heart border.

- Absence or very small size of the thymic shadow in the first day of life is highly suggestive of microdeletion 22q11.2 syndrome.

- Blurred diaphragmatic contour with air-filled lungs extending below the cardiac silhouette on a frontal radiograph suggests significant air trapping in the lungs with flat or inverted diaphragm.

- Rib notching is an infrequent manifestation of coarctation of the aorta in children. Asymmetrically increased sclerosis of the lower margins of the ribs is more commonly seen.

References

1. Yoo SJ, Bradley TJ. Vascular rings, pulmonary artery sling and related conditions. In: Anderson RH, Baker EJ, Penny DJ, et al, eds. Pediatric Cardiology, 3rd ed. Philadelphia: Elsevier; in press

2. Kim YM, Yoo SJ, Kim TH, et al. Tracheal compression by elongated aortic arch in patients with congenitally corrected transposition of the great arteries. Pediatr Cardiol 2001;22:471–477

3. Kim YM, Yoo SJ, Kim WH, Kim TH, Joh JH, Kim SJ. Bronchial compression by posteriorly displaced ascending aorta in patients with congenital heart disease. Ann Thorac Surg 2002;73:881–886

4. Dodge-Khatami A, Tulevski II, Hitchcock JF, de Mol BA, Bennink GB. Vascular rings and pulmonary arterial sling: from respiratory collapse to surgical cure, with emphasis on judicious imaging in the hi-tech era. Cardiol Young 2002;12:96–104

5. Philip S, Chen SY, Wu MH, Wang JK, Lue HC. Retroesophageal aortic arch: diagnostic and therapeutic implications of a rare vascular ring. Int J Cardiol 2001;79:133–141

6. Berdon WE, Baker DH, Bordiuk J, Mellins R. Innominate artery compression of the trachea in infants with stridor and apnea. Radiology 1969;92:272–278

7. Strife JL, Baumel AS, Dunbar JS. Tracheal compression by the innominate artery in infancy and childhood. Radiology 1981;139:73–75

8. Weinberger M, Abu-Hasan M. Pseudo-asthma: when cough, wheezing, and dyspnea are not asthma. Pediatrics 2007;120:855–864

9. Wells TR, Gwinn JL, Landing BH, Stanley P. Reconsideration of the anatomy of sling left pulmonary artery: the association of one form with bridging bronchus and imperforate anus. Anatomic and diagnostic aspects. J Pediatr Surg 1988;23:892–898

10. Fiore AC, Brown JW, Weber TR, Turrentine MW. Surgical treatment of pulmonary artery sling and tracheal stenosis. Ann Thorac Surg 2005;79:38–46, discussion 38–46

11. Ghaye B, Szapiro D, Fanchamps JM, Dondelinger RF. Congenital bronchial abnormalities revisited. Radiographics 2001;21:105–119

12. Doolittle AM, Mair EA. Tracheal bronchus: classification, endoscopic analysis, and airway management. Otolaryngol Head Neck Surg 2002;126:240–243

13. O'Sullivan BP, Frassica JJ, Rayder SM. Tracheal bronchus: a cause of prolonged atelectasis in intubated children. Chest 1998;113:537–540

14. Moncada RM, Venta LA, Venta ER, Fareed J, Walenga JM, Messmore HL. Tracheal and bronchial cartilaginous rings: warfarin sodium-induced calcification. Radiology 1992;184:437–439

15. Brunnée T, Graf K, Kastens B, Fleck E, Kunkel G. Bronchial hyperreactivity in patients with moderate pulmonary circulation overload. Chest 1993;103:1477–1481

16. Worsley DF, Alavi A, Aronchick JM, Chen JT, Greenspan RH, Ravin CE. Chest radiographic findings in patients with acute pulmonary embolism: observations from the PIOPED Study. Radiology 1993;189:133–136

17. Williamson WA, Tronic BS, Levitan N, Webb-Johnson DC, Shahian DM, Ellis FH Jr. Pulmonary venous infarction. Chest 1992;102:937–940

18. Freedom RM, Yoo SJ, Goo HW, Mikailian H, Anderson RH. The bronchopulmonary foregut malformation complex. Cardiol Young 2006;16:229–251

19. Griffin N, Mansfield L, Redmond KC, et al. Imaging features of isolated unilateral pulmonary artery agenesis presenting in adulthood: a review of four cases. Clin Radiol 2007;62:238–244

20. Figa FH, Yoo SJ, Burrows PE, Turner-Gomes S, Freedom RM. Horseshoe lung—a case report with unusual bronchial and pleural anomalies and a proposed new classification. Pediatr Radiol 1993;23:44–47

21. Yoo SJ, Al-Otay A, Babyn P. The relationship between scimitar syndrome, so-called scimitar variant, meandering right pulmonary vein, horseshoe lung and pulmonary arterial sling. Cardiol Young 2006;16:300–304

22. Pearl W. Scimitar variant. Pediatr Cardiol 1987;8:139–141

23. Heyneman LE, Nolan RL, Harrison JK, McAdams HP. Congenital unilateral pulmonary vein atresia: radiologic findings in three adult patients. AJR Am J Roentgenol 2001;177:681–685

24. Kataoka H. Pericardial and pleural effusions in decompensated chronic heart failure. Am Heart J 2000;139:918–923

25. Woodring JH. Distribution of pleural effusion in congestive heart failure: what is atypical? South Med J 2005;98:518–523

26. Kouerinis IA, Hountis PA, Loutsidis AK, Bellenis IP. Spontaneous pneumothorax: are we missing something? Interact Cardiovasc Thorac Surg 2004;3:272–273

27. Yamagishi H. The 22q11.2 deletion syndrome. Keio J Med 2002;51:77–88

28. Chen CM, Yu KY, Lin HC, Yeh GC, Hsu HH. Thymus size and its relationship to perinatal events. Acta Paediatr 2000;89:975–978

29. Glavina-Durdov M, Springer O, Capkun V, Saratlija-Novaković Z, Rozić D, Barle M. The grade of acute thymus involution in neonates correlates with the duration of acute illness and with the percentage of lymphocytes in peripheral blood smear. Pathological study. Biol Neonate 2003;83:229–234

30. Matzinger MA, Briggs VA, Dunlap HJ, Udjus K, Martin DJ, McDonald P. Plain film and CT observations in prostaglandin-induced bone changes. Pediatr Radiol 1992;22:264–266

31. Nadroo AM, Shringari S, Garg M, al-Sowailem AM. Prostaglandin induced cortical hyperostosis in neonates with cyanotic heart disease. J Perinat Med 2000;28:447–452

32. Davies MK, Mackintosh P, Cayton RM, Page AJ, Shiu MF, Littler WA. The straight back syndrome. Q J Med 1980;49:443–460

33. Basu PS, Elsebaie H, Noordeen MH. Congenital spinal deformity: a comprehensive assessment at presentation. Spine 2002;27:2255–2259

34. Kawakami N, Mimatsu K, Deguchi M, Kato F, Maki S. Scoliosis and congenital heart disease. Spine 1995;20:1252–1255, discussion 1256

35. Herrera-Soto JA, Vander Have KL, Barry-Lane P, Myers JL. Retrospective study on the development of spinal deformities following sternotomy for congenital heart disease. Spine 2007;32:1998–2004

III Individual Heart Diseases

Chest radiographs may show characteristic findings in some heart diseases or nonspecific findings such as cardiomegaly and an abnormal vascular pattern in others. They play a limited role in the diagnosis of heart diseases. Nevertheless, the assessment of disease severity and recognition of the unusual manifestations of known disease as well as identification of unrecognized conditions require knowledge os radiographic manifestations of individual heart diseases. Using a bulleted format, basic pathologic features, clinical manifestations, and radiographic findings are summarized in this section.

12 Lesions with Left-to-Right Shunt

With Christian J. Kellenberger

Definition and Classification

- A spectrum of lesions with either an intracardiac or extracardiac communication whose fundamental abnormality is allowing blood to shunt from the higher pressure systemic circulation to the lower pressure pulmonic circulation, resulting in oxygenated blood recirculating through the lungs
- Levels of shunt
  - Intracardiac
    - *Atrial septal defects* (**Fig. 12.1**)
      - Patent foramen ovale: persistence of fetal pathway from the right atrium to the left atrium
      - Fossa ovalis defect (also called secundum defect): one or more holes in the floor of the fossa ovalis
      - Primum defect: a form of atrioventricular septal defect with the bridging leaflets of the common atrioventricular valve attached to the ventricular septal crest
      - Sinus venosus defect: a defect involving the most posterior and cranial part of the wall between the right and left atria; usually associated with an anomalous connection of the right upper pulmonary vein to the superior vena cava.
      - Coronary sinus defect: primarily a defect of the wall between the left atrium and the coronary sinus. The coronary sinus ostium appears and functions as an atrial septal defect. It is often associated with a persistent left superior vena cava. When the wall between the left atrium and the coronary sinus is completely unroofed, the coronary sinus ostium is an interatrial communication channel and the left superior vena cava appears to connect directly to the roof of the left atrium.
    - *Atrioventricular septal defects* (endocardial cushion defects) (**Fig. 12.2**)
      - With both interatrial and interventricular shunts: The bridging leaflets of the common

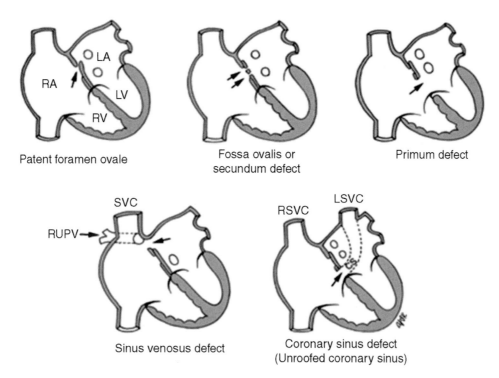

Patent foramen ovale

Fossa ovalis or secundum defect

Primum defect

Sinus venosus defect

Coronary sinus defect (Unroofed coronary sinus)

Fig. 12.1 Atrial septal defects. RUPV, right upper pulmonary vein; SVC, superior vena cava; CS, coronary sinus; LSVC, left superior vena cava; RSVC, right superior vena cava; RA, right atrium; LA, left atrium; RV, right ventricle; LV, left ventricle.

Atrioventricular septal defects

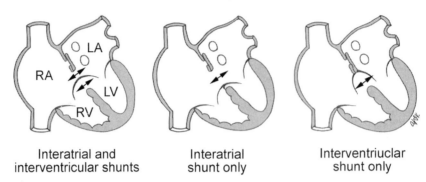

| Interatrial and interventricular shunts | Interatrial shunt only | Interventriuclar shunt only |

Fig. 12.2 Atrioventricular septal defects. LA, left atrium; LV, left ventricle; RA, right atrium; RV, right ventricle.

atrioventricular valve are free floating across the defect or have chordal attachment to the ventricular septal crest.

○ With interatrial shunt only: The bridging leaflets are completely attached to the ventricular septal crest, leaving the defect exclusively between the atria.

○ With interventricular shunt only: Very rarely, the bridging leaflets are attached to the defective atrial septal margin, leaving the defect exclusively between the ventricles.

– *Ventricular septal defects* (**Fig. 12.3**). Classified according to the location of the defect within the septum seen from the right ventricle and its relationships to the membranous septum, atrioventricular valves, and semilunar valves.

○ Perimembranous defects: the most common type and involves the membranous septum and adjacent muscular septum

○ Muscular defects: completely surrounded by the muscle

○ Doubly committed juxtaarterial defect: involves the most cranial part of the septum. The aortic

and pulmonary valves are in fibrous continuity in the roof of the defect.

○ Non-perimembranous, juxtatricuspid defect: exceedingly rare defect involving the inlet part of the muscular ventricular septum along the tricuspid annulus

• Extracardiac arterial

– Ruptured sinus of Valsalva

– Coronary artery-cameral fistulas

– Anomalous coronary artery arising from the pulmonary artery

– Aortopulmonary window

– Patent ductus arteriosus

• Extracardiac venous

– Partial anomalous pulmonary venous connections

□ Atrial, atrioventricular, and ventricular septal defects as well as patent ductus arteriosus, which constitute most left-to-right shunt lesions, are discussed below.

Pathophysiology

□ Distinguished by different anatomic communications: The common denominator is that the pulmonary flow is greater than systemic flow.

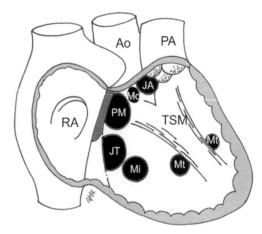

Modified Soto's classification of ventricular septal defects

Perimembranous (PM) defect
Muscular defects:
- In inlet septum (Mi)
- In trabecular septum (Mt)
- In outlet septum (Mo)
Doubly-committed
juxta-arterial (JA) defect
Juxtatricupsid (JT),
non-perimembranous defect

Fig. 12.3 Ventricular septal defects. RA, right atrium; Ao, ascending aorta; PA, pulmonary artery; TSM, trabecular septomarginalis.

□ Coexisting cardiac lesions may significantly affect shunt volume.

□ Hemodynamic severity varies according to the site of the defect.

- *Atrial septal defect*
  - Hemodynamics of an atrial septal defect are determined by the relative filling resistances of the right and left ventricles rather than the size of the defect.
  - Right ventricular compliance increases, resulting in right ventricular dilatation.
- *Atrioventricular septal defect*
  - Hemodynamics of an atrioventricular septal defect depend on the type and extent of the anomaly and include shunting of blood across the interatrial and interventricular components of the defect and the regurgitation of blood into atria through incompetent atrioventricular valves.
- *Ventricular septal defect*
  - Hemodynamics of a ventricular septal defect are determined by the size of the defect and the pressure difference between the left and right ventricles, with the right ventricular pressure reflecting the pulmonary vascular resistance.
  - Secondary complications associated with a ventricular septal defect
    ○ Adherent tricuspid valve tissue resulting in left ventricle–right atrial shunting
    ○ Obstructive right ventricular muscle bundles
    ○ Subaortic ridge with stenosis
    ○ Aortic valve prolapse with aortic regurgitation
    ○ Dilatation of sinus of Valsalva with aortic-right ventricular fistula
- *Patent ductus arteriosus*
  - Hemodynamics of a patent ductus arteriosus are determined by the size of the defect and pulmonary/aortic systolic pressure gradient.
  - Blood flow may be right-to-left with persistent fetal circulation.
  - Closure is delayed in premature infants with respiratory distress and hypoxia.

□ Over time, pulmonary arterial vasculature responds to high flow and high pressures by undergoing medial hypertrophy and endothelial thickening, leading to increased pulmonary vascular resistance and ultimately irreversible pulmonary hypertension.

□ Eisenmenger's physiology occurs when the pulmonary artery pressure equals or exceeds aortic pressure resulting in a right-to-left shunt.

Clinical Manifestations

□ Variable age of presentation depending on size and location of communication
- *Atrial septal defect*
  - Even large defects may be asymptomatic and go undetected into adulthood.
  - Clinically significant lesions may cause exercise limitation, dyspnea, fatigue due to right heart volume and sometimes pressure overload.
  - Rare cause of congestive heart failure or pulmonary infections
  - Long-standing lesions may lead to pulmonary arterial hypertension and Eisenmenger's physiology.
  - Associated with several syndromes including Holt-Oram and Ellis-van Creveld
- *Atrioventricular septal defect*
  - May present at birth or within first few days of life depending on degree of shunting and atrioventricular valve regurgitation
  - Defect with interatrial shunt only (so-called primum defect) may simply cause exercise limitation, dyspnea, fatigue due to right heart volume, and sometimes pressure overload.
  - Defect with both interatrial and interventricular shunts may present with congestive heart failure and recurrent pulmonary infections.
  - Tendency to develop premature pulmonary vascular disease and pulmonary arterial hypertension
  - Most commonly diagnosed congenital heart defect with trisomy 21
  - Frequently associated with isomerism syndromes
- *Ventricular septal defect*
  - Small defect, asymptomatic
  - Neonates are often asymptomatic due to high pulmonary vascular resistance.
  - Moderate defect associated with irritability, fatigue, poor feeding, and recurrent pulmonary infections
  - Large defect usually symptomatic at 4 to 6 weeks of age with congestive heart failure due to a decrease in pulmonary vascular resistance
  - Long-standing large defects may lead to pulmonary hypertension and Eisenmenger's physiology.
  - Most common lesion associated with other congenital defects and an important part of more complex anomalies
  - Occurs with various trisomy chromosomal syndromes
- *Patent ductus arteriosus*
  - May be silent and asymptomatic
  - May present with a continuous asymptomatic murmur
  - May present early with congestive heart failure in premature infants when there is a decrease in pulmonary vascular resistance
  - May present later with congestive heart failure or failure to thrive in full-term infants
  - May result in substantial pulmonary hypertension and Eisenmenger's physiology
  - Complications of an aneurysm of the ductus arteriosus include embolization of thrombi, rupture,

infection, and phrenic and recurrent laryngeal nerve palsy.

Chest Radiographic Findings

□ Depicts the physiology of the lesion, but is not diagnostic of the individual lesion (**Table 12.1**)
□ Depicts a lesion only if there is at least a 2:1 left-to-right shunt
  • *Atrial septal defect* (Cases 12.1, 12.2)
    – Increased pulmonary vasculature with an overcirculation pattern
    – Proportionate or often marked enlargement of main pulmonary artery
    – Normal to slightly enlarged cardiac size
    – Right ventricle and right atrium enlarged
    – Left atrium not enlarged
    – Marked cardiomegaly indicates additional complication of atrioventricular valve regurgitation or right heart failure
    – Aortic knob appears small due to the prominent pulmonary artery and rotation of the heart from right ventricular enlargement.
    – Superior vena cava may be inapparent due to mediastinal rotation.
  • *Atrioventricular septal defect* (Cases 12.3, 12.4)
    – With interatrial shunt only (so-called primum defect)
      ○ Increased pulmonary vasculature with an overcirculation pattern
      ○ Proportionate enlarged main pulmonary artery
      ○ Normal to slightly enlarged cardiac size
    – With both interatrial and interventricular shunts
      ○ Markedly increased pulmonary vasculature with mixed overcirculation pattern and pulmonary venous hypertension with edema
      ○ Proportionate enlargement of main pulmonary artery
      ○ Moderate to severe cardiomegaly
      ○ Biventricular enlargement
      ○ Biatrial or right atrial enlargement
      ○ Aortic knob inapparent
      ○ Large shunt with reduced pulmonary compliance causes marked overinflation of the lungs.
  • *Ventricular septal defect* (Cases 12.5, 12.6, 12.7)
    – Increased pulmonary vasculature with an overcirculation pattern
    – Pulmonary venous hypertension with edema in infants with large shunts
    – Proportionate enlargement of main pulmonary artery
    – Degree of cardiomegaly proportionate to size of shunt
    – Biventricular enlargement and left atrial enlargement
    – Right atrium not enlarged unless complicated by a left ventricle-to-right atrial shunt

– Aortic knob is normal to unapparent unless complicated by aortic insufficiency.
– Large shunt with reduced pulmonary compliance causes overinflation of lungs.
– Left lower lobe atelectasis complication of bronchial compression with severe left atrial enlargement
– Decrease in pulmonary overcirculation and heart size may result from spontaneous closure of the ventricular septal defect, development of obstructive right ventricular muscle bundles or development of pulmonary hypertension.
  • *Patent ductus arteriosus* (Cases 12.8, 12.9)
    – Premature infant best diagnosed by evaluating a series of chest radiographs
      ○ Increasing ill-defined ground glass parenchymal densities due to interstitial pulmonary edema
      ○ Increasing heart size
    – Full-term infant
      ○ Mildly to moderately increased pulmonary vasculature with overcirculation pattern
      ○ Proportionate enlargement of main pulmonary artery
      ○ Mild to moderate cardiomegaly
      ○ Left ventricular and left atrial enlargement
      ○ Right heart not enlarged
      ○ Prominent bulge below aortic knob due to enlarged ductus
      ○ Enlarged ascending aorta and aortic knob in older children
    – Aneurysm of the ductus arteriosus (Case 12.10)
      ○ Focal mass in the left mediastinum in the region of the aorticopulmonary window
□ Long-standing Eisenmenger's physiology
  • Decreased size of peripheral pulmonary vessels
  • Disproportionately enlarged main pulmonary artery and tortuous hilar arteries
  • Cardiac size becomes smaller.
  • Left atrial enlargement disappears.
  • Right ventricular enlargement
  • Right atrium may be enlarged due to tricuspid regurgitation with right heart failure.
  • Aortic knob normal to unapparent

Table 12.1   Summary of Chamber Enlargement in Common Shunt Lesions

	RA	RV	LA	LV	AO	PA
ASD	↑	↑	-	-	-	↑↑
AVSD	↑↑	↑	↑ or -	↑	-	↑↑
VSD	-	↑	↑	↑	-	↑
PDA	-	-	↑	↑	↑	↑

Abbreviations: RA, right atrium; RV, right ventricle; LA, left atrium; LV, left ventricle; AO, ascending aorta; PA, pulmonary artery; ASD, atrial septal defect; AVSD, atrioventricular septal defect; VSD, ventricular septal defect; PDA, patent ductus arteriosus

Pearls

- Neonatal presentation of patent ductus arteriosus is found in premature infants.

- Infant presentation of ventricular septal defect is usually with additional left-sided obstructive lesion or complete atrioventricular septal defect.

- Older infant or childhood presentation is found in cases of atrial septal defect, small ventricular septal defect, patent ductus arteriosus, or atrioventricular septal defect with an interatrial shunt only.

- Enlarged left atrium suggests that the atrial septum is intact and the shunt is at the ventricular or supracardiac level.

- Difficult to distinguish patent ductus arteriosus from ventricular septal defect

- Normal left atrium suggests an atrial level shunt.

- Enlarged aorta indicates supracardiac shunt.

- Both right and left isomerisms are commonly associated with an atrioventricular septal defect.

Case 12.1

Atrial septal defect in a 17-year-old patient. Chest radiographs show moderate cardiomegaly with increased pulmonary vascularity. The retrosternal clear space on the lateral view is obliterated by the dilated right ventricle and main pulmonary artery. There are no signs of left atrial enlargement. Right atrial enlargement is also not obvious on chest radiographs despite obvious dilatation of the right atrium (RA) and right ventricle (RV) in magnetic resonance images. The left atrium (LA) and left ventricle (LV) are not dilated. Note a defect (D) in the central part of the interatrial septum in axial image. The estimated pulmonary-to-systemic flow ratio (Qp/Qs) was 2.5. Ao, ascending aorta; PA, pulmonary artery.

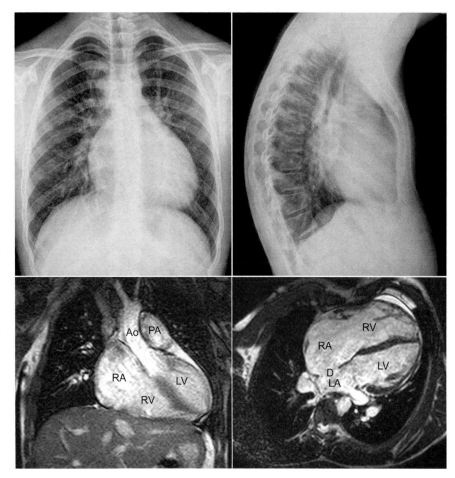

Case 12.2

Atrial septal defect. Chest radiograph obtained at age 9 years shows mild cardiomegaly with a moderately enlarged main pulmonary artery and mildly increased pulmonary vasculature due to shunting across a secundum atrial septal defect. A follow-up study at age 15 years shows further enlargement of the heart and dilation of the pulmonary vasculature.

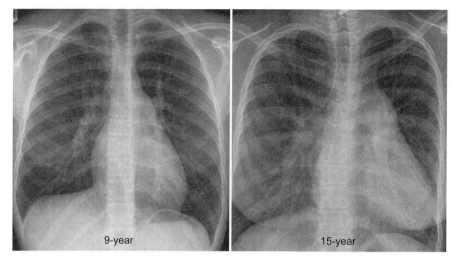

Case 12.3

Atrioventricular septal defect in a 15-day-old infant. Chest radiographs show moderate cardiomegaly with specific right atrial enlargement, enlarged main pulmonary artery, increased pulmonary vasculature, and interstitial pulmonary edema. Aortic knob is inapparent. There is hypersegmentation of the sternal manubrium, which is a skeletal stigma of trisomy 21.

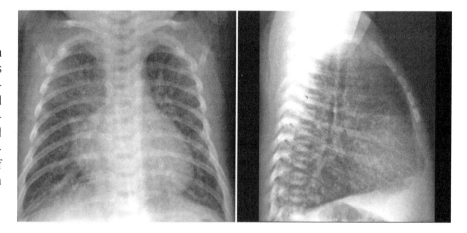

Case 12.4

Atrioventricular septal defect in a 5-month-old infant. Chest radiographs show moderate cardiomegaly with biventricular and right atrial enlargement, enlarged main pulmonary artery with increased pulmonary vasculature, and hyperinflation of both lungs.

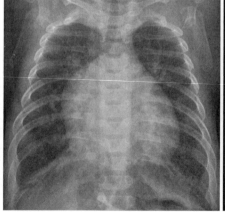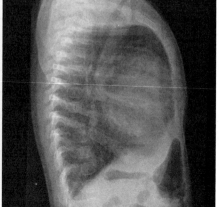

Case 12.5

Moderate-sized perimembranous ventricular septal defect in a 2-day-old infant. Chest radiograph shows moderate cardiomegaly, enlarged main pulmonary artery, and increased pulmonary vasculature. A follow-up study at age 2 weeks shows congestive heart failure with pulmonary edema due to a decrease in pulmonary vascular resistance.

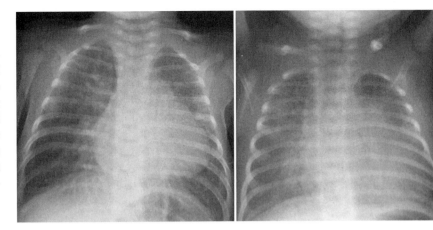

Case 12.6

Moderate-sized perimembranous ventricular septal defect in a 2-year-old child. Chest radiographs show moderate cardiomegaly, enlarged main pulmonary artery, and increased pulmonary vasculature with hyperinflation and no associated pulmonary edema.

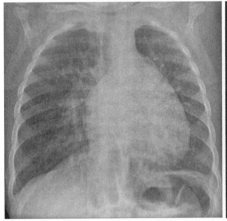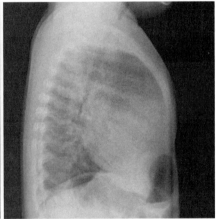

Case 12.7

Ventricular septal defect in an 11-year-old child. Chest radiographs show long-standing Eisenmenger stage defect with normal heart size, disproportionately enlarged main pulmonary artery, and tortuous hilar arteries with decreased peripheral pulmonary vasculature.

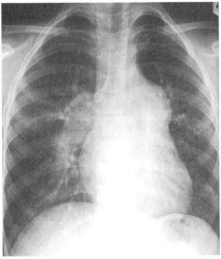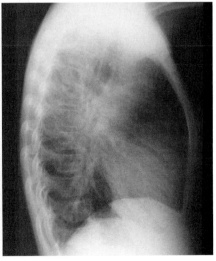

Case 12.8

Patent ductus arteriosus in a premature infant at 2 days of age. Chest radiographs shows mild cardiomegaly with small granular lungs appearing as respiratory distress syndrome (left panel). Several days later, a follow-up study shows progressive cardiomegaly and extensive pulmonary edema resulting from shunting across a patent ductus arteriosus (right panel).

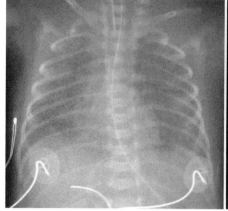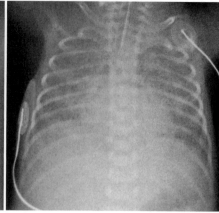

Case 12.9

Patent ductus arteriosus in an 8-year-old child. Chest radiographs show mild cardiomegaly, moderately enlarged main pulmonary artery, increased pulmonary vasculature, and an enlarged aortic knob.

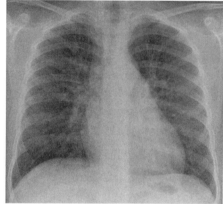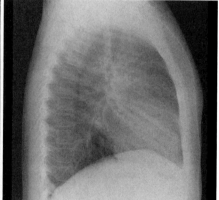

Case 12.10

Aneurysm of ductus arteriosus in an 11-day-old infant. Chest radiograph shows a focal mass (*arrows*) in the region of the aorticopulmonary window in the left upper mediastinum. Reconstructed computed tomography (CT) images show the aneurysm of the ductus at the aortic end. The pulmonary arterial end was occluded. asc, ascending; desc, descending.

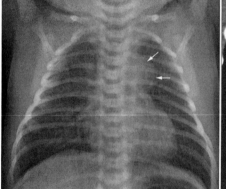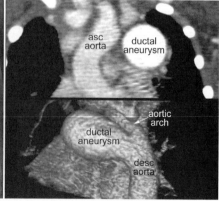

13 Truncus Arteriosus
With Christian J. Kellenberger

Definition and Classification

- Characterized by a single great artery arising from the base of the heart, which gives origin to systemic, pulmonary, and coronary arteries
- Presence of only one arterial trunk is necessary for the diagnosis without any remnant of an atretic pulmonary artery or aorta.
- Almost always centered over a large ventricular septal defect
- Commonly used synonyms: persistent truncus arteriosus and common arterial trunk
- Collett and Edwards's classification relates to the site of origin of the pulmonary arteries from the common arterial trunk (**Fig. 13.1**, upper panel)
  - *Type I:* Origin of a short main pulmonary artery from the base of the truncus
  - *Type II:* Separate posterior origins of pulmonary artery branches from the truncus
  - *Type III:* Separate lateral origins of pulmonary artery branches from the truncus

- *Type IV:* Branches to the lungs originating from descending aorta; this type is regarded as a variant of tetralogy of Fallot with pulmonary atresia in which each lung is supplied by a major aortopulmonary collateral artery.
- Van Praagh and Van Praagh's modification (**Fig. 13.1**, lower panel)
  - *Type A1:* Origin of a main pulmonary artery from the base of the truncus
  - *Type A2:* Separate origins of pulmonary artery branches from the truncus
  - *Type A3:* Absent left, right, or both pulmonary arteries, with the absent pulmonary artery originating from a ductus arteriosus or collateral artery
  - *Type A4:* With obstructive lesion of the aortic arch

Pathophysiology

- Intracardiac admixture lesion at ventricular septal defect level due to similar pressures in both ventricles

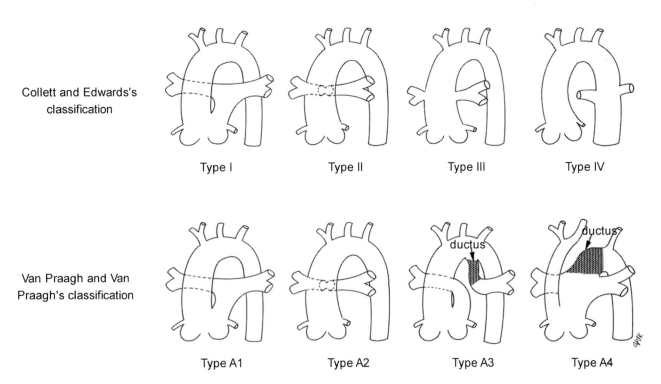

Collett and Edwards's classification

Type I   Type II   Type III   Type IV

Van Praagh and Van Praagh's classification

Type A1   Type A2   Type A3   Type A4

Fig. 13.1 Collett and Edwards's (*top panel*) and Van Praagh and Van Praagh's (*bottom panel*) classification systems.

□ Extracardiac left-to-right shunt at truncal level with a significant increase in pulmonary flow when pulmonary vascular resistance decreases

□ Occasionally the pulmonary blood flow may be restrictive when there is associated obstruction
  • Ostial stenosis from an obstructive truncal leaflet
  • Pulmonary artery may be underdeveloped and hypoplastic or have an intrinsic stenosis.

□ Truncal valve composed of one to six cusps with thickened and dysplastic leaflets, which may function normally or be stenotic, regurgitant, or both, resulting in left and right ventricular pressure and volume overload

□ Coronary artery circulation has a variable pattern of origins, and a coronary ostium may be congenitally stenotic or obstructed by a truncal valve leaflet, resulting in an ischemic cardiomyopathy.

Clinical Manifestations

□ Classically characterized as a cyanotic heart lesion

□ Infants and small children with low pulmonary resistance present with early congestive heart failure, frequent respiratory infections, and growth retardation, and cyanosis may be minimal or absent.

□ High mortality rate in early infancy due to congestive heart failure, often with an ischemic cardiomyopathy

□ Protective pulmonary vascular obstructive disease or pulmonary artery obstruction prolongs survival.

□ Frequent association with DiGeorge syndrome

□ Slightly increased incidence with maternal diabetes

□ Uncommonly associated with atrioventricular septal defect, tricuspid atresia, other forms of univentricular atrioventricular connection, hypoplastic left ventricle, and total anomalous pulmonary venous return

Chest Radiographic Findings

□ Clinical and radiographic findings, when correlated together, are often diagnostic.

□ Findings may range from being highly suggestive of truncus arteriosus to mimicking more common forms of heart disease, often with complete transposition of the great vessels or a large ventricular septal defect in failure.

□ In the first few days of life, pulmonary vasculature is markedly increased with mixed pulmonary overcirculation and pulmonary venous hypertension with edema as pulmonary vascular resistance decreases.

□ Branch pulmonary arteries can be seen as discrete structures arising at a higher level than normal.

□ Abnormally high left hilum is uncommon but is valuable when present.

□ Rarely, the pulmonary vasculature may be decreased or asymmetric due to hypoplasia, stenosis, or absence of a branch pulmonary artery.

□ In an older child with normal or only slightly increased pulmonary vasculature and lack of significant cardiomegaly, development of pulmonary vascular disease should be suspected.

□ Substantial cardiomegaly with enlargement of both ventricles and left atrium due to central shunting across the ventricular septal defect and an extracardiac left-to-right shunt

□ Left atrium, significantly enlarged due to increased pulmonary venous return

□ Cardiac enlargement may increase with development of an ischemic cardiomyopathy.

□ Typically, an oval cardiac configuration due to biventricular enlargement, absence or hypoplasia of the right ventricular outflow tract

□ Occasionally boot-shaped configuration

□ Concave main pulmonary artery segment

□ Occasionally, a well-defined convexity of the pulmonary arterial segment due to a pseudopulmonary artery trunk or a prominent left pulmonary artery arising from the left lateral aspect of the truncus

□ Aortic arch is often right-sided

□ Truncal root may be quite dilated when there is stenosis or regurgitation of the truncal valve

□ Mediastinum is narrow due to absence of the pulmonary trunk and a small thymus, which may be stress related or due to hypoplasia or aplasia in association with DiGeorge syndrome.

□ Associated bronchial compression from the truncal root or pulmonary arteries may result in uneven lung aeration with hyperaeration and segmental atelectasis.

□ Associated with a high incidence of pneumonia

□ High incidence of associated skeletal anomalies

Pearls

□ Truncus arteriosus should be highly suspected with findings of moderate to severe cardiomegaly showing an egg-on-side or boot-shaped appearance, a small thymic shadow, and a right aortic arch occurring with prominent pulmonary vascularity of the overcirculation type.

Case 13.1

Truncus arteriosus in a 4-day-old infant. Chest radiographs show moderate cardiomegaly with a typical oval configuration, concave pulmonary arterial segment of the left heart border, and increased pulmonary vascularity with mild venous congestion. The superior mediastinum is narrow in the frontal view, and the retrosternal space is devoid of tissue in the lateral view, suggesting thymic hypoplasia or aplasia associated with DiGeorge syndrome.

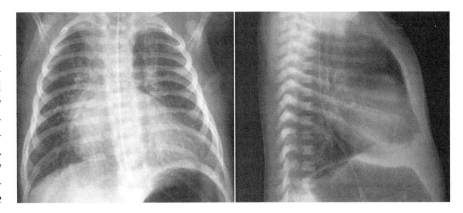

Case 13.2

Truncus arteriosus in a 1-day-old infant. Chest radiograph shows mild cardiomegaly with an oval configuration and a straight left upper heart border, narrow mediastinum with a concave main pulmonary artery, pulmonary overcirculation with mild venous congestion, and a left aortic arch. The findings are indistinguishable from those of complete transposition of the great arteries.

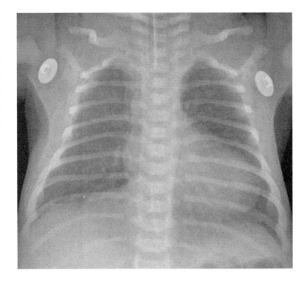

Case 13.3

Truncus arteriosus in a 1-month-old infant. Chest radiographs show moderate cardiomegaly with an oval configuration, high prominent hilar pulmonary arteries, increased pulmonary overcirculation with pulmonary venous hypertension, and a narrow mediastinum. Lungs are hyperinflated with an interstitial pattern of pulmonary edema.

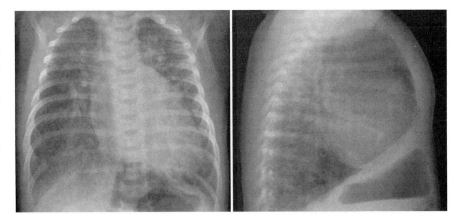

Case 13.4

Truncus arteriosus in a 6-day-old infant. Chest radiograph shows a boot-shaped heart with round cardiac apex and concave pulmonary arterial segment of the left heart border. The pulmonary vascularity is markedly increased.

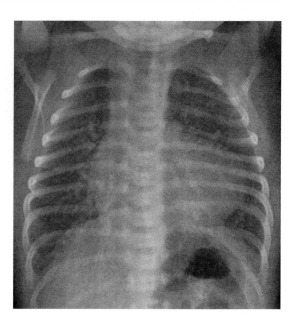

14 Ebstein's Malformation and Other Forms of Congenital Tricuspid Regurgitation

With Christian J. Kellenberger

Definition and Classification

- Any abnormality of the tricuspid valve resulting in congenital tricuspid regurgitation of varying severity
- Ebstein's malformation (**Fig. 14.1**) results from downward displacement of tricuspid valve tissue attachment below the normal annulus and dividing the right ventricle into a proximal atrialized portion and a distal functional right ventricle. Displaced attachment typically involves the septal and posterior leaflets of the valve. The anterior leaflet does not usually show displaced attachment but is usually large and sail-like. As the leaflet edges are not aligned properly, varying degree of tricuspid regurgitation (**Fig. 14.1,** *arrows*) characterizes this malformation. Occasionally, the enlarged anterior leaflet may fuse with the displaced leaflets to form a sac of atrialized right ventricle, causing tricuspid stenosis or atresia. The latter form can be associated with functional or anatomic pulmonary atresia.
- Similar hemodynamic consequences in other congenital tricuspid valve malformations, with variable dysplasia having deficient leaflets, extra leaflets, unguarded tricuspid orifice, and isolated clefts
- Transient tricuspid insufficiency in infants caused by myocardial dysfunction most often secondary to pulmonary hypertension

- Isolated giant right atrial aneurysm a rare condition with idiopathic dilatation of the right atrium associated with tricuspid annular dilation and tricuspid regurgitation
- Associated lesions include congenitally corrected transposition, a variety of left heart lesions, and conduction anomalies

Pathophysiology

- Other than Ebstein's malformation, most anomalies of the tricuspid valve do not occur in isolation.
- Combination of displacement, dysplasia, and abnormal attachments of valve tissue produces tricuspid regurgitation
- The atrialized portion of the right ventricle is a thin-walled venous reservoir devoid of myocardium with ineffective contractions similar to Uhl's malformation of the right ventricle.
- The atrialized portion of the right ventricle and the true right atrium is a common chamber receiving the regurgitant flow.
- To-and-fro motion may cause functional obstruction of the right atrial outlet.
- Impeding right atrial emptying results in increased right atrial pressure and right-to-left atrial shunting

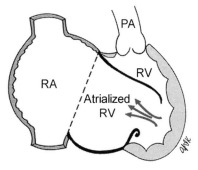

Non-stenotic form

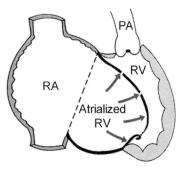

Stenotic form

Fig. 14.1 Ebstein's malformation of the right tricuspid valve. PA, pulmonary artery; RA, right atrium; RV, right ventricle.

with an associated patent foramen ovale or atrial septal defect.

□ Severity of right-to-left shunt across an atrial septal defect depends on the amount of tricuspid regurgitation and pulmonary vascular resistance.

□ The atrialized portion of the right ventricle reduces the size of the functional right ventricle.

□ Degree of impaired right ventricular function relates to the size of the atrialized portion.

Clinical Manifestations

□ Broad spectrum of clinical symptoms, which depend on degree of right ventricular atrialization, degree of tricuspid regurgitation, degree of right ventricular hypoplasia, and status of atrial septum

□ Mild form with good-sized functional right ventricle and minimal symptoms

□ Moderately symptomatic in later childhood or adolescence with variable degrees of cyanosis, cardiac arrhythmias, and exercise intolerance

□ Severe form presents in infancy with dyspnea, cyanosis, and right-sided heart failure

Chest Radiographic Findings

□ Variable depending on severity of malformation

□ Mild minimal findings

□ Moderate to severe proportionate findings related to degree of tricuspid regurgitation, right outflow tract obstruction, and right-to-left atrial shunting

□ Pulmonary vascularity tends to be normal or reduced when there is a significant right-to-left atrial shunt.

□ Small pulmonary arteries may also relate to hypoplastic lungs resulting from cardiac enlargement.

□ Flat main pulmonary artery segment

□ May be massive cardiomegaly due to right atrial enlargement

□ Cardiac configuration "box-like" from right atrial enlargement and an abnormal left cardiac contour due to a dilated right ventricular outflow tract, which is the only functional part of the right ventricle

□ Sharply defined right atrial border due to reduced contraction

□ Underdeveloped lungs and compressive atelectasis from the enlarged right heart chambers

---

Pearls

□ Common malformation in neonates or infants with severe cyanosis producing severe cardiomegaly in the first few days of life

□ Elevated right atrial pressures producing a right-to-left shunt across a patent foramen ovale or

associated atrial septal defect causes cyanosis

□ Severe form with characteristic wall-to-wall heart with massive right atrial enlargement

---

Case 14.1

Ebstein's malformation in a 9-day-old infant. Chest radiographs show a characteristic "wall-to-wall" heart due to massive dilatation of the right atrium and right ventricle related to tricuspid regurgitation. The lungs are underdeveloped with compressive atelectasis, and pulmonary vascularity is reduced related to small pulmonary arteries and right-to-left atrial shunting.

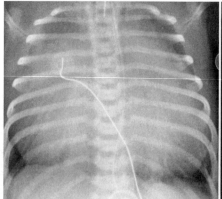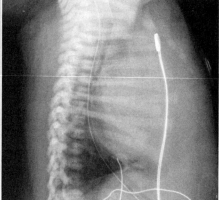

Case 14.2

Ebstein's malformation in a 2-year-old child with cyanosis. Chest radiographs show marked cardiomegaly with right atrial enlargement due to tricuspid regurgitation and dilatation of the right ventricular outlet that correlate very well with right atrial and right ventricular angiograms. Note that the retrosternal space is obliterated by the dilated right ventricular outflow tract. The pulmonary vascularity is mildly decreased indicating a right-to-left atrial shunt.

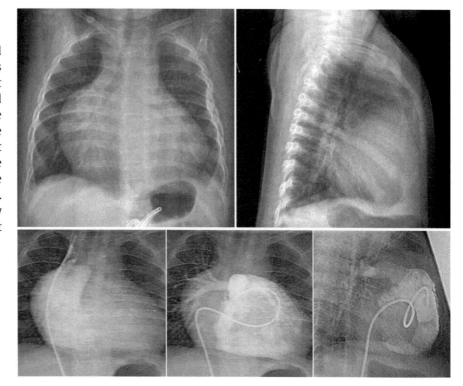

Case 14.3

Ebstein's malformation in a 2-year-old child. Chest radiographs show marked cardiomegaly with a "box-like" configuration due to massive right atrial enlargement and elevation of an enlarged right ventricular outflow tract and decreased pulmonary vascularity.

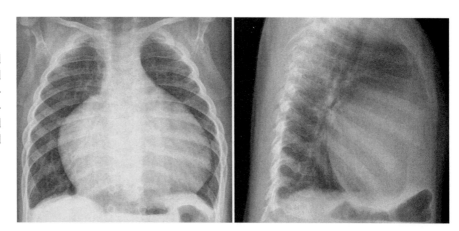

Case 14.4

Stenotic Ebstein's malformation with pulmonary stenosis in a 4-day-old infant. Chest radiographs show only mild cardiomegaly and diminished pulmonary vascularity. As there was no significant tricuspid regurgitation, the right atrial volume overload is only mild to moderate.

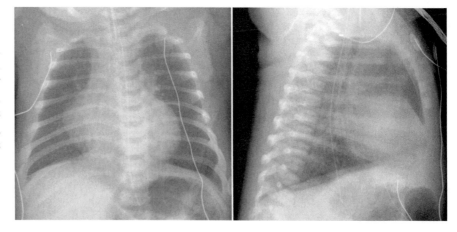

Case 14.5

Isolated giant right atrial aneurysm in a 1-week-old infant. Chest radiographs show marked cardiomegaly due to right atrial dilatation, which fills much of the right hemithorax, and normal pulmonary vascularity.

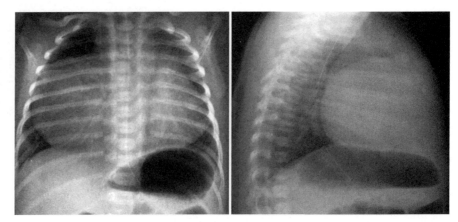

15 Tetralogy of Fallot and Related Conditions

With Christian J. Kellenberger

Definition and Classification

- Tetralogy of Fallot is composed of a constant set of the following four features, which result from anterior, superior, and leftward displacement of the outlet or infundibular septum relative to the rest of the septum (**Fig. 15.1**). The displaced outlet septum (door) encroaches on the right ventricular outflow tract (RVOT).
  - Large unrestricted ventricular septal defect
  - RVOT obstruction, predominantly subpulmonary muscular obstruction often with associated valvar and supravalvar stenosis
  - Overriding aorta
  - Right ventricular hypertrophy
- In severe form, tetralogy is associated with pulmonary atresia. The pulmonary arterial anatomy varies and the blood flow to the pulmonary arteries is through either a patent ductus arteriosus or collateral arteries arising from the aorta or its branches (**Fig. 15.2**). The collateral arteries are of congenital origin and called major aortopulmonary collateral arteries (MAPCAs) in contrast to acquired collateral arteries such as dilated bronchial and intercostal arteries.
- Tetralogy of Fallot is rarely associated with absent pulmonary syndrome in which the RVOT is guarded by vestigial valve tissue causing free pulmonary regurgitation from in utero life. The proximal pulmonary arteries in the mediastinum and lung hila are aneurysmally dilated.

- A large ventricular septal defect can be associated with an obstructing aberrant muscle bundle within the right ventricle above the septal defect, causing a hemodynamic effect similar to that in tetralogy of Fallot. This condition is called two- or double-chambered right ventricle.

Pathophysiology

- Hemodynamics of tetralogy are dependent on the degree of pulmonary stenosis and pulmonary arterial anatomy.
- Right-to-left shunt through the ventricular septal defect
- The more severe the pulmonary stenosis, the greater the right-to-left shunt through the ventricular septal defect, allowing blood flow from the right ventricle into the overriding aorta and reducing pulmonary blood flow.
- Mild pulmonary stenosis with a large ventricular septal defect resembles an isolated ventricular septal defect. This mild form is termed an acyanotic or pink tetralogy of Fallot.
- Atretic pulmonary outflow tract may be considered a severe form of tetralogy of Fallot and may involve the pulmonary valve and variable portions of the pulmonary arteries. In severe forms, the branch pulmonary arteries are involved, and the continuity between right and left pulmonary arteries is interrupted (**Fig. 15.2**).
- In pulmonary atresia, pulmonary circulation may be supplied through a patent ductus arteriosus or systemic

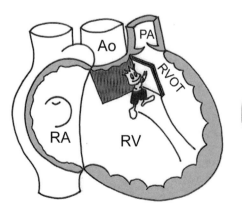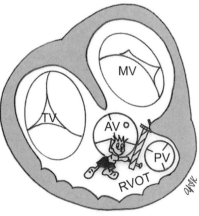

Fig. 15.1 Features of tetralogy of Fallot. Ao, ascending aorta; AV, aortic valve; MV, mitral valve; PA, main pulmonary artery; PV, pulmonary valve; RA, right atrium; RV, right ventricle; RVOT, right ventricular outflow tract.

193

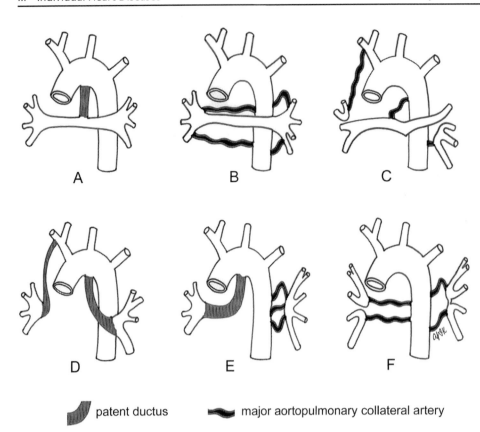

Fig. 15.2 In severe form, tetralogy is associated with pulmonary atresia. Pulmonary circulation may be supplied by a patent ductus arteriosus or major aortopulmonary collateral arteries. The right and left pulmonary arteries can be confluent (A–C) or nonconfluent (D–F). Not infrequently, branch pulmonary arteries in the mediastinum are not formed (E and F).

▰ patent ductus   ∿ major aortopulmonary collateral artery

collateral arteries. In most cases, the patent ductus arteriosus and the MAPCAs do not coexist in supplying the same lung. Patent ductus arteriosus or MAPCAs are rarely seen in cases without pulmonary atresia. Morphology of pulmonary arterial tree and supply are the central features (**Fig. 15.2**).

- Absent pulmonary valve variant is characterized by severe pulmonary regurgitation and severely dilated central pulmonary arteries, which cause significant compression of the main and segmental bronchi.
- Peripheral pulmonary arteries show arborization abnormalities and may compress more distal bronchi, leading to distal air trapping
- Central bronchi may have deficient or defective cartilage also leading to bronchomalacia.
- Tetralogy of Fallot is often associated with deletion of chromosome 22q11, and less commonly with the VACTERL association (vertebral abnormalities, anal atresia, cardiac abnormalities, tracheoesophageal fistula, esophageal atresia, renal agenesis, and limb defects) or trisomy 21.

Clinical Manifestations

- Age of presentation depends on degree of right ventricular outflow tract obstruction.
- Central feature is cyanosis, which is mostly continuous but can be intermittent.

- Most common cause of cyanosis at 1 month
- Severe obstruction presents usually after first week or month of life.
- Less severe obstruction is usually progressive, resulting in a later presentation.
- Polycythemia develops as cyanosis worsens.
- Squatting position after exercise to increase systemic resistance, which forces more blood into pulmonary circulation, increasing peripheral oxygen saturation
- Hypercyanotic spells are due to a transient increase in pulmonary resistance and may result in loss of consciousness.
- Pink tetralogy may present with congestive heart failure.
- When the ductus arteriosus is the only source of the pulmonary blood flow, symptoms and signs of hypoxia and cyanosis develop early with closure of the ductus. When the source of pulmonary blood flow is MAPCAs, presentation may vary according to the amount of blood flow through the MAPCAs.
- Absent pulmonary valve presents with severe respiratory symptoms and less severe symptoms of cyanosis.

Chest Radiographic Findings

- Normal or slightly enlarged cardiac size
- Cardiac contour is often boot-shaped due to leftward rotation of the cardiac axis, uplifted or elevated cardiac apex, and small or absent main pulmonary arterial segment of the left heart border. A boot-shaped heart

is not a feature of two- or double-chambered right ventricle.

- Cardiomegaly is unusual but can be seen in the following:
  - Pink tetralogy
  - Tetralogy with atrioventricular septal defect
  - Pulmonary atresia with increased pulmonary blood flow
  - Absence of the pulmonary valve
- Marked concavity of main pulmonary artery segment with pulmonary atresia due to underdeveloped infundibulum and main pulmonary artery
- Prominent hilar and intrapulmonary arteries with mild pulmonary stenosis and left-to-right shunt
- Aneurysmal main and proximal branch pulmonary with absence of pulmonary valve
- Normal to moderately reduced pulmonary vascularity correlates with degree of pulmonary stenosis.
- Asymmetric pulmonary vascularity with associated pulmonary artery stenosis or an anomalous origin of a pulmonary artery from an arterial duct or ascending aorta
- In tetralogy of Fallot with pulmonary atresia, the vascularity is typically reduced when the source of pulmonary

blood supply is a patent ductus arteriosus. When MAPCAs are the source, the pulmonary vascularity varies according to the size and degree of stenosis of the MAPCAs.

- Disorganized hilar and intrapulmonary arteries with an unusual reticular pattern, often giving the impression of increased pulmonary vascularity with associated MAPCAs; the vascularity may show asymmetric distribution between the lungs and uneven distribution within a lung.
- Prominent ascending aorta, which correlates with the degree of pulmonary stenosis
- Right aortic arch in up to 30% of cases; a higher incidence with pulmonary atresia and absence of pulmonary valve
- Hyperinflation with increasing cyanosis
- Multifocal lung hyperinflation and atelectasis with absence of pulmonary valve
- Thymic hypoplasia or atrophy; a small or absent thymic shadow with narrow superior mediastinum in the newborn is suggestive of microdeletion of the chromosome 22q11. Normally formed thymus may become atrophic with postnatal stress.
- Rarely collateral vessels cause rib notching.

Pearls

- Decreased pulmonary vascularity with normal heart size favors tetralogy of Fallot.
- Cardiomegaly suggests a tetralogy of Fallot variant, associated defects, or ventricular dysfunction.
- Increased pulmonary overcirculation may be seen with an acyanotic tetralogy of Fallot, and with pulmonary atresia with pulmonary circulation supplied by large MAPCAs.
- Aneurysmal central pulmonary arteries with associated airway obstruction and multifocal lung

hyperinflation and atelectasis are characteristic of absence of the pulmonary valve.

- Bizarre uneven vascularity with associated uneven lung aeration relates to arterial collateral supply.
- Degree of enlargement of the ascending aorta relates to degree of pulmonary stenosis.
- Right aortic arch more common with pulmonary atresia and absence of the pulmonary valve

---

Case 15.1

Tetralogy of Fallot in a 4-month-old infant. Chest radiographs show characteristic findings of tetralogy of Fallot with a normal heart size with an uplifted apex, deficient main pulmonary artery segment of the left heart border, a prominent right aortic arch, and reduced pulmonary vascularity. Thymic atrophy is seen with cyanosis and stress.

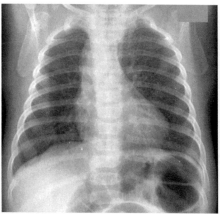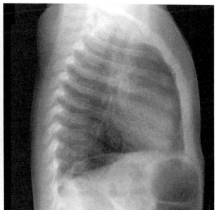

Case 15.2

Mild acyanotic form of tetralogy of Fallot (pink tetralogy) in a 5-month-old infant. Chest radiographs show findings mimicking a ventricular septal defect with moderate cardiomegaly, dilated main pulmonary artery, and increased pulmonary vascularity with a normal left aortic arch and a prominent thymus. The cardiac apex is rounded and slightly uplifted.

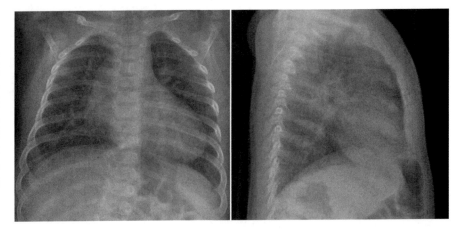

Case 15.3

Tetralogy of Fallot with atrioventricular septal defect in a 2-week-old infant. Chest radiographs show moderate disproportionate cardiomegaly with specific right atrial dilatation due to an associated atrioventricular septal defect. The main pulmonary arterial segment of the left heart border is slightly small. Pulmonary vascularity appears mildly reduced only in the lateral view.

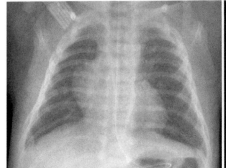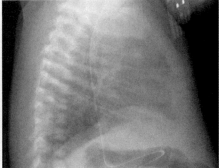

Case 15.4

Tetralogy of Fallot with major aortopulmonary collateral arteries. Chest radiograph in a 2-month-old *(left panel)* shows asymmetrically increased pulmonary vascularity and moderate cardiomegaly due to the presence of additional pulmonary blood supply from multiple major aortopulmonary collateral arteries (MAPCAs). Following coil embolization of several MAPCAs the chest radiograph at 11 months of age *(right panel)* shows a decrease in the reticular pattern due to occlusion of superimposed collaterals and decreased cardiomegaly with a reduction in pulmonary overcirculation.

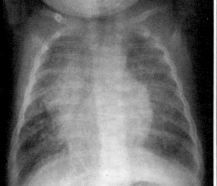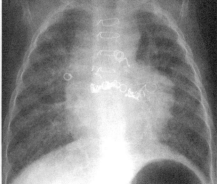

Case 15.5

Tetralogy of Fallot with stenosis of the left pulmonary artery in a 9-month-old infant. Chest radiograph shows findings of tetralogy of Fallot with normal heart size and an uplifted apex, concave main pulmonary artery, and asymmetric pulmonary vascularity. The vascularity is reduced throughout the left lung, which is due to juxtaductal stenosis of the left pulmonary artery. Contrast-enhanced computed tomography (CT) images show stenosis *(arrow)* of the origin of the left pulmonary artery (LPA). Note that the left lower pulmonary vein (LLPV) is small as compared with the right lower pulmonary vein (RLPV) due to reduced blood flow to the left lung. Ao, ascending aorta; ao, descending aorta; D, ventricular septal defect; LA, left atrium; LV, left ventricle; MPA, main pulmonary artery; RA, right atrium; RPA, right pulmonary artery; RV, right ventricle.

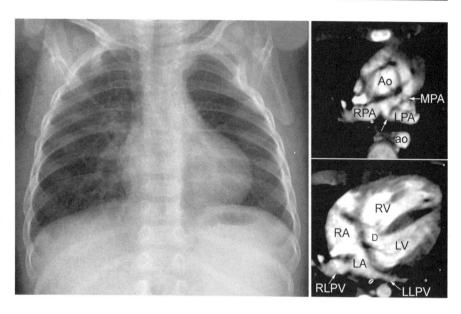

Case 15.6

Tetralogy of Fallot with isolated origin of the left pulmonary artery from the ductus arteriosus in a 5-month-old infant. Initial chest radiographs *(upper panels)* show mildly decreased pulmonary vascularity in the left lung, mild cardiomegaly, and a right aortic arch. Following palliation with implantation of stents in the left ductus arteriosus *(lower panels)*, there is increased left pulmonary vascularity.

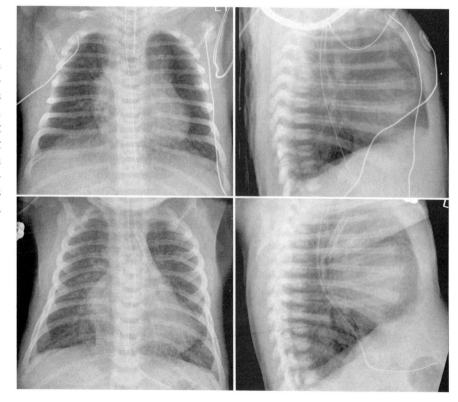

Case 15.7

Tetralogy of Fallot with pulmonary atresia and patent ductus arteriosus in a newborn with microdeletion of the chromosome 22q11. Chest radiographs show mild cardiomegaly with rounded and uplifted cardiac apex. The pulmonary vascularity is only mildly reduced. The aortic arch is right-sided. A left patent ductus arteriosus was the only source of blood supply to both lungs. The superior mediastinum is narrow in the frontal view and retrosternal space is empty due to thymic hypoplasia.

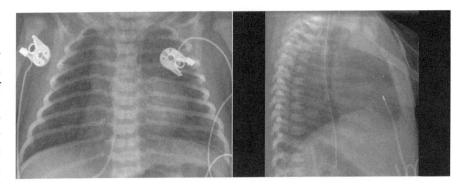

Case 15.8

Tetralogy of Fallot with pulmonary atresia and multiple major aortopulmonary collateral arteries in a 9-week-old infant. Chest radiograph shows moderate cardiomegaly, marked concavity of the main pulmonary artery segment of the left heart border, and uneven size of intrapulmonary arteries. The left lower lung is particularly underperfused. The diagram is the pulmonary arterial anatomy seen at angiography. LLL, left lower lobe; LUL, left upper lobe; RML, right middle lobe; RUL, right upper lobe.

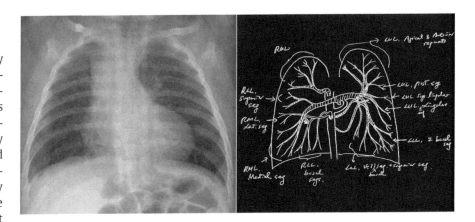

Case 15.9

Tetralogy of Fallot with pulmonary atresia and major aortopulmonary collateral arteries in a 4-month-old infant. Chest radiographs show moderate cardiomegaly and uneven distribution of peripheral pulmonary vascularity. The pulmonary vessels are prominent, tortuous, and disorganized. Lungs are hyperinflated.

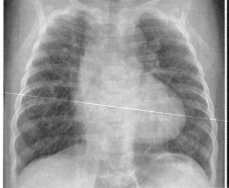
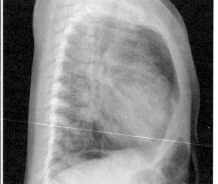

Case 15.10

Various manifestations of tetralogy of Fallot with absent pulmonary valve syndrome in four infants. The central pulmonary vessels are aneurysmally dilated. The lungs show variable degree of aeration with multifocal hyperinflation and atelectasis resulting from central bronchial compression due to the aneurysmal pulmonary arteries.

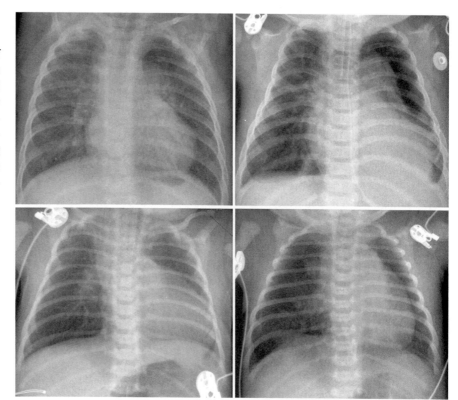

16 Pulmonary Valvar Stenosis

With Christian J. Kellenberger

Definition and Classification

- Pulmonary valvar stenosis occurs with a reduced orifice of the pulmonary valve due to fusion of the thickened valve leaflets. The valve can also be bicuspid and have a hypoplastic annulus. Stenosis of the dysplastic valve is typically seen in Noonan syndrome.
- Isolated or associated with subvalvar, supravalvar, or peripheral branch pulmonary artery stenosis
- Critical pulmonary stenosis refers to obstruction resulting in suprasystemic right ventricular systolic pressures, tricuspid regurgitation, and a right-to-left shunt across the atrial septum, and often pulmonary circulation is dependent on the flow through the ductus arteriosus.

Pathophysiology

- Increased impedance to right ventricular outflow requires increased right ventricular pressure to maintain pulmonary circulation.
- Increasing pressure results in concentric hypertrophy of the right ventricle and loss of compliance with impaired diastolic filling.
- Systolic pressure in the right ventricle and degree of hypertrophy are proportional to the degree of obstruction in the absence of heart failure.
- Severity of the lesion is generally classified according to the right ventricular systolic pressure.
- Less severe obstruction is well tolerated with gradual hypertrophy and dilatation of the right ventricle and preserved right ventricular function.
- More severe obstruction leads to suprasystemic right ventricular pressures, moderate dilatation of the right ventricle, and right heart failure.
- Right atrium may also become hypertrophied and dilated with tricuspid valve regurgitation.

- Increasing right atrial pressures leads to right-to-left shunting at atrial level if foramen ovale is patent or an atrial defect is present.

Clinical Manifestations

- Often well compensated and asymptomatic for years
- Asymptomatic murmur may be the presentation
- Symptoms of fatigue and dyspnea with greater cardiac output demands by growth in later childhood or with moderate exercise
- Severe stenosis may result in right ventricular failure with systemic venous congestion.
- Critical stenosis will lead to hypoxia.
- Cyanosis may occur due to right-to-left shunting across an associated atrial septal defect or a patent foramen ovale.

Chest Radiographic Findings

- Poststenotic dilatation of the main and usually left pulmonary arteries due to a high-velocity jet effect through the stenotic valve
- High position of the dilated main pulmonary artery, which may overlap the aortic knuckle
- Dilated main pulmonary artery may not be seen due to overlying thymus gland.
- Degree of poststenotic dilatation is not related to the severity of obstruction, with mild stenosis often having marked dilation.
- Poststenotic dilatation is not seen when obstruction is subvalvar or supravalvar.
- Small main pulmonary artery with dysplastic valve, and subvalvar and supravalvar stenosis
- Peripheral pulmonary vascularity usually normal
- Decreased pulmonary vascularity with associated right-to-left atrial shunts
- Heart size is usually normal.
- Right ventricular hypertrophy may result in obliteration of the retrocardiac clear space.

□ Mild cardiac enlargement may develop due to hypertrophy, with dilatation not occurring until significant heart failure develops.

□ Dilating right ventricle indicates heart failure with a decompensating right ventricle and enlargement of right atrium with tricuspid insufficiency.

□ Normal size aorta

Pearls

□ Isolated pulmonary valvar stenosis shows characteristic poststenotic dilatation of the main and left pulmonary arteries.

□ Poststenotic dilatation does not occur with subvalvar stenosis.

□ Localized dilatation of the main pulmonary artery is not possible to distinguish from idiopathic pulmonary artery dilation.

□ Peripheral pulmonary vascularity is normal when there is no right-to-left shunt.

□ With associated right-to-left shunts or right heart failure, peripheral pulmonary vascularity is decreased.

Case 16.1

Pulmonary valve stenosis in a 2-year-old child. Chest radiographs show mild cardiomegaly, high position of a dilated main pulmonary artery *(arrows)*, dilatation of the left pulmonary artery, and normal peripheral pulmonary vascularity. Right ventriculograms show a thickened pulmonary valve *(arrows)* which is doming in ventricular systole. The main pulmonary artery (MPA) shows poststenotic dilatation. For differential diagnosis of convex bulge of the main pulmonary arterial segment of the left heart border, see **Fig. 8.37.** RV, right ventricle.

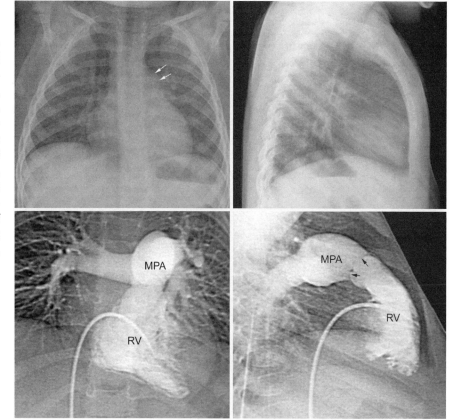

Case 16.2

Critical pulmonary valve stenosis in a 5-day-old infant. Chest radiographs show moderate cardiomegaly from right ventricular hypertrophy and an enlarged right atrium due to tricuspid regurgitation. Decreased pulmonary vascularity is associated with right-to-left atrial shunting. The findings are similar to those seen in pulmonary atresia with intact ventricular septum (see **Fig. 17.1**).

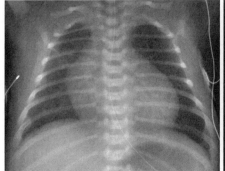
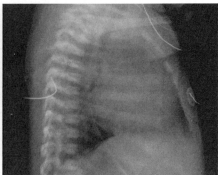

Case 16.3

Pulmonary valve stenosis and multiple peripheral pulmonary arterial stenosis in a 4-year-old child with Williams syndrome. Chest radiographs show normal heart size, mildly dilated main and left pulmonary arteries often not present with a dysplastic pulmonary valve, and uneven peripheral vascularity with regions of oligemia most marked in the right lung and left upper lobe due to variable degrees of peripheral branch stenosis.

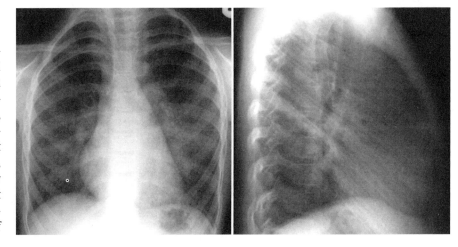

17 Pulmonary Atresia with Intact Ventricular Septum

With Christian J. Kellenberger

Definition and Classification

- Extreme form of pulmonary valve stenosis with imperforate valve resulting in complete obstruction to right ventricular outflow
- Not a simple isolated lesion but considered part of the more complex hypoplastic right heart anomalies
- Tricuspid valve apparatus is almost always abnormal and often hypoplastic.
- Classification relates to a spectrum of right ventricular dimensions (**Fig. 17.1**):
  - *Classic hypertrophic form*: small hypertrophied right ventricle with small, not severely incompetent tricuspid valve, often associated with fistulous communications between the right ventricle and the coronary arterial systems
  - *Dilated form*: large right ventricle with large and incompetent tricuspid valve, typically with Ebstein malformation or dysplasia of the leaflets

Pathophysiology

- Life-threatening complete obstruction of right ventricular outflow
- Obligatory interatrial communication with right-to-left shunting and complete admixture of systemic and pulmonary venous return
- Pulmonary blood flow is dependent on left-to-right flow through the ductus arteriosus.
- Patency of the ductus arteriosus is critical.
- Systemic collateral arteries are rare.
- Right ventricular pressures are exceedingly high.
- Dysplasia of tricuspid valve apparatus and annulus small tricuspid valve with variable degrees of regurgitation.
- Fistulous communications exist between endocardial surface of right ventricle and coronary arteries in hypertrophic form.
- Retrograde coronary blood flow with desaturated blood from right ventricle leads to ventricular ischemia, myocardial necrosis, and fibrosis.
- Left ventricle provides total cardiac output.

Clinical Manifestations

- Varied clinical findings relate to size of right ventricle, competence of tricuspid valve, and size of ductus arteriosus.
- Tricuspid regurgitation with right-to-left shunting results in cyanosis.
- Rapid presentation of severe neonatal cyanosis and hypoxemia with closure of ductus arteriosus

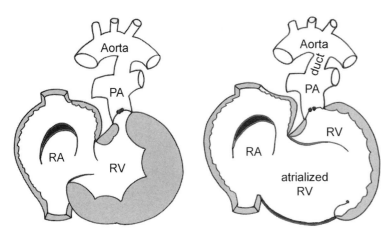

Classic hypertrophic form   Dilated form

Fig. 17.1 Classification of pulmonary atresia. PA, pulmonary artery; RA, right atrium; RV, right ventricle.

Chest Radiographic Findings

- Size of ductus arteriosus determines the magnitude of pulmonary blood flow and the size of the pulmonary arteries.
- Main pulmonary arteries are usually normal.
- Pulmonary vascularity is typically decreased but can be normal when the ductus is large.
- Variable heart size; the degree of cardiomegaly correlates with the degree of tricuspid valve regurgitation.

- Primarily right atrial and left ventricular enlargement
- Right atrial enlargement can be enormous with severe tricuspid regurgitation.
- Overall cardiac contour may mimic an egg-on-side because of the hypoplastic right ventricular outflow tract and right atrial enlargement.
- Ascending aorta and isthmus enlarged receiving total cardiac output

Pearls

- Neonate with severe cyanosis and massive cardiomegaly with disproportionately enlarged right atrium due to severe tricuspid regurgitation indistinguishable from Ebstein's anomaly
- Pulmonary vascularity may appear normal initially, with decreasing vascularity indicating a closing ductus arteriosus.

- May show an egg-on-side configuration
- Prominent aortic arch due to increased left cardiac output.

Case 17.1

Pulmonary atresia with intact ventricular septum in a 1-day-old infant. Chest radiographs show moderate cardiomegaly primarily with right atrial and left ventricular enlargement. Pulmonary vascularity is decreased, correlating with a restricted amount of blood flow across the ductus arteriosus.

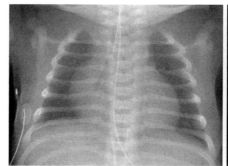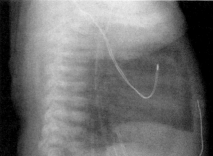

Case 17.2

Pulmonary atresia with intact ventricular septum in a new-born infant. Chest radiograph shows a typical egg-on-side appearance with dilated right atrium and flat left upper heart border, and markedly diminished pulmonary vascularity.

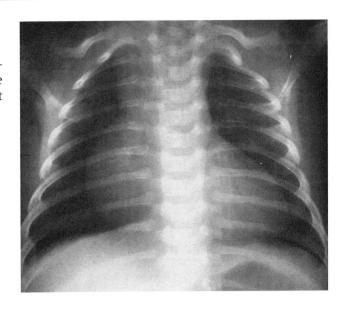

Case 17.3

Pulmonary atresia with intact ventricular septum and mild tricuspid regurgitation in a 1-day-old infant. Chest radiographs show only mild cardiomegaly and decreased pulmonary vascularity. Right atrium is not enlarged, which would indicate an unrestrictive atrial septal defect with right-to-left shunting.

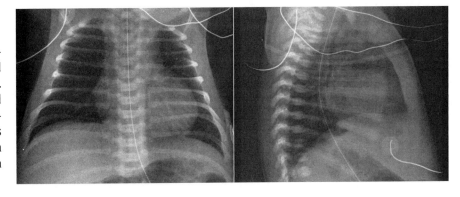

18 Partial and Total Anomalous Pulmonary Venous Connections

With Monica Epelman

Definition

□ Abnormal connection of some or all of the pulmonary veins to a systemic vein or the right atrium (**Fig. 18.1**).

□ Isolated or associated with other cardiac anomalies

□ Partial and total anomalous drainage are described as two distinct entities, as the classification, pathophysiology, and diagnosis are quite different.

□ Partial anomalous venous connection

   • Anomalous connection of one or more pulmonary veins, which may be unilateral or bilateral

   • Uncommonly mixed drainage to multiple sites with anomalous connection of more than one pulmonary vein

   • Anomalous drainage of right pulmonary veins significantly more common

   • Partial anomalous drainage of a right pulmonary vein to superior or inferior vena cava is associated with a sinus venosus atrial septal defect.

   • Partial anomalous drainage of a right pulmonary vein to right atrium can also be associated with a secundum atrial septal defect.

   • Partial anomalous drainage of right pulmonary veins to the inferior vena cava–right atrial junction is associated with the scimitar syndrome (hypogenetic right lung syndrome, congenital venolobar syndrome) (**Fig. 18.2**).

   – Hypoplasia or aplasia of one or more lobes of the right lung with lobation, segmentation, and fusion abnormalities, and hypoplasia and abnormal branching pattern of the right pulmonary artery and bronchus

   – Systemic arterial blood supply to the right lung in most cases. True pulmonary sequestration with disconnected bronchial supply is rare.

   – Occasionally with horseshoe lung or crossover lung

   – Anomalies of right hemidiaphragm

   – Anomalies of bony thorax and soft tissues with excess extrapleural areolar tissue

   • Partial anomalous drainage of a left pulmonary vein(s) is usually into the left innominate vein or coronary sinus and often associated with a secundum atrial septal defect.

   • Partial anomalous drainage is common in left isomerism.

□ Total anomalous pulmonary venous connection

   • Anomalous connection of all pulmonary veins directly to one of the systemic veins or right atrium

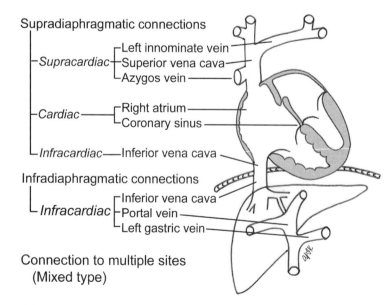

Supradiaphragmatic connections

┌─Supracardiac ─┬─ Left innominate vein
│   ├─ Superior vena cava
│   └─ Azygos vein
│
├─Cardiac ──────┬─ Right atrium
│   └─ Coronary sinus
│
└─Infracardiac ── Inferior vena cava

Infradiaphragmatic connections

└─Infracardiac ─┬─ Inferior vena cava
                ├─ Portal vein
                └─ Left gastric vein

Connection to multiple sites
(Mixed type)

Fig. 18.1 Classification of anomalous pulmonary venous connections according to the site of abnormal connection.

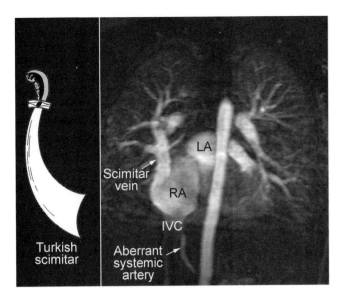

Fig. 18.2 Scimitar syndrome. IVC, inferior vena cava; LA, left atrium; RA, right atrium.

- Classification based on the site of insertion of the pulmonary veins (**Fig. 18.1**)
- Most commonly all the pulmonary veins drain collectively through a confluence to a single site and rarely to multiple sites.
- Total anomalous connection is associated with visceral heterotaxies, most commonly right isomerism.

Pathophysiology

- Depends on how much of the pulmonary circulation empties into the systemic circulation, presence of pulmonary venous obstruction, and associated cardiac anomalies
- Partial anomalous pulmonary venous connection
    - Basically a left-to-right shunt increasing the pulmonary-to-systemic flow ratio proportional to the number of veins connected to the right-sided circulation and to the presence of an associated atrial septal defect
    - Mild physiologic abnormality with a hemodynamically relevant left-to-right shunt usually with complete return of all veins from one lung or with an associated atrial septal defect
    - Right atrium and ventricle dilate, leading to right heart volume overload.
    - Increased pulmonary blood flow rarely leads to pulmonary artery hypertension.
- Total anomalous pulmonary venous connection
    - Unobstructed pulmonary venous return causes a left-to-right shunt, and with all blood bypassing the left atrium, an obligatory interatrial right-to-left shunt is necessary for survival.
    - Complete mixing of systemic and pulmonary venous blood within the heart, resulting in identical oxygenation in all four chambers and produces cyanosis
    - Right ventricular volume overload with increased pulmonary vascularity; may lead to right heart failure
    - Left atrium and ventricle receive less than normal flow and may show some degree of underdevelopment.
    - Obstructed pulmonary venous return results in pulmonary venous and arterial hypertension, pulmonary edema, and diminished pulmonary return, leading to low cardiac output.
    - Severe pulmonary venous congestion results in increased pulmonary lymphatic flow and increased flow through available alternative venous pathways.
    - Reflex pulmonary arterial vasoconstriction leads to increased pulmonary vascular resistance and decrease in pulmonary blood flow.
    - Increased right-sided pressure overload leads to right heart failure.
    - Restriction to flow may result from an obstruction of the pulmonary venous circuit or across the atrial septum.
    - *Infracardiac type* is almost always obstructed and is a result of a combination of factors:
        - Following closure of the ductus venosus, the pulmonary venous flow is forced through the portal sinusoid system, resulting in significant impedance of blood flow by the hepatic parenchyma.
        - Extrinsic obstruction of the descending anomalous draining vein passing through the diaphragm hiatus
        - Length of the descending anomalous draining vein
        - Stenosis at connection of anomalous vein with portal vein
    - Supracardiac type, seldom obstructed
        - Intrinsic stenosis at connection of common pulmonary vein with vertical vein or its attachment to the innominate vein
        - Extrinsic obstruction as vertical vein passes through a triangular space between left pulmonary artery, left ductus arteriosus, and left main bronchus, called anatomical vice
        - Intrinsic stenosis of vertical vein
    - Cardiac type, rarely obstructed
        - Stenosis at connection of common vein to coronary sinus

Clinical Manifestations

☐ Partial anomalous pulmonary venous connection
- Symptoms usually do not occur unless more than half of the pulmonary flow is connected to the right-sided circulation.
- Typically an acyanotic lesion
- Exertional dyspnea may be the only symptom.
- Scimitar syndrome often discovered on a chest radiograph performed for recurrent respiratory infections

☐ Total anomalous pulmonary venous connection
- Three major clinical patterns depending on the size of the atrial communication and the presence of pulmonary venous obstruction
  - Severe obstruction
    - Neonatal period with severe tachypnea and respiratory distress
    - Marked cyanosis
    - Pulmonary arterial hypertension progresses
  - Mild or moderate obstruction
    - Early in life overload of right ventricle leads to congestive heart failure.
    - Mild cyanosis
    - Pulmonary arterial hypertension develops.
  - No obstruction
    - Minimal symptoms in infancy with increased respiratory effort, or recurrent respiratory infections. Occasionally failure to thrive.
    - Mild or absent cyanosis
    - Pulmonary arterial hypertension is absent.

Chest Radiographic Findings

☐ Varies according to the site of abnormal venous drainage and whether it is obstructed

☐ Partial anomalous pulmonary venous connection
- Mildly to moderately increased pulmonary vascularity with an overcirculation pattern
- Anomalous pulmonary vein may be seen as an unusual intraparenchymal vessel.
- Dilated superior vena cava when receives anomalous venous drainage
- Dilated azygos vein when receives anomalous venous drainage
- Mild to moderate cardiomegaly with right heart dilatation
- Scimitar syndrome (hypogenetic right lung syndrome, congenital venolobar syndrome)
  - Right lung hypoplasia with mediastinal shift and elevation of the right hemidiaphragm, often associated with scoliosis
  - Rightward displacement of the heart with obscuration of right heart border
  - Retrosternal soft tissue density with severe right lung hypoplasia
  - Characteristic anomalous vein appearing as a Turkish scimitar
  - Right pulmonary artery small or absent
  - Bizarre right lung vascular pattern due to arborization anomalies and associated systemic arterial collateral typically to a portion of the right lower lung
  - Right lower lung extending to the left with associated horseshoe lung; abnormal horizontal vessels in the medial aspect of the left lower lung region are characteristic. The abnormal lung is demarcated by a vertical fissure.

☐ Total anomalous pulmonary venous connection
- Supracardiac unobstructed
  - Snowman configuration is the most characteristic sign.
    - Frontal image consists of left vertical vein and dilated superior vena cava as the upper half and the body is the enlarged heart: rarely seen before 2 years of age
    - Lateral radiograph may show pretracheal density made up of a dilated right superior vena cava and left vertical vein. This finding differentiates a venous circuit from thymus located in the anterior mediastinum
  - Anomalous circuit in infants is small and not well visualized.
  - Localized dilation of superior vena cava or azygos vein
  - Increased pulmonary vascularity with an overcirculation pattern
  - Large main pulmonary artery may be hidden in the superior mediastinal silhouette.
  - Cardiomegaly due to right heart enlargement
  - Left-sided chambers are small or not enlarged.
- Cardiac unobstructed
  - Increased pulmonary vascularity with an overcirculation pattern
  - Large main pulmonary artery
  - Moderate cardiomegaly due to right heart enlargement
  - Right atrial enlargement may be marked
- Infracardiac obstructed
  - Pulmonary venous hypertension with a diffuse reticular pattern due to interstitial edema, dilated pulmonary veins, and lymphatics
  - Normal main pulmonary artery size

– Lung volumes are usually large in contrast to respiratory distress syndrome.
– Normal heart size due to reduced pulmonary blood flow
– Small aorta
– Overinflated lung parenchyma

– Small pleural effusions
– Thymic atrophy
• Mixed
  – Asymmetric uneven pattern of vascularity depending on the presence of localized obstruction

---

Pearls

▫ Partial anomalous pulmonary venous connection closely mimics an atrial septal defect.

▫ Scimitar syndrome is a characteristic entity with a constellation of findings.

▫ Unobstructed total anomalous pulmonary venous connection closely mimics a large left-to-right shunt.

▫ Most characteristic lesion is the supracardiac circuit producing the snowman configuration, but rarely seen in infants.

▫ Supracardiac vascular circuit on the lateral view is a pretracheal density and not located in the retrosternal window, which helps differentiate from a large left-to-right shunt with a large thymus.

▫ Obstructed infracardiac total anomalous pulmonary venous connection presents in a neonate acutely with severe cyanosis and respiratory distress.

▫ Neonatal chest radiograph with findings of diffuse reticular opacities due to obstructed total anomalous pulmonary venous connection may be confused with primary pulmonary disease, including respiratory distress syndrome, pneumonia, meconium aspiration, and pulmonary lymphangiectasia.

▫ Air bronchograms are absent with obstructed veins.

Case 18.1

Unilateral partial anomalous connection of the right upper pulmonary veins to the superior vena cava in a 2-year-old child. Chest radiographs show mild cardiomegaly with right heart dilatation, mildly increased pulmonary vasculature with unusual right central intraparenchymal vessels, and a dilated superior vena cava. The pulmonary vascularity is more prominent in the right lung than in the left lung.

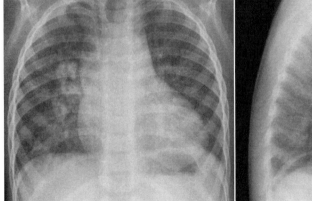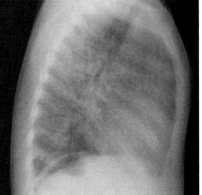

Case 18.2

Partial anomalous pulmonary venous connection to the superior vena cava in a 3-year-old child. Chest radiograph shows mild cardiomegaly and increased pulmonary vascularity with slightly more prominent right hilar vessels and clear lungs. There is a rounded structure along the lower trachea and above the right main bronchus. This proved to be the anomalous pulmonary vein (PV) connecting to the superior vena cava (SVC) as shown on the contrast-enhanced magnetic resonance (MR) angiogram. The right lower pulmonary veins (RLPV) and left pulmonary veins have normal connections to the left atrium (LA); left ventricle (LV); right pulmonary artery (RPA).

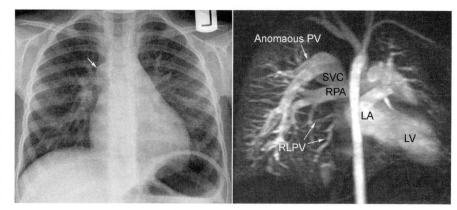

Case 18.3

Partial anomalous pulmonary venous connection to the left innominate vein in a 5-year-old child. Chest radiograph shows mild cardiomegaly with slight prominence of the right atrium and superior vena cava. The pulmonary vascularity is slightly increased, appearing similar to an atrial septal defect. Contrast-enhanced MR angiogram shows an anomalous left pulmonary vein *(arrow)* coursing along the left side of the mediastinum draining upward toward the left innominate vein. The anomalous vein correlates with the abnormal vessel seen on the chest radiograph *(arrows)*. Ao, ascending aorta; LPA, left pulmonary artery; SVC, superior vena cava.

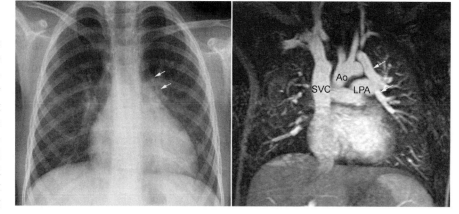

Case 18.4

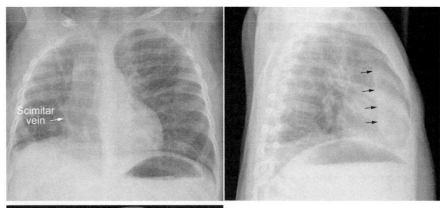

Scimitar syndrome in a 15-month-old child. Frontal chest radiograph shows hypoplasia of the right lung with displacement of the heart and mediastinal structures to the right and elevation of the right hemidiaphragm. The right lung shows abnormally arranged pulmonary vessels. A scimitar vein is seen in the right lower lung. Lateral chest radiograph shows a retrosternal band of tissue *(arrows)*. Contrast-enhanced computed tomography (CT) image shows that the space between the displaced heart and the right anterior chest wall is filled with tissue *(asterisk)*. The interface between this tissue and the right lung (*arrows* in CT) is the posterior margin of the restrosternal band on the lateral chest radiograph.

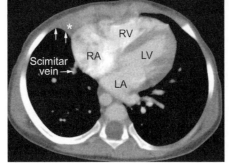

Case 18.5

Various degrees of right lung hypoplasia in scimitar syndrome. The *arrows* indicate the scimitar vein.

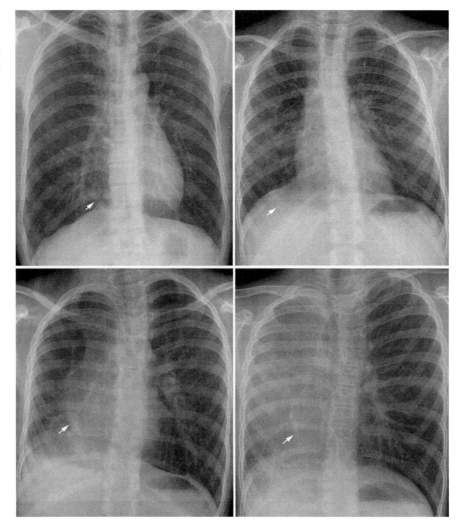

Case 18.6

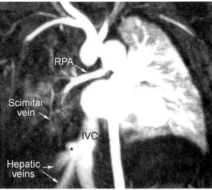

Scimitar syndrome with complete obstruction of the scimitar vein in a 3-month-old infant. Chest radiograph shows hypoplasia of the right lung with displacement of the heart to the right. The hypoplastic right lung shows diffuse haziness and a reticular pattern. The left lung shows increased vascularity and interstitial pulmonary edema. Contrast-enhanced MR angiogram shows hypoperfused right lung with a small right pulmonary artery (RPA). There is a tiny vertical channel in the right lower lung, which courses toward the inferior vena cava (IVC) from where a diverticular outpouching *(asterisk)* arises. The outpouching is considered a remnant of the scimitar vein.

Case 18.7

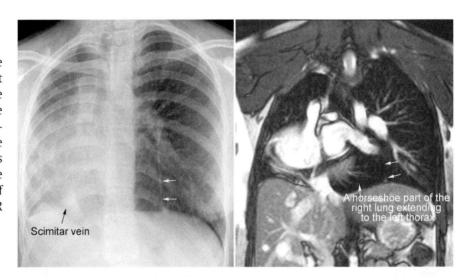

Scimitar syndrome with horseshoe lung in a 17-year-old boy. The right lung is severely hypoplastic and the mediastinal structures including the heart are displaced into the right thorax. There is a vertical fissure *(arrows)* in the left lower lung. This fissure is consistent with the fissure demarcating the horseshoe part of the right lung as seen on an MR image.

Case 18.8

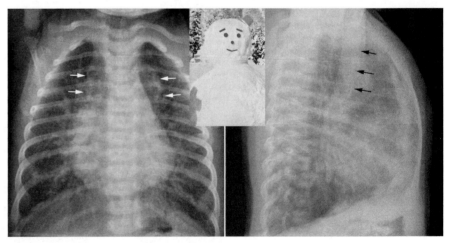

Total anomalous pulmonary venous connection to the left innominate vein in a 5-week-old infant. Frontal chest radiograph shows a snowman or figure-of-8 appearance. This finding is rarely seen in infancy. The upper part of the snowman is formed by the dilated vertical vein and right superior vena cava *(white arrows)*. The vertical veins and superior vena cava are superimposed on one another on the lateral chest radiograph and seen as a band of haziness *(black arrows)* in the pretracheal region, which differentiates it from thymus located in the retrosternal window.

Case 18.9

Total anomalous pulmonary venous connection to the left innominate vein in a 5-day-old infant. Chest radiograph shows mild cardiomegaly with increased pulmonary vascularity and widening of the right superior mediastinal contour *(arrows)*. Contrast-enhanced CT image shows the individual pulmonary veins *(asterisks)* forming a confluence behind the left atrium, which drains through a left vertical vein to the left innominate vein. The vertical vein is not visible on the chest radiograph. The superior vena cava (SVC) is dilated, causing widening of the right superior mediastinum.

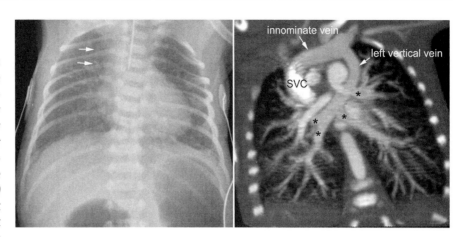

Case 18.10

Total anomalous pulmonary venous connection to the left-sided azygos vein in a 5-year-old child with right atrial isomerism and atrioventricular septal defect. Chest radiographs show an unusual anomalous pulmonary venous circuit (traced with *dots*) with a common pulmonary vein hidden behind the heart. Contrast-enhanced CT images nicely show the anomalous pulmonary venous route. A large atrioventricular septal defect (D) is seen. L-A, left-sided atrium; LV, left ventricle; R-A, right-sided atrium; RV, right ventricle.

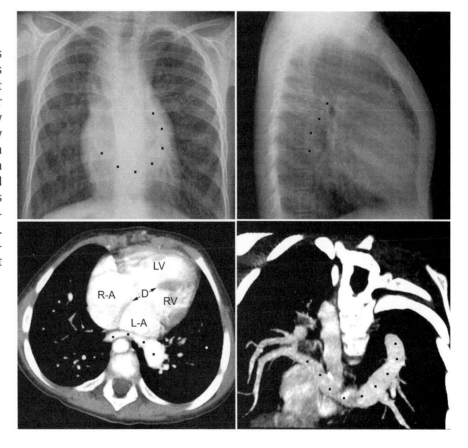

Case 18.11

Total anomalous pulmonary venous connection to the coronary sinus in a 1-month-old infant. Chest radiographs show moderate cardiomegaly with specific right heart enlargement, increased pulmonary vascularity with an overcirculation pattern and edema, and hyperinflation.

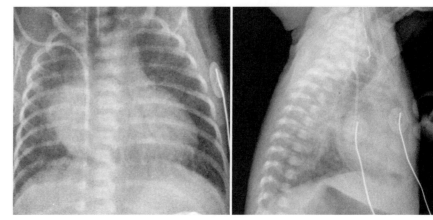

Case 18.12

Total anomalous pulmonary venous connection to portal vein. Chest radiographs at birth *(left panel)* and a follow-up at 8 days old *(right panel)* show progressive pulmonary venous hypertension and a normal-sized heart.

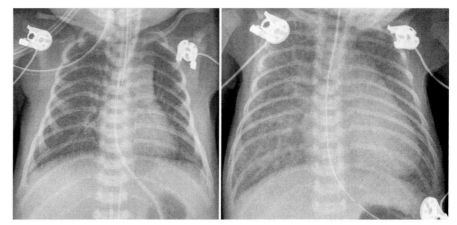

Case 18.13

Mixed type of total anomalous pulmonary venous connection in a 1-year-old child with dextrocardia and atrioventricular septal defect. Chest radiographs show asymmetric interstitial edema due to stenosis of the right pulmonary venous drainage. The pulmonary vascularity is increased in both lungs.

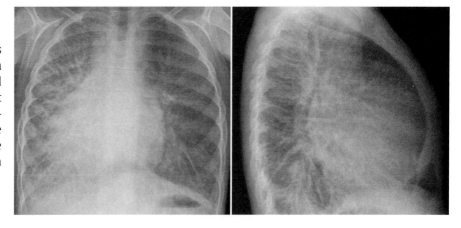

19 Congenital Stenosis and Atresia of the Individual Pulmonary Veins

With Anne Geoffray

Definition and Classification

□ Stenosis represents narrowing of the pulmonary veins of varying degree, usually involving multiple veins unilaterally or bilaterally. It can be tubular, with extension into the lung, or discrete, tending to form at the junction of the veins with the left atrium.

□ Atresia is a complete occlusion of the pulmonary veins that requires a coexisting anomalous pathway through intraparenchymal pulmonary or pulmonary-to-systemic venous anastomoses. It should be differentiated from pulmonary veno-occlusive disease (PVOD) in which obstructive intimal fibrosis involves the pulmonary venules and small veins, causing pulmonary hypertension.

Pathophysiology

□ Congenital obstruction of the pulmonary veins without anomalous drainage can cause long-standing pulmonary venous hypertension.

□ Over time, the pulmonary veins become markedly thickened, often resulting in obliteration of the lumina, leading to increased pulmonary capillary pressures and ultimately pulmonary arterial hypertension.

□ Unilateral pulmonary vein obstruction may decompress through venous connections to the contralateral normal lung as well as to pulmonary-to-systemic venous collaterals and lymphatics.

□ Pulmonary arterial blood flow is redistributed to the unaffected parts of the lungs.

Clinical Manifestation

□ Bilateral pulmonary vein stenosis or atresia presents with severe respiratory distress and rapidly progressive heart failure soon after birth.

□ Cyanosis results from right-to-left shunting through an atrial septal defect or persistent foramen ovale.

□ Unilateral pulmonary vein obstruction often presents late with complaints of recurrent infections or hemoptysis due to systemic arterial collaterals or bronchial varices.

□ Unilateral pulmonary vein obstruction results in impaired growth of the ipsilateral pulmonary artery due to preferential perfusion of the normal lung.

□ Severe pulmonary venous obstruction may lead to development of systemic-to-pulmonary arterial collaterals.

Chest Radiographic Findings

□ The affected lung shows a pattern of pulmonary venous hypertension with increased interstitial markings and generalized ground-glass haziness due to pulmonary edema and interlobular septal thickening from engorged lymphatics.

□ Dilated tortuous intraparenchymal pulmonary venous collaterals may be seen.

□ Unilateral involvement may show a small lung volume with ipsilateral mediastinal shift and a small pulmonary artery.

□ Abnormal mediastinal, perihilar, and pleural soft tissue thickening due to pulmonary-to-systemic venous collaterals, lymphatic engorgement, and systemic arterial collaterals

□ Recurrent pulmonary infections or pulmonary hemorrhage

□ Heart size is usually normal unless pulmonary arterial hypertension has resulted in right heart dilatation.

- The radiographic findings vary according to the number of vessels involved, their distribution, and the degree of stenosis.
- The findings of bilateral pulmonary vein obstruction are indistinguishable from those of obstructed total anomalous pulmonary venous connection.
- Unilateral involved lung is hypoplastic and reticulated due to chronic pulmonary venous hypertension

with subpleural septal lines and transpleural systemic-to-pulmonary arterial collateral vessels.
- Prone to recurrent infections or pulmonary hemorrhage
- Pulmonary vein obstruction should be considered in all infants with suspected pulmonary arterial hypertension.

Case 19.1

Bilateral pulmonary vein stenosis in a 7-week-old infant. Chest radiographs show moderate reticular interstitial markings throughout both lungs due to chronic edema and lymphatic dilatation. Heart size is normal. Contrast-enhanced computed tomography (CT) images show a variable pattern of individual pulmonary vein stenosis with discrete narrowing of the right lower pulmonary vein (RLPV), a longer segment narrowing of the left lower pulmonary vein (LLPV). The right upper pulmonary vein (RUPV) is nearly atretic. The left upper pulmonary vein was also stenotic. RA, right atrium; LA, left atrium; RV, right ventricle; LV, left ventricle; Ao, ascending aorta; PA, pulmonary artery.

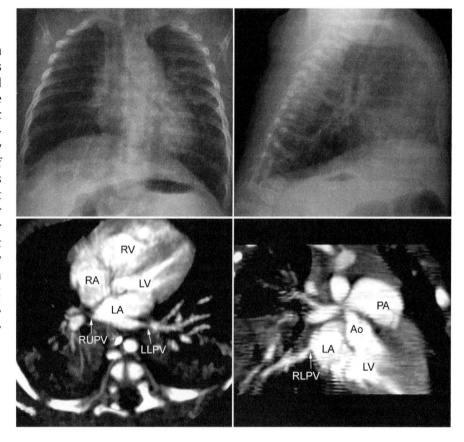

Case 19.2

Unilateral left pulmonary vein stenosis in a 1-month-old infant. Chest radiograph shows a unilateral reticulonodular pattern in the left lung due to chronic pulmonary venous hypertension and lymphatic dilatation. Small left pleural effusion is present. Right lung has an unrelated finding of upper lobe atelectasis. Contrast-enhanced magnetic resonance (MR) angiographic image shows severe stenosis of the left lower pulmonary vein (LLPV) as it connects to the left atrium (LA). The left upper pulmonary vein was not identified. The right pulmonary vein (RPV) appears unobstructed. Note that the left pulmonary artery (LPA) is much smaller than the right pulmonary artery (RPA), suggesting preferential pulmonary arterial blood flow to the unaffected right lung.

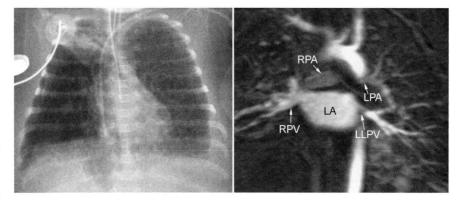

Case 19.3

Unilateral left pulmonary vein stenosis in a 1-week-old infant. Chest radiograph shows significantly reduced vascularity in the left lung and increased vascularity in the right lung.

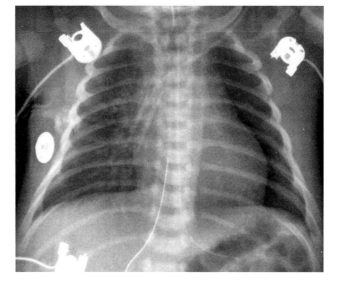

Case 19.4

Right pulmonary vein atresia in a 2-year-old child. The right lung volume is reduced and shows diminished vascularity with a reticular pattern. Axial CT image shows a large left pulmonary vein (LPV) connecting to the left atrium. No vein from the right lung was found to connect to the left atrium. The patient had hemoptysis from bronchial varices. RA, right atrium; LA, left atrium; RV, right ventricle; LV, left ventricle. (Courtesy of L.P. Koopman and N. de Graaf, Erasmus Medical Center, Sophia Children's Hospital, Rotterdam, the Netherlands.)

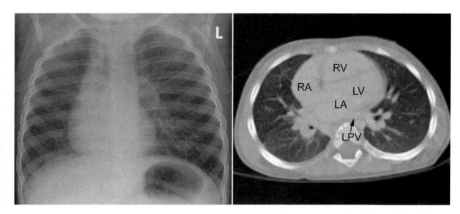

Case 19.5

Pulmonary veno-occlusive disease in a 16-year-old child with severe pulmonary hypertension. Chest radiograph shows a mildly enlarged heart and a markedly dilated main pulmonary arterial segment. Both lungs show generalized increase in interstitial markings with blurring of vessel margins. Contrast-enhanced CT images show thickened interstitial markings extending to the pleural surface. The lung parenchyma shows a mosaic pattern with a ground-glass appearance. The visualized pulmonary veins were not obstructed.

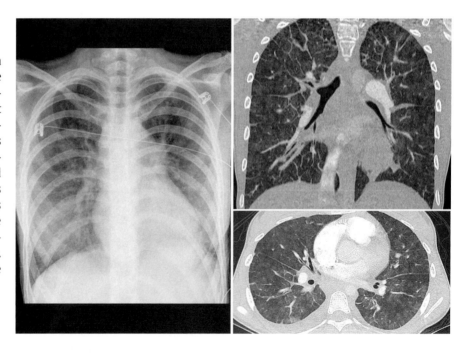

20 Abnormalities of the Mitral Valve and Related Anomalies

With Anne Geoffray

Definition and Classification

- Various anatomic lesions result in obstruction to flow from the left atrium to left ventricle.
- Congenital mitral stenosis is a malformed valve of variable morphology, including hypoplasia of the annulus, fusion of leaflets, double orifice valve, shortened or thickened chordae tendineae, and abnormal papillary muscles.
- Cor triatriatum versus supramitral stenosing ring (**Fig. 20.1**):
  - Cor triatriatum is an intraatrial membrane with one or more potentially restrictive ostia dividing the left atrium into a distal chamber containing the left atrial appendage (LAA) and mitral valve, and a proximal chamber that receives the pulmonary veins.
  - Supramitral stenosing ring is a circumferential membrane arising from the left atrial wall overlying the mitral valve. The atrial appendage is above and behind the membrane, and therefore belongs to the proximal chamber.
- Shone's syndrome is the concurrence of both left ventricular inflow and outflow tract obstructions. The left ventricular inflow obstructions include supravalvar mitral ring, mitral arcade, and parachute mitral valve. The left ventricular outflow obstructions include subvalvar stenosis, bicuspid aortic valve, and aortic coarctation.

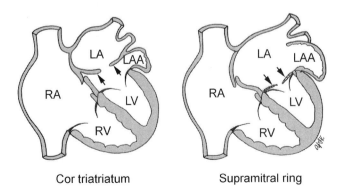

Fig. 20.1 Comparison of cor triatriatum and supramitral stenosing ring. LA, left atrium; LAA, left atrial appendage; LV, left ventricle; RA, right atrium; RV, right ventricle.

- Mitral regurgitation can rarely be due to a congenitally dysplastic mitral valve.

Pathophysiology

- To maintain left ventricular filling, obstruction at the mitral valve level results in increasing left atrial pressure proportional to the severity of stenosis.
- Restriction of blood flow from lungs to left ventricle, which results in decreased cardiac output
- Restriction of pulmonary venous return increases pulmonary venous and capillary pressure, resulting in pulmonary edema.
- Chronic pulmonary edema may lead to pulmonary hemosiderin deposition and fibrosis.
- Pulmonary hypertension develops, resulting in increased pulmonary vascular resistance.
- In response to increased afterload, the right ventricle hypertrophies and eventually fails.
- Severely restrictive intraatrial membrane with cor triatriatum is associated with various forms of anomalous pulmonary venous drainage with development of pulmonary-to-systemic venous communications as alternate pathways for drainage.

Clinical Presentation

- Variable age of presentation depending on the severity of the obstruction
- Frequent initial symptoms from pulmonary venous hypertension include dyspnea, tachypnea, wheezing, and recurrent respiratory tract infections mimicking primary pulmonary disease.
- General symptoms from heart failure and reduced cardiac output include poor feeding, failure to thrive, and fatigue.

Chest Radiographic Findings

- Pulmonary venous hypertension with increased interstitial markings and generalized ground-glass haziness due to pulmonary edema
- Chronic reticular interstitial pattern with hemosiderin deposition, fibrosis, and lymphatic engorgement

219

□ Variable cardiomegaly with right ventricular enlargement depending on the degree of pulmonary arterial hypertension

□ Signs of left atrial enlargement; in cor triatriatum, the left atrial appendage is not enlarged because it is distal to the obstruction.

□ Dilatation of the central pulmonary arteries with development of pulmonary arterial hypertension

□ Small aorta with decreased cardiac output

Pearls

□ Pattern of diffuse pulmonary venous hypertension and pulmonary edema is proportionate to the severity of stenosis.

□ Specific finding of left atrial enlargement with supramitral or mitral valvar stenosis

□ Development of pulmonary arterial hypertension results in marked right ventricular enlargement and prominent central pulmonary arteries.

Case 20.1

Mitral valve stenosis in a 6-year-old child. Chest radiographs show specific left atrial enlargement with prominence of the left atrial appendage contour and mild pulmonary venous hypertension.

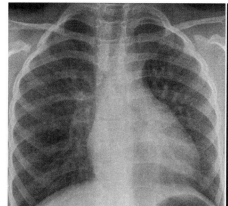
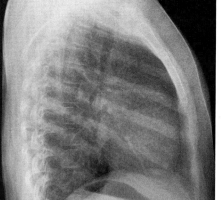

Case 20.2

Cor triatriatum in a 2-month-old infant. Chest radiographs show mild cardiomegaly with prominence of the right heart contour without left atrial enlargement and mild pulmonary venous hypertension. There was mild restriction across the cor triatriatum.

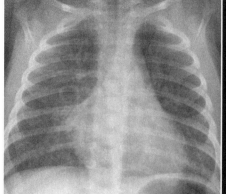
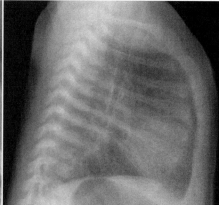

Case 20.3

Cor triatriatum in a 2-year-old child. Chest radiographs show moderate cardiomegaly, pulmonary venous hypertension with central airspace edema, and dilatation of the central pulmonary arteries that hides the small aorta due to pulmonary arterial hypertension. The left atrial appendage segment of the left heart border is not prominent. The patient had a severely restrictive form of cor triatriatum.

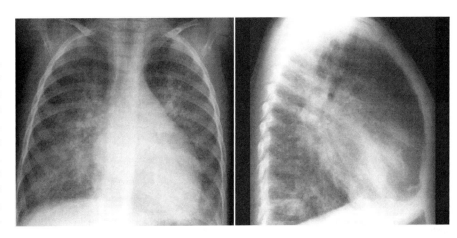

Case 20.4

Dysplastic mitral valve regurgitation in a 16-day-old infant with coarctation of the aorta. Chest radiograph shows moderate cardiomegaly with a globular appearance. Both lungs show diffusely increased interstitial markings due to pulmonary venous hypertension.

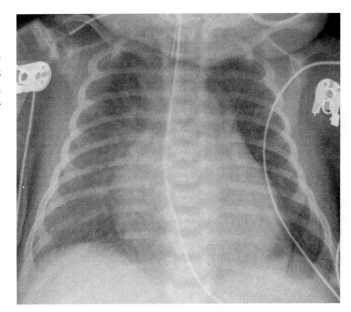

Case 20.5

Dysplastic mitral valve regurgitation with atrial septal defect and patent ductus arteriosus in an 11-week-old infant. The left atrial appendage segment (arrows) shows a severe bulge. Both lungs shows findings of severe pulmonary venous hypertension.

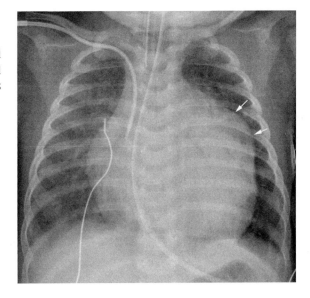

21 Obstructive Lesions of the Left Ventricular Outflow Tract

With Monica Epelman

Classification and Definitions

□ Valvar
- Variable deformity of the cusps and leaflets
  - Hypoplastic: small
  - Dysplastic: thickened and nodular
  - Abnormal number: fusion of commissures
□ Supravalvular stenosis
- Congenital narrowing of ascending aorta localized or diffuse
- Aortic dysplasia with thickening of the aortic wall resulting in an hourglass deformity
- Commonly associated with Williams syndrome, which is the result of microdeletion of chromosome 7q11.23, characterized by an elfin face, neurodevelopmental retardation, and multisystem manifestations with obstruction of major arteries to varying degrees, and often associated with hypercalcemia
□ Subvalvular stenosis
- Discrete membranous thickened ridge, diaphragm, or fibromuscular tunnel
- Hypertrophic cardiomyopathy with asymmetric septal hypertrophy: with or without abnormal anterior motion of the mitral valve

Pathophysiology

□ Disturbs normal blood flow, resulting in further thickening of the aortic valve leaflets and increasing obstruction
□ Valvar stenosis commonly progresses with a variable rate.
□ Increased pressure overload in systole leads to left ventricular hypertrophy.
□ Left ventricular decompensation may result in reduced contractility and heart failure.
□ Compromised blood supply to myocardium may lead to ventricular dysrhythmia.
□ Severe obstruction leads to underdevelopment of the left ventricle.
□ Supravalvar stenosis is usually progressive, and aortic regurgitation is common.

□ Supravalvar stenosis is often associated with systemic arterial and coronary ostial stenosis, which may worsen with time.
□ Supravalvar stenosis is often associated with peripheral pulmonary artery stenosis, which may resolve spontaneously.
□ Systemic hypertension is common.
□ Subvalvar stenosis often progresses with a variable rate; often associated with aortic regurgitation damaged by subvalvar jet
□ Muscular subaortic obstruction is associated with a small aortic root.

Clinical Manifestations

□ Critical aortic valve stenosis presents in early infancy with congestive heart failure and circulatory collapse.
□ Acute ischemia may result in a dysrhythmia and sudden death during physical activity.
□ Complication of bacterial endocarditis
□ Asymptomatic systolic murmur
□ Well tolerated unless severe
□ Dyspnea, easy fatigability, or chest pain may develop
□ Syncope in severe obstruction

Chest Radiographic Findings

□ Variable findings, which reflect the degree of stenosis and left ventricular decompensation
□ Pulmonary vasculature is normal until left ventricular decompensation with pulmonary venous hypertension and pulmonary edema.
□ Mild to moderate cardiomegaly with specific left ventricular enlargement
□ Dilatation of ascending aorta due to poststenotic dilatation from abnormal jetting across stenotic valve
□ Aortic valve contour may be small with supravalvar stenosis.
□ Aortic valve calcification extremely rare in children

Case 21.1

Critical aortic valve stenosis in a 4-week-old infant. Chest radiographs show marked cardiomegaly with pulmonary edema due to left ventricular decompensation and congestive heart failure. Aorta is not enlarged.

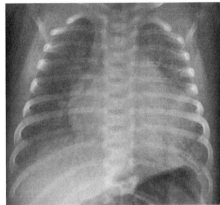 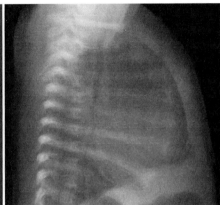

Case 21.2

Aortic valve stenosis in a 12-year-old child. Chest radiographs show mild cardiomegaly and normal pulmonary vascularity. The dilated ascending aorta results in a convex right upper mediastinal border.

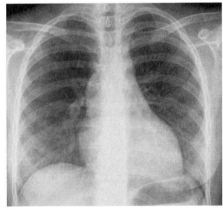 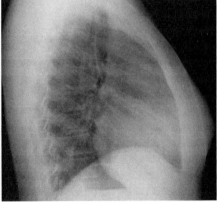

Case 21.3

Aortic valve stenosis and regurgitation in a 15-year-old patient. Chest radiographs show moderate cardiomegaly with specific left ventricular enlargement and pulmonary venous hypertension. The ascending aortic contour and aortic knob are enlarged.

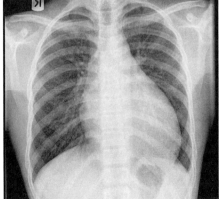 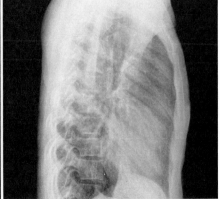

Case 21.4

Subaortic stenosis in a 4-year-old child. Chest radiographs show mild cardiomegaly with signs of left ventricular and left atrial enlargement. The ascending aorta and aortic knob are not dilated. The pulmonary vascularity is normal.

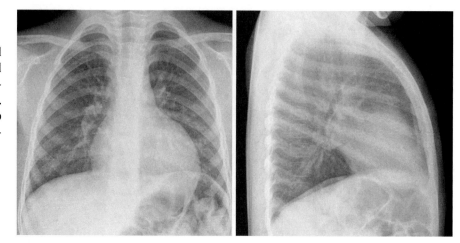

22 Hypoplastic Left Heart Syndrome

With Monica Epelman

Definition and Classification

- Not a single lesion but a constellation of cardiac anomalies characterized by underdevelopment of the left heart with normally related and connected great vessels
- Most marked cases show severe stenosis or atresia of the aortic and mitral valves with the left atrium, left ventricle, and ascending aorta markedly underdeveloped (**Fig. 22.1**).
- In some cases only the aortic valve is atretic, and the left ventricle is small and thickened, with the left atrium normal or enlarged.
- Hypoplasia of the aortic arch is variable and there is usually a juxtaductal coarctation.
- Ventricular septum is usually intact.
- Presence of a ventricular septal defect results in a relatively large left ventricle.
- Survival requires an atrial septal defect and patent ductus arteriosus.

Pathophysiology

- Distinguished by different degrees of underdevelopment of the left side of the heart and hypoplasia of the ascending aorta
- An interatrial communication through a stretched patent foramen ovale or true atrial septal defect is needed to decompress the left atrium and provide left-to-right shunting of blood.
- Cases with unrestricted atrial septal defect show less severe pulmonary venous hypertension (**Fig. 22.1**, left panel). Cases with intact atrial septum or restrictive atrial septal defect have severe impairment of blood flow from the left heart, and there is marked pulmonary venous hypertension (**Fig. 22.1**, right panel). A decompressing vein, called a levoatriocardinal vein, can be present.
- Decreased left ventricular compliance results in most of the pulmonary venous blood returning to the left atrium shunting left to right into the right atrium.
- A small amount of left atrial blood may cross a patent mitral valve and be ejected into a tiny ascending aorta.
- Total mixing of saturated pulmonary with desaturated systemic venous blood in right atrium
- Blood flows into the right ventricle and out through an enlarged pulmonary artery.
- Right ventricle maintains both pulmonary and systemic circulations, with blood reaching the aorta through a patent ductus arteriosus.
- An adequate-size ductus arteriosus is needed, permitting a right-to-left shunt during ventricular systole, sending blood from the right ventricle to the descending aorta.
- Major hemodynamic abnormality is inadequate maintenance of the systemic circulation, which depends on the size of the ductus arteriosus.
- Difficulties develop with higher systemic than pulmonary vascular resistance and closure of the ductus arteriosus, resulting in systemic hypoperfusion and shock.
- Right ventricular function deteriorates, resulting in systemic hypoperfusion.
- Abnormal ventricular wall motion may result from endocardial fibroelastosis or ischemic damage.

Clinical Manifestations

- Symptoms vary depending on the severity of the lesion.
- Most common cause of congestive heart failure in the first few days of life
- Signs of heart failure with tachycardia, dyspnea, tachypnea, hepatomegaly
- Restrictive atrial communication presents in the first few hours of life with severe hypoxemia.

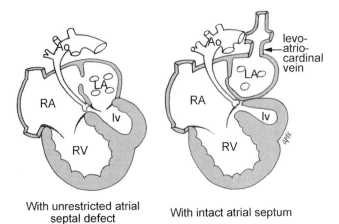

With unrestricted atrial septal defect   With intact atrial septum

Fig. 22.1 Types of hypoplastic left heart syndrome. Ao, ascending aorta; LA, left atrium; lv, rudimentary left ventricle; RA, right atrium; RV, right ventricle.

225

- Ductus arteriosus partially closes, resulting in systemic hypoperfusion and shock.
- Signs of low cardiac output with weak peripheral pulses and vasoconstricted extremities
- Cyanosis due to right-to-left shunting through a patent ductus arteriosus
- Grayish-blue color denoting a mix of cyanosis and hypoperfusion

Chest Radiographic Findings

- Variety of findings may be seen depending on anatomic variables
- In first hours of life, normal heart and pulmonary vascularity
- Cardiomegaly develops rapidly and is associated with increased pulmonary vascularity.
- Pulmonary vasculature may demonstrate a variety of flow patterns.
- Pulmonary vascularity varies with the degree of shunting across the atrial communication and ductus arteriosus.
- Pulmonary vascularity may be normal or increased, with a mixed pattern of pulmonary venous hypertension and overcirculation.

- When there is a nonrestrictive atrial defect, pulmonary vasculature is increased, with an overcirculation pattern as more blood enters the pulmonary arteries.
- When the atrial defect is restrictive, increased left atrial pressure results in severe pulmonary venous and arterial hypertension.
- Pattern of pulmonary venous hypertension and pulmonary edema is variable.
- Pulmonary edema may range from minimal to severe.
- Atypical pattern of homogeneously hazy lungs resulting from pulmonary edema
- Heart size varies according to the degree of left-to-right shunt across the atrial septum and ductus arteriosus. With restrictive interatrial communication and severe pulmonary arterial and venous hypertension, the heart may be normally sized. With a large left-to-right shunt and reduced pulmonary vascular resistance, the heart enlarges and pulmonary vascularity increases.
- Heart may not be enlarged with high-grade pulmonary venous obstruction.
- An underdeveloped small aorta is difficult to detect as the pulmonary artery is large and positioned high, mimicking an aortic knob.
- Thymus is commonly hypoplastic secondary to postnatal stresses.

Pearls

- Pulmonary vasculature demonstrates a variety of flow relationships, reflecting important anatomic

changes, namely in the size of the atrial communication and the size of the ductus arteriosus.

Case 22.1

Hypoplastic left heart syndrome with mitral stenosis, aortic atresia, an unrestricted atrial septal defect, and a large patent ductus arteriosus. Chest radiographs obtained at day 1 and 4 days later show increasing heart size and pulmonary overcirculation with mild edema due to a decrease in pulmonary vascular resistance.

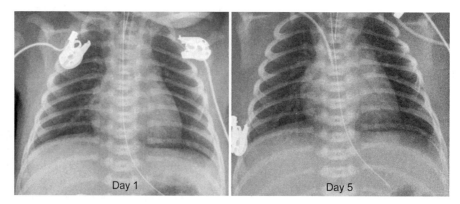

Day 1

Day 5

Case 22.2

Hypoplastic left heart syndrome with mitral and aortic atresia and intact atrial septum in a 1-day-old infant. Chest radiograph *(left panel)* shows a normal heart size and an extensive reticulonodular interstitial pattern as a result of severe pulmonary venous hypertension due to the intact atrial septum. The radiographic findings are indistinguishable from obstructed total anomalous pulmonary venous connection. The hypertensive left atrium was decompressed through a levoatriocardinal vein, which is a vertical venous channel between the left upper pulmonary vein and left innominate vein (see **Fig. 22.1**). A follow-up study at 4 weeks of age *(right panel)* with stenting of the decompressing levoatriocardinal vein and balloon atrial septostomy shows improvement with moderate cardiomegaly and improved pulmonary edema.

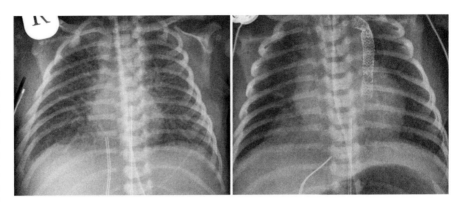

Case 22.3

Hypoplastic left heart syndrome with long-term prostaglandin administration. Chest radiograph in a newborn *(left upper panel)* shows mild cardiomegaly with normal pulmonary vascularity. A follow-up study at 4 months of age *(right upper panel)* shows increased cardiomegaly with right heart enlargement and increased pulmonary vascularity with pulmonary edema. On long-term prostaglandins awaiting heart transplantation, subtle periosteal reaction has developed along the clavicles, ribs, and proximal humeri. Radiographs of the lower extremities show extensive symmetric cortical hyperostosis.

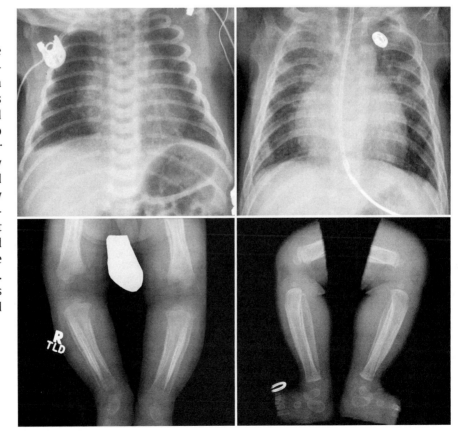

Case 22.4

Hypoplastic left heart syndrome with critical aortic stenosis, who underwent balloon dilatation of the aortic valve on three days of life. Chest radiograph at 1 month of age shows moderate cardiomegaly associated with mild edema. A follow-up study at 4 months of age shows deterioration with congestive heart failure and progressive diffuse pulmonary edema.

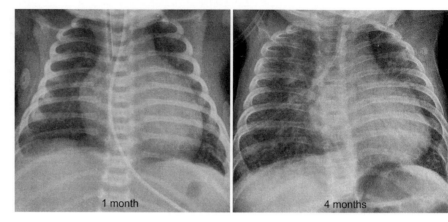

23 Obstructive Lesions of the Aortic Arch

With Monica Epelman

□ Obstructive lesions of the aortic arch include the following varieties:
- Discrete coarctation of the aorta
- Tubular hypoplasia of the aortic arch
- Combined hypoplasia and discrete coarctation
- Interruption of the aortic arch

■ Coarctation and Tubular Hypoplasia of the Aortic Arch

Definition and Classification

□ Congenital stenosis of the thoracic aorta of variable severity
□ Severe forms leave only a small residual lumen, with mild forms producing only minimal narrowing.
□ The terms *preductal* and *postductal* as well as *infantile* and *adult type* are misleading.
□ Coarctation versus tubular hypoplasia (**Fig. 23.1**)

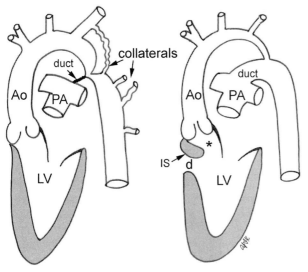

Isolated coarctation

Tubular hypoplasia of the aortic arch

Fig. 23.1 Coarctation and tubular hypoplasia of the aortic arch. Tubular hypoplasia of the aortic arch is usually associated with left ventricular outflow flow tract obstruction (asterisk) due to posterior malalignment of the infundibular septum (IS). Ao, ascending aorta; d, ventricular septal defect; LV, left ventricle; PA, pulmonary artery.

□ Simple aortic coarctation refers to discrete coarctation in the absence of other intracardiac lesions, with the exception of a bicuspid aortic valve.
□ Localized ridge-like infolding almost always in a juxtaductal position
□ Diffuse with a long hypoplastic segment proximal to the ductus arteriosus
□ Complex aortic coarctation refers to coarctation in the presence of other intracardiac anomalies and almost always includes a patent ductus arteriosus. The right panel of Fig. 23.1 shows an example with a posterior malalignment type of ventricular septal defect causing subaortic stenosis.
□ Other associations include Berry aneurysms of the circle of Willis.
□ Association with Turner syndrome

Pathophysiology

□ Simple aortic coarctation is not associated with cardiac defects, and collateral circulation develops gradually over time.
□ Complex aortic coarctation is almost always associated with conditions that decrease antegrade flow through the ascending aorta and increase right-to-left shunting across the ductus arteriosus in utero, including ventricular septal defect and left-sided obstructive lesion, such as subaortic stenosis and mitral valve anomalies (**Fig. 23.1**, right panel).
□ Discrete juxtaductal aortic narrowing results in systolic overloading and hypertrophy of the left ventricle.
□ In weeks to months as the left ventricle hypertrophies and dilates, the ejection fraction improves and the cardiac output reaches the high normal range.
□ At rest left ventricular pressures are normal or mildly increased, but they increase to abnormal levels when afterload is increased with exercise.
□ Progressive development of a collateral circulation between the proximal high pressure and the distal low pressure aorta below the coarctation
□ Usual vessels developing a collateral circulation are from the subclavian arteries and arteries around the scapula, internal mammary arteries, and the intercostal arteries.
□ Blood flow through renal, splanchnic, and leg arteries is normal at rest, but may not increase appropriately with exercise.

- Complex and long segment hypoplasia results in systolic overloading of the left ventricle as well as pulmonary hypertension.
- Right ventricular systolic overloading, right ventricular hypertrophy, and elevated right-sided pressures develop.
- Good collateral circulation has not yet developed, with blood being delivered to the descending aorta from a patent ductus arteriosus.
- Ductal lumen provides additional space to the narrowed aorta.
- Hemodynamic deterioration occurs rapidly at the time of ductal closure.
- Cardiac decompensation, cardiac enlargement, and congestive heart failure develop.

Clinical Manifestations

- Age of symptoms depends on the type and severity of the coarctation, the presence of associated cardiovascular anomalies, and most importantly the patency of the ductus arteriosus.
- Simple aortic coarctation is often asymptomatic in children and diagnosed late:
  - Asymptomatic hypertension in the upper extremities with lower pressures in the legs
  - Absent, diminished or delayed peripheral pulses
  - Leg discomfort on exertion
  - Chest pain and syncope
- Complex aortic coarctation presents early in infancy toward the end of the first week of life due to severe obstruction:
  - Patent ductus acts as a bypass for blood around the coarctation with good collateral circulation not yet developed, and closure causes increasing obstruction resulting in early congestive heart failure.
  - Differential cyanosis may be present, with the lower half of the body cyanotic due to the right-to-left ductal shunt.
  - Other symptoms include poor feeding, weight gain, respiratory distress, acute circulatory shock, and renal failure.

Chest Radiographic Findings

- Findings vary depending on the anatomy and severity of the obstruction as well as the presence of associated congenital heart lesions.
- Simple aortic coarctation
  - Normal pulmonary vascularity
  - Heart size is normal.
  - Prominent cardiac apex with left ventricular hypertrophy
  - Variable abnormal configuration of aortic arch and descending aorta

- Thymus frequently obscures diagnostic characteristics of aorta
- Convexed prominent leftward curvature of descending aorta due to poststenotic dilatation may be the only visible finding.
- 'Figure-of-3' configuration consisting of an upper convexity due to pre-stenotic part of the aortic knob and origin of left subclavian artery, lower convexity due to poststenotic dilatation of the descending aorta and the waist at the actual site of stenosis
- Ascending aorta normal or dilated; moderately dilated ascending aorta when the aortic valve is bicuspid with or without stenosis or insufficiency
- Rib notching represents pressure erosion from dilated or tortuous intercostal arteries due to a collateral circulation. Irregular asymmetric sclerosis is a more common finding.
- Rib sclerosis and notching is usually bilateral involving the inferior aspects of the third to eighth ribs posteriorly.
- First to third ribs are not notched because the intercostal arteries arise from the thyrocervical trunk originating from the aorta above the coarctation.
- Occasionally an aberrant right subclavian artery distal to the site of coarctation prevents development of right-sided rib notching.
- Atretic left subclavian artery or one arising distal to coarctation prevents left-sided rib notching.
- Dilated, tortuous internal mammary arteries cause scalloping of retrosternal soft tissues.
- Superior mediastinal widening due to extensive collateral formation
- Rib notching is rarely seen in children under the age of 7.
- Lack of rib notching does not always mean a mild gradient or the lack of a good collateral network.
- Complex aortic coarctation
  - Increased pulmonary overcirculation with pulmonary venous hypertension and pulmonary edema due to left ventricular failure
  - Moderate to marked cardiomegaly with global enlargement of the left atrium, left ventricle, and right ventricle due to left ventricular failure and increased pulmonary arterial pressures
  - Enlarged central pulmonary arteries with pulmonary hypertension
  - Aorta is normal or small and the 'figure-of-3' configuration is not present.
  - Rib notching is not seen due to lack of a developed collateral circulation.
- Pseudocoarctation is an asymptomatic variant with a tortuous, dilated, and kinked aorta that is not associated with a pressure gradient across the lesion.
  - Exaggerated abnormal aortic contour and a classic 'figure-of-3' configuration may be seen.
  - Absence of cardiomegaly and rib notching

- Aortic coarctation is divided into simple and complex types.
- Simple lesion, asymptomatic in infancy
- Descending aorta may simply lie more lateral than usual with a leftward convexity or show the 'figure-of-3' configuration

- Rib notching cannot be relied upon and is often absent.
- Complex lesion symptomatic in infancy and must be considered with findings of congestive heart failure in the first week of life

■ Interruption of the Aortic Arch

Definition and Classification

- An extreme form of aortic obstruction characterized by complete discontinuity of the arch between the proximal ascending aorta and the distal descending aorta with a segment of the arch absent
- Anatomic distinction from aortic arch atresia where continuity of the aorta is maintained and an obstruction is due to an imperforate fibrous strand of variable length
- Anatomically a variable length of aortic arch is absent and blood is delivered to the descending aorta through a patent ductus arteriosus.
- Classification depends on the location of the interruption (**Fig. 23.2**):
  - Type A: the interruption is distal to the left subclavian artery, similar to coarctation.
  - Type B: the interruption is between the left carotid and left subclavian arteries, with an aberrant right subclavian artery being common.
  - Type C: the interruption is between the right innominate and left carotid arteries.
- Almost always associated with a ventricular septal defect and patent ductus arteriosus
- Other common associated lesions are bicuspid aortic valve, mitral valve deformity, subaortic stenosis, truncus arteriosus, complete and corrected transposition, aorticopulmonary window, and double-outlet right ventricle.

- Type B interruption is commonly associated with DiGeorge syndrome.

Pathophysiology

- Aortic arch interruption is most often a consequence of an intracardiac conotruncal malformation causing subaortic obstruction, which compromises blood flow to the ascending aorta during fetal life.
- Ductal dependent left-sided obstructive lesion with the descending thoracic aorta receiving blood from the pulmonary artery

Clinical Manifestations

- Similar to extreme form of complex tubular hypoplasia of the aortic arch, as discussed in Chapter 22
- Acute cardiovascular collapse or heart failure after spontaneous closure of the ductus arteriosus, which may occur in the first days of life.
- Commonly congestive heart failure toward the end of the first week of life
- May present with respiratory distress, variable degrees of cyanosis, poor peripheral pulses

Chest Radiographic Findings

- Increased pulmonary overcirculation with associated left-to-right shunts
- Pulmonary venous hypertension with increased interstitial markings and generalized ground-glass haziness due to pulmonary edema

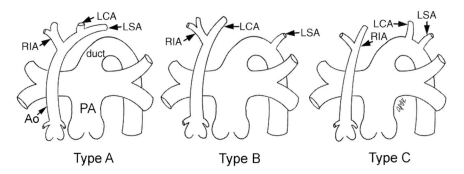

Fig. 23.2 Classification of interruption of the aortic arch. Ao, ascending aorta; LCA, left common carotid artery; LSA, left subclavian artery; PA, pulmonary artery; RIA, right innominate artery.

□ Mixed pattern of pulmonary edema and overcirculation with pulmonary edema predominating

□ Mild to moderate cardiomegaly with biventricular and left atrial enlargement

□ Moderate to marked enlargement of the main pulmonary artery often in a higher position

□ Midline trachea down to bifurcation due to complete interruption and absence of the transverse aortic arch

□ Inconspicuous appearance of aortic knob

□ Termination of descending aorta at level of main pulmonary artery

□ Narrow superior mediastinum due to hypoplasia or aplasia of thymus with DiGoerge syndrome or due to postnatal stress.

□ Rib notching is rare. When present, it indicates a stenotic or closed ductus arteriosus.

Pearls

□ Large heart with increased pulmonary vascularity and pulmonary edema in a critically ill newborn

□ Midline trachea and inconspicuous aortic knob due to complete interruption and absence of the transverse aortic arch

---

Case 23.1

Coarctation of the aorta in a 16-year-old patient. Chest radiographs show a characteristic 'figure-of-3' aortic contour with the indentation (*arrow* in **A**) formed by the infolding wall of the aorta and poststenotic dilatation of the descending aorta. Bilateral subtle notching involving the third to sixth ribs is seen due to development of arterial collaterals with erosions from dilated intercostal arteries. A thin band of soft tissue (*arrows* in **B**) is seen behind the sternum on the lateral radiograph considered to be dilated internal mammary arteries. Prominent ascending aorta is related to a bicuspid aortic valve. (**C**) Contrast-enhanced magnetic resonance (MR) angiogram shows a tight aortic coarctation with a small residual lumen and a posterior ridge-like shelf distal to the origin of the left subclavian artery. A well-developed network of arterial collaterals is present to bypass the obstruction through the intercostal arteries. The internal mammary artery (IMA) is dilated.

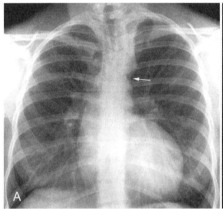
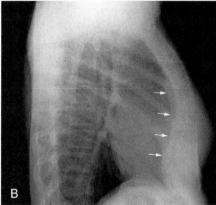
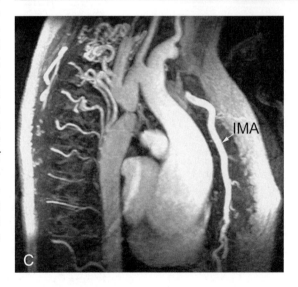

Case 23.2

Coarctation of the aorta in a 10-year-old patient. Chest radiograph shows an outward convexity *(black arrows)* of the poststenotic part of the descending aorta. The aortic knob is not clearly defined. There is mild cardiomegaly with a prominent cardiac apex. There is subtle irregularity and sclerosis of the inferior surfaces of the ribs, which is best shown in the left fifth rib *(white arrows).*

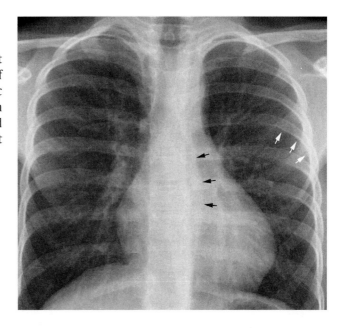

Case 23.3

Tubular hypoplasia of the aortic arch and discrete coarctation of the aorta with a large perimembranous ventricular septal defect and a patent ductus arteriosus in a neonate. Chest radiograph obtained on 4th day of life shows moderate cardiomegaly with pulmonary overcirculation and interstitial edema. A follow-up study at 14 days of age shows progressive cardiac enlargement and congestive heart failure. Hemodynamic deterioration occurred rapidly with closure of the ductus arteriosus.

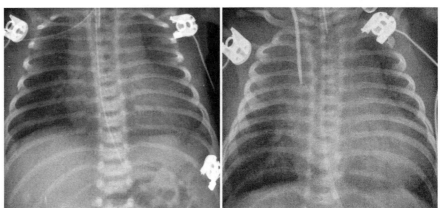

Case 23.4

Interrupted aortic arch with a ventricular septal defect in a 4-day-old infant. Chest radiograph shows moderate cardiomegaly with pulmonary overcirculation and edema, which are suggestive of an obligatory left-to-right shunt in an early neonate. There are pleural effusions.

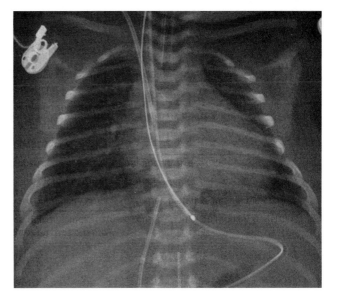

24 Transpositions of the Great Arteries

With Kevin S. Roman

□ *Transposition* is a term to describe ventriculoarterial connection. It refers to discordant ventriculoarterial connection: the right ventricle connects to the aorta and the left ventricle to the pulmonary artery. Transposition occurs with various types of atrioventricular connections:
  • With concordant atrioventricular connection: complete transposition
  • With discordant atrioventricular connection: congenitally corrected transposition
  • With various forms of univentricular atrioventricular connections
  • With various forms of atrioventricular connections in the presence of right or left atrial isomerism
□ There are two classic types of transposition:
  • Complete transposition
  • Congenitally corrected transposition

■ Complete Transposition

Definition and Classification (Fig. 24.1)

□ Characterized by normal atria, normally related ventricles, normal atrioventricular connections, and abnormal discordant ventriculoarterial connections
  • Right atrium connects to morphologic right ventricle, which gives rise to the aorta

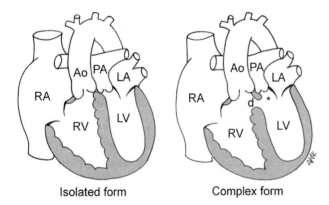

Isolated form   Complex form

Fig. 24.1 Complete transposition. Asterisk indicates subpulmonary outflow tract, which is often narrowed in the complex form. Ao, ascending aorta; d, ventricular septal defect; LA, left atrium; LV, left ventricle; PA, pulmonary artery; RA, right atrium; RV, right ventricle.

  • Left atrium connects to morphologic left ventricle, which gives rise to the pulmonary artery
□ Also called D-transposition, as it occurs with D-loop ventricles (the morphologically right ventricle on the right side of the morphologically left ventricle) and, in the majority of cases, with a right-sided and anterior aorta. It is a confusing term because of variations in ventricular loop and great arterial relationship.
□ Complete transposition as a simple form: about 50% of patients are without associated defects other than a patent foramen ovale or a small patent ductus arteriosus.
□ Associated lesions in 50%: ventricular septal defect, left ventricular outflow tract obstruction, and obstructive lesion of the aortic arch.

Pathophysiology

□ Concordant atrioventricular and discordant ventriculoarterial connections result in two isolated parallel circulations:
  • Deoxygenated systemic venous blood returns to the right atrium, enters the right ventricle, and exits into the aorta, only to return to the right atrium.
  • Oxygenated pulmonary venous blood returns to the left atrium, enters the left ventricle, and exits into the pulmonary artery, only to return to the left atrium.
□ Survival depends on mixing between these circulations, which may be across a patent foramen ovale or atrial septal defect, additional ventricular septal defect, or patent ductus arteriosus.
□ As the pulmonary vascular resistance falls postnatally, there is increased pulmonary blood flow unless an associated pulmonary stenosis is present.

Clinical Manifestations

□ Varies according to the presence of associated defects
□ Soon after birth with closure of ductus arteriosus there is severe hypoxemia.
□ Cyanosis is the most common presentation and is often seen within the first hours of life.
□ Mild cyanosis with associated lesions that permit good mixing
□ Heart failure is seen with associated large ventricular septal defects.

Chest Radiographic Findings

- Neonates often have normal heart size and pulmonary vascularity.
- Increased pulmonary vasculature with an overcirculation pattern with decreasing pulmonary vascular resistance
- Over time, heart size enlarges.
- An oblong egg-on-side appearance due to rightward displacement of the right ventricular outflow tract and combined right atrial and left ventricular dilatation
- Narrow vascular pedicle due to parallel course of anteroposteriorly related great arteries and small thymus as it atrophies with postnatal stress
- Decreased pulmonary vasculature with associated severe pulmonary stenosis
- Aortic arch usually left sided

Pearls

- Most common cyanotic lesion presenting in newborn period
- Classic findings seen over time with decreasing pulmonary vascular resistance

- Increased pulmonary overcirculation
- Heart enlarges with a typical egg-on-side configuration.
- Narrow vascular pedicle with thymic atrophy

■ Congenitally Corrected Transposition

Definition and Classification (Fig. 24.2)

- Characterized by normal atria with inverted ventricles, resulting in abnormal discordant atrioventricular connections and abnormal discordant ventriculoarterial connections
  - Right atrium is connected to the left ventricle, which gives rise to the pulmonary artery.
  - Left atrium is connected to the right ventricle, which gives rise to the aorta.
- Also called L-transposition because it occurs with L-loop ventricles (the morphologically right ventricle on the left side of the morphologically left ventricle)

and, in the majority of cases, with a left-sided and anterior aorta. It is a confusing term because of variations in ventricular loop and great arterial relationship.
- Most patients have additional malformations that determine presentation, radiographic findings, and management:
  - Ventricular septal defect
  - Pulmonary stenosis
  - Ebstein's malformation or dysplastic tricuspid valve; often associated with an obstructive lesion of the aortic arch when tricuspid regurgitation is severe
  - Dextrocardia
  - Conduction disturbances

Pathophysiology

- Discordant connections at two levels result in physiologically correct circulation and therefore are considered to be congenitally corrected.
  - Desaturated systemic venous blood returns to the right atrium, passes through the right-sided morphologic left ventricle, and into the pulmonary artery.
  - Oxygenated pulmonary venous blood returns to the left atrium, passes through the left-sided morphologic right ventricle, and into the aorta.
- Associated lesions result in a spectrum of hemodynamic abnormalities.

Clinical Manifestations

- Widely variable and relate to associated lesions
- Without associated lesions, symptoms may be absent if there is no significant functional or conduction disturbance.

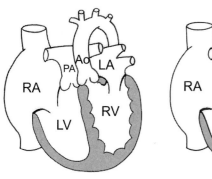

Isolated form   Complex form

Fig. 24.2 Congenitally corrected transposition. Asterisk indicates subpulmonary outflow track which is often narrowed in the complex form. Ao, ascending aorta; d, ventricular septal defect; LA, left atrium; LV, left ventricle; PA, pulmonary artery; RA, right atrium; RV, right ventricle.

- Congestive heart failure with an unobstructed pulmonary outflow and ventricular septal defect
- Cyanosis with pulmonary stenosis and ventricular septal defect
- Overtime progression of conduction defects to complete heart block results in cardiac failure.
- Progressive tricuspid regurgitation and right ventricular failure may lead to pulmonary arterial hypertension.

Chest Radiographic Findings

- Variable depending on the associated anomalies
- High incidence of dextrocardia or mesocardia
- Isolated anomaly with no hemodynamic abnormality may appear normal.
- Variable pulmonary vascularity related to associated lesions:
  - Increased pulmonary vascularity with left-to-right shunts in cases with a ventricular septal defect and unobstructed pulmonary outflow

- Decreased pulmonary vascularity with right-to-left shunts with a ventricular septal defect and pulmonary stenosis
- Pulmonary venous hypertension and pulmonary edema with tricuspid regurgitation and right ventricular failure
- Inapparent main pulmonary artery due to rightward and posterior positioning
- Normal to moderate cardiomegaly
  - Associated shunts with variable chamber enlargement
  - Associated tricuspid valve anomaly and regurgitation with left atrial enlargement
  - Progression of right ventricular failure with global cardiac enlargement
- Ascending aorta arising from the right ventricle is the most leftward and anterior great vessel, forming a relatively straight or convex fullness of the upper left heart border and superior mediastinum

---

Pearls

- Strongly suspected when dextrocardia or mesocardia is present with situs solitus or when levocardia or mesocardia is present with situs inversus.
- Hallmark finding of a prominent convexity of the upper left cardiac border
- Lesions of tricuspid valve almost considered a basic part of the entity and result in specific marked enlargement of the left atrium

---

- Variable pulmonary vascularity and heart size related to associated lesions
- Permanent pacemaker is often needed due to progressive conduction disturbances

---

Case 24.1

Complete transposition of the great arteries. Chest radiograph in a neonate *(left panel)* shows normal heart size with a narrow vascular pedicle giving rise to the so-called egg-on-side appearance and mild pulmonary overcirculation. The superior mediastinum appears narrow due to the anteroposterior relationship of the transposed great vessels and small thymus due to the stress of hypoxia. In follow-up at 3 days of age *(right panel)*, there is increased heart size and pulmonary overcirculation due to decreasing pulmonary vascular resistance.

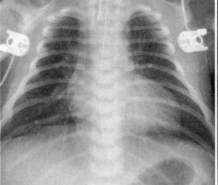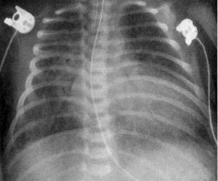

Case 24.2

Complete transposition of the great arteries in a 5-day-old neonate. Chest radiographs show characteristic findings of a mildly enlarged heart with a typical egg-on-side appearance, concave main pulmonary artery with a narrow vascular pedicle, and pulmonary overcirculation with mild venous congestion.

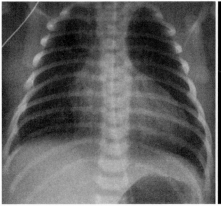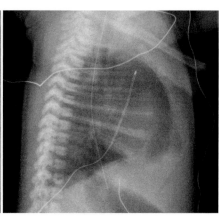

Case 24.3

Complete transposition of the great arteries with a ventricular septal defect in a 3-day-old neonate. Chest radiograph shows a characteristic heart with an egg-on-side configuration, a narrow superior mediastinum, and pulmonary overcirculation with congestive heart failure.

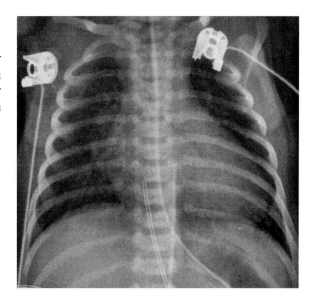

Case 24.4

Complete transposition of the great arteries with ventricular septal defect and coarctation of the aorta in a 13-day-old neonate. Chest radiographs show marked cardiomegaly, pulmonary overcirculation with congestive heart failure due to an associated large ventricular septal defect or aortic coarctation.

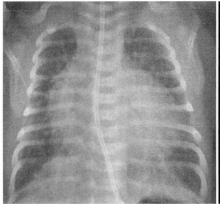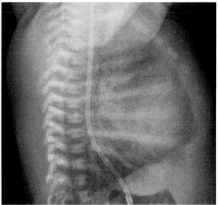

Case 24.5

Untreated complete transposition of the great arteries with a ventricular septal defect and patent ductus arteriosus in a 7-year-old child. Chest radiographs show moderate cardiomegaly, concave main pulmonary artery with disproportionately enlarged hilar vessels, and mildly prominent peripheral vasculature without venous congestion. The patient had pulmonary hypertension.

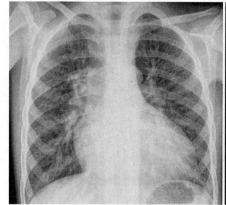
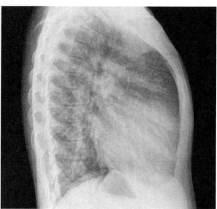

Case 24.6

Congenitally corrected transposition of the great arteries with a ventricular septal defect and mild pulmonary stenosis in a 3-year-old child. Chest radiograph shows situs solitus and levocardia with a prominent left upper and mid-cardiac border, which is formed by the right ventricular outflow tract (RVOT) and ascending aorta (Ao) as shown on a contrast-enhanced magnetic resonance (MR) angiogram. There is mild cardiomegaly and pulmonary vascularity is normal with a balanced circulation. PA, pulmonary artery; RV, right ventricle.

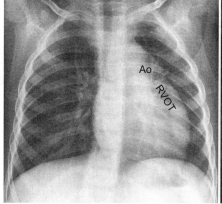
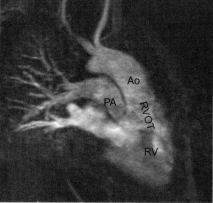

Case 24.7

Congenitally corrected transposition of the great arteries with Ebstein's malformation of the left-sided tricuspid valve in a 17-year-old patient. Chest radiographic findings correlate very well with MR findings. The left mid-heart border shows characteristic prominence formed by the right ventricular outflow tract (RVOT) that connects to the ascending aorta (Ao), which ascends along the left anterior aspect of the main pulmonary artery. MR image in a four-chamber plane shows offset attachments *(double-headed arrow)* of the right-sided mitral and left-sided tricuspid valves. LA, left atrium; LV, left ventricle; RA, right atrium; RV, right ventricle.

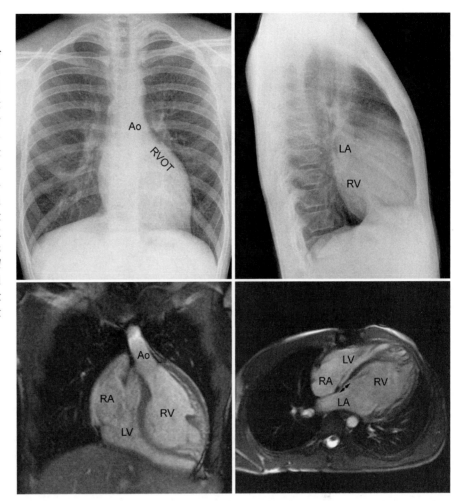

Case 24.8

Congenitally corrected transposition of the great arteries with ventricular septal defect and pulmonary stenosis in a 17-month-old child with isolated dextrocardia. Chest radiograph shows situs solitus and dextrocardia. The prominent convex left upper cardiac border is the ascending aorta (Ao) as shown on an accompanying angiogram. The aortic arch is right sided with the aortic knob (descending aorta, ao) on the right side of the trachea. The aortic arch has an unusually long transverse course from left to right. The aortic arch may compress the trachea. The pulmonary vascularity is mildly reduced. LV, left ventricle; PA, pulmonary artery; RV, right ventricle.

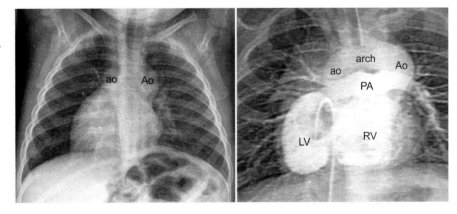

Case 24.9

Congenitally corrected transposition of the great arteries in a 10-month-old infant with situs inversus and levocardia. Levocardia in this patient with situs inversus is highly suggestive of congenitally corrected transposition. The aortic arch is right sided. The heart is normal in size and the pulmonary vascularity is normal.

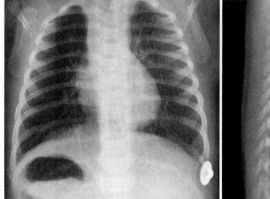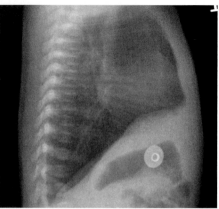

Case 24.10

Congenitally corrected transposition of the great arteries with regurgitation of a dysplastic tricuspid valve and heart block. Chest radiograph at 15 months of age *(left panel)* shows moderate cardiomegaly with left atrial enlargement and pulmonary venous congestion due to left-side tricuspid regurgitation. The left upper and mid-heart border shows characteristic prominence (*white arrows*). A postoperative follow-up at 17 months old *(right panel)* shows a pulmonary artery band (*black arrow*) across the midline-positioned main pulmonary artery to prepare for a double switch operation and a permanent pacemaker system.

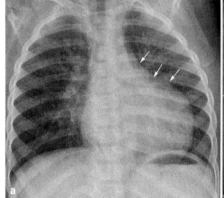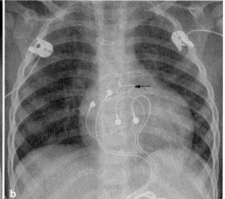

25 Double-Outlet Ventricles

With Kevin S. Roman

Definition

- A type of ventriculoarterial connection in which both great arteries arise completely or predominantly from either the right or the left ventricle. Double outlet left ventricle is exceedingly rare.
- Almost always associated with a ventricular septal defect

Classification of Double-Outlet Right Ventricle

- Classification is based on the location of the ventricular septal defect relative to the aortic and pulmonary valves (**Fig. 25.1**).

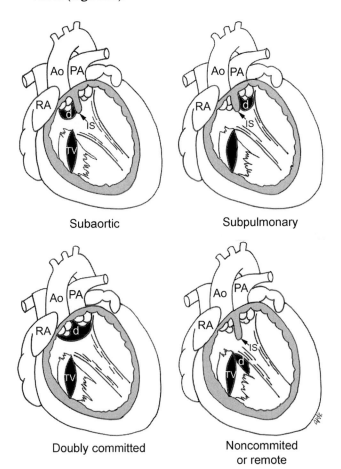

Subaortic

Subpulmonary

Doubly committed

Noncommited or remote

Fig. 25.1 Classification of double-outlet right ventricle according to the location of the ventricular septal defect relative to the arterial valves. Ao, ascending aorta; d, ventricular septal defect; IS, infundibular septum; PA, pulmonary artery; RA, right atrium; TV tricuspid valve.

Pathophysiology

- Variable anatomic lesion with a spectrum of physiologic changes that closely mimic other congenital heart defects
- Hemodynamics depend mostly on the position of the ventricular septal defect relative to the great vessels and the presence or absence of outflow tract stenosis.
  - Subaortic defect without associated pulmonary stenosis: physiology is similar to a large ventricular septal defect.
  - Subaortic defect with associated pulmonary stenosis: physiology is similar to tetralogy of Fallot.
  - Subpulmonic defect: physiology is similar to complete transposition of the great arteries with a ventricular septal defect.
  - Doubly committed defect: mixing of unsaturated and saturated blood flowing into great arteries
  - Noncommitted defect: atrioventricular septal defect or perimembranous inlet ventricular septal defect with mixing of saturated and unsaturated blood
- Early-onset pulmonary vascular disease may occur with marked pulmonary overcirculation.

Clinical Symptoms

- Presentation varies with the type of anatomy and depends on the direction of streaming of blood.
- Mild to marked cyanosis with pulmonary stenosis in cases with subaortic ventricular septal defect
- Severe cyanosis in cases with subpulmonary ventricular septal defect
- Congestive heart failure without pulmonary stenosis

Chest Radiographic Findings

- Variable; largely determined by the presence of pulmonary or aortic obstruction
- Presence of pulmonary stenosis: mild cardiomegaly, decreased pulmonary vascularity, and a concave main pulmonary artery segment
- Absence of pulmonary stenosis: moderate cardiomegaly, increased pulmonary vascularity, and dilated main pulmonary artery
- Presence of aortic stenosis, moderate cardiomegaly, increased pulmonary vascularity, pulmonary venous hypertension with edema, and dilated main pulmonary artery

Case 25.1

Double-outlet right ventricle with a subaortic ventricular septal defect and pulmonary stenosis in a 2-week-old neonate. Chest radiographs show mild cardiomegaly with an upturned rounded apex, decreased pulmonary vascularity, and a concave main pulmonary artery, indistinguishable from tetralogy of Fallot. In fact, the type of ventriculoarterial connection in tetralogy of Fallot with more than 50% overriding of the aorta is double-outlet right ventricle.

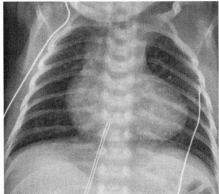
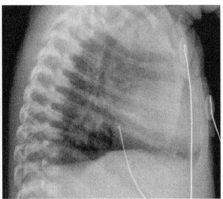

Case 25.2

Double-outlet right ventricle with a subpulmonary ventricular septal defect in a 2-day-old newborn. The heart is mildly enlarged and the pulmonary vascularity is increased for a newborn infant. The heart shows an egg-on-side appearance, as in complete transposition of the great arteries.

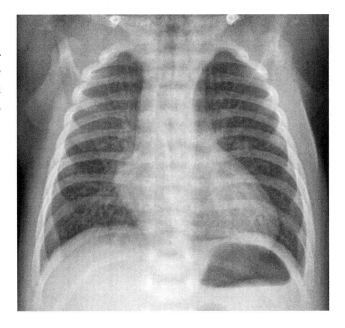

26 Hearts with Single-Ventricle Physiology

With Kevin S. Roman

Definition and Classification

- So-called single-ventricle physiology refers to a situation in which both pulmonary and systemic circulations are maintained entirely or mainly by the work of one ventricle. Despite morphologic variations, fundamental hemodynamic physiology is similar and requires univentricular repair.
- Pathologic conditions that cause single-ventricle physiology (**Fig. 26.1**):
  - Double-inlet left ventricle (so-called single left ventricle)
  - Double-inlet right ventricle (so-called single right ventricle)
  - Double-inlet indeterminate ventricle (so-called common ventricle)
  - Absent right atrioventricular connection is synonymous with tricuspid atresia when the absent connection involves the morphologic right ventricle.
  - Absent left atrioventricular connection
  - Also included are the following:
    - Hypoplastic right heart with pulmonary atresia or critical stenosis (Chapter 17)
    - Hypoplastic left heart syndrome (Chapter 22)
    - Unbalanced atrioventricular septal defects
- In most cases there are two ventricular chambers present, with one well formed and a second rudimentary, although on occasion there are two equally dominant ventricles.
- Atrioventricular valves guarding the inlet can be two separate valves, one patent valve with one atretic valve or a common valve.
- Tricuspid atresia: often associated with left juxtaposition of the atrial appendages

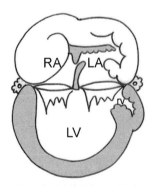

Double inlet left ventricle

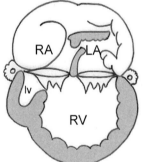

Double inlet right ventricle

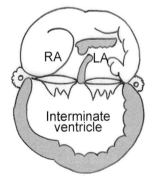

Double inlet indeterminate or common ventricle

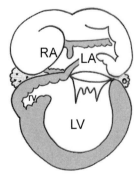

Absent right atrioventricular connection

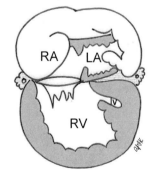

Absent left atrioventricular connection

Fig. 26.1 Types of univentricular atrioventricular connections. LA, left atrium; LV, left ventricle; RA, right atrium; RV, right ventricle.

243

□ Great artery origins vary and may be concordant, discordant, or double outlet from the main or rudimentary chamber

□ Great artery connections may be patent or obstructed

Pathophysiology

□ Variable depending on the associated cardiac anomalies

□ Each atrium drains entirely or mainly to the major ventricular chamber in double-inlet ventricles.

□ In tricuspid atresia, the right atrium drains to the left atrium through the atrial communication. The left atrium then drains to the left ventricle.

□ Admixture lesion that is not affected by the ventricular type

□ Major determinant of hemodynamics is the presence and severity of pulmonary outflow tract obstruction and less commonly of aortic outflow tract obstruction.

□ When the rudimentary ventricular chamber gives rise to an arterial trunk, the ventricular septal defect is a part of the outflow tract to that arterial trunk. A restrictive ventricular septal defect causes obstruction to the arterial trunk that arises from the rudimentary chamber. The ventricular septal defect may become increasingly restrictive over time.

□ Ideal anatomy is a well-balanced circulation with some degree of pulmonic stenosis.

Clinical Manifestations

□ Association with pulmonary stenosis or atresia: presents with cyanosis

□ Without pulmonary outflow obstruction: presents with heart failure and minimal cyanosis
  • Tachypnea, dyspnea, failure to thrive, and recurrent pulmonary infections in early infancy
  • Over time, development of pulmonary vascular disease, which reduces pulmonary blood flow and increases cyanosis

□ Less common is left outflow obstruction, which presents with symptoms of poor perfusion and circulatory shock.

Chest Radiographic Findings

□ Variable pulmonary vascularity
  • Normal flow with a balanced anomaly
  • Decreased flow with pulmonary obstruction
  • Increased flow with absence of pulmonary obstruction
  • Rarely, pulmonary venous hypertension and pulmonary edema with left outflow obstruction
  • Pulmonary hypertension pattern with long-standing unobstructed pulmonary outflow

□ Variable heart size
  • Normal heart size with moderate restriction of pulmonary outflow
  • Moderate cardiomegaly with unobstructed pulmonary outflow

□ Variable heart contour
  • Most typical is a double inlet left ventricle with a rudimentary outflow chamber producing a bulge on the upper left heart border. A similar feature is also seen in congenitally corrected transposition of the great arteries.
  • Right atrial dilatation in tricuspid atresia with restrictive atrial septum
  • Sigmoid configuration of the right heart with convex right upper and concave right lower heart border is characteristic of left juxtaposition of the atrial appendages. Prominent left upper heart border is formed by two overlapped atrial appendages.

□ Absent main pulmonary artery due to the posterior and medial origin

□ Variable aortic contour
  • Enlarged with severe pulmonary obstruction
  • Convexity of ascending aorta toward the side of the morphologic right ventricle
  • Right aortic arch most common with severe pulmonary stenosis

---

Pearls

□ Extremely variable findings, depending on the ventricular type and associated lesions

□ Unusual straight or convex left upper cardiac contour suggests double-inlet left ventricle with transposition of the great arteries.

□ Decreased pulmonary vascularity, normal heart size, and enlarged aorta with pulmonary obstruction

□ Increased pulmonary vascularity, moderate cardiomegaly with unobstructed pulmonary outflow

Case 26.1

Double-inlet left ventricle with straddling left atrioventricular valve and transposition of the great arteries in a 3-year-old child. Chest radiograph shows a rounded bulging contour of the left upper heart border, which is formed by the rudimentary right ventricle (rv) and the ascending aorta as shown on contrast-enhanced magnetic resonance (MR) angiogram. This configuration is also seen in congenitally corrected transposition of the great arteries, which is a related malformation (see Case 24.6). Ao, ascending aorta; D, ventricular septal defect; LV, left ventricle; RA, right atrium.

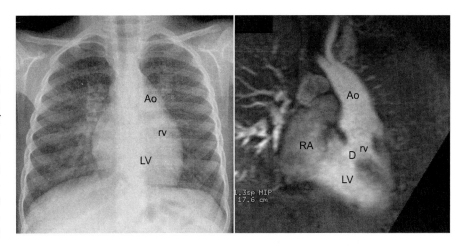

Case 26.2

Double-inlet left ventricle with transposition and pulmonary stenosis in a 5-week-old infant. Chest radiograph shows mesocardia with mild cardiomegaly, decreased pulmonary vascularity, and an enlarged aorta (Ao).

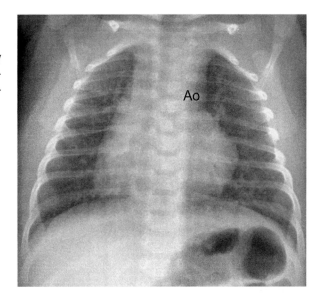

Case 26.3

Double-inlet right ventricle without pulmonary stenosis in a 5-year-old child. Chest radiograph shows nonspecific moderate cardiomegaly and increased pulmonary vascularity.

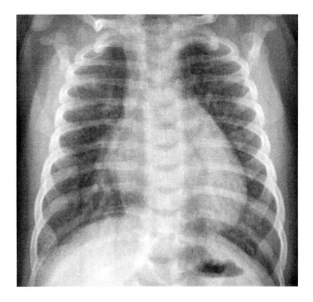

Case 26.4

Tricuspid atresia with double-outlet right ventricle in a newborn. Chest radiograph shows mild cardiomegaly. The right heart border shows a sigmoid configuration with the rounded superior vena cava (SVC) and concave right atrial border (RA). The shoulder part of the left heart border is prominent. IVC, inferior vena cava; LAA, left atrial appendage; RAA, right atrial appendage.

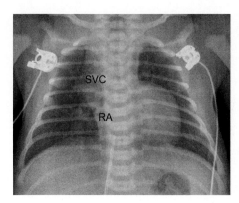

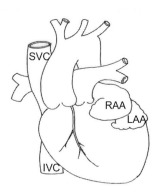

27 Abnormal Situs and Cardiac Malposition

With Kevin S. Roman

Definition and Classification

- Normally, body organs show asymmetric arrangement (**Table 27.1**). Situs refers to the pattern of arrangement of the body organs relative to the midline.
- Situs of the abdominal organs, bronchopulmonary system, and atria should be designated separately. The types of situs at three levels are concordant in the majority of cases (visceroatrial concordance rule), but there are rare exceptions (**Fig. 27.1**).
  - Situs solitus: usual arrangement
  - Situs inversus: mirror-image arrangement
  - Heterotaxy: neither solitus nor inversus
    - Characterized by jumbled arrangement of the abdominal organs
    - Bronchopulmonary anatomy is symmetric or isomeric, both sides resembling the arrangement of the normal right or left side: bronchopulmonary right and left isomerisms.
    - Atrial anatomy is also symmetric or isomeric, both sides showing the characteristic morphologies of the normal right or left atrium: right or left atrial isomerisms.
- Right isomerism refers to bilateral right-sided anatomy and is associated with asplenia.
- Left isomerism refers to bilateral left-sided anatomy and is almost always associated with polysplenia.
- Cardiac position is independent of body situs. Any cardiac position can be associated with any type of body situs.

- Cardiac malposition is defined as any combination of situs and cardiac position other than a combination of situs solitus and levocardia.
- Incidence of congenital heart diseases according to types of situs and position of the heart:
  - Situs solitus: 8–10/1000
    - Almost always in situs solitus with dextrocardia or mesocardia in which congenitally corrected transposition of the great arteries is the most common
  - Situs inversus: frequent
    - Approximately 10 to 50% in situs inversus with dextrocardia
    - Almost always in situs inversus with levocardia or mesocardia
  - Right isomerism: 100%
  - Left isomerism: almost always (**Tables 27.2, 27.3**)

Clinical Manifestations

- Asplenia syndrome with right isomerism:
  - 100% incidence of congenital heart disease, almost always cyanotic heart disease, which presents early in the neonatal period
  - Majority show single-ventricle physiology with pulmonary stenosis or atresia
  - Worst outcome with early death when associated with obstructive type of total anomalous pulmonary venous connection

Table 27.1 Features Characterizing Normal Asymmetry of Body Organs

	Right	Left
Abdominal organs	• Larger lobe of the liver	• Spleen and stomach
Lung lobation	• Three lobes	• Two lobes
Main bronchus	• Short, eparterial	• Long, hyparterial
Pulmonary artery	• Transverse course in front of the right main bronchus	• Oblique course crossing over the left main bronchus (epbronchial course)
	• Origin of the first branch proximally in the mediastinum	• Origin of the first branch distally at the hilum
Atrium	• Triangular appendage with wide junction demarcated by crista terminalis	• Finger-like appendage with narrow junction not demarcated by crista terminalis
	• Pectinate muscles extending to the atrioventricular junction	• Pectinate muscles confined to the appendage
	• Fossa ovalis with limbus	• No fossa ovalis

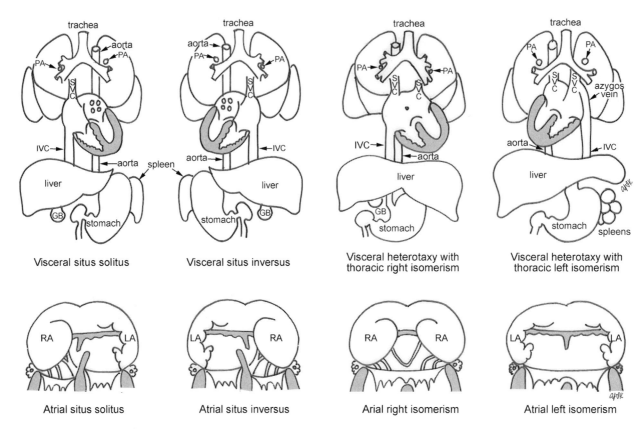

Fig. 27.1 Types of visceral and atrial situs; GB, gallbladder; IVC, inferior vena cava; LA, left atrium; PA, pulmonary artery; RA, right atrium; SVC, superior vena cava.

Table 27.2   Common Congenital Cardiac Defects in Right and Left Isomerism

	Right Isomerism	Left Isomerism
Bilateral superior venae cavae	45%	45%
Bilateral systemic venous drainage	70%	60%
Absence of coronary sinus	~100%	~60%
Interruption of the inferior vena cava	<2.5%	80%
Juxtaposition of the aorta and inferior vena cava	~90%	Uncommon
Extracardiac type of total anomalous pulmonary venous connection with/without obstruction	50%, with obstruction in 50%	Rare
Pulmonary venous connection to ipsilateral atriums	4%	45%
Atrioventricular septal defect	90%	50%
Atrial septum Functionally common atrium in 50%	Usually better formed, intact in ~20%	
Atrioventricular connection	Univentricular in 70%	Biventricular in ~75%
Ventriculoarterial connection	Concordant only in 4%	Concordant in ~70%
Pulmonary atresia or stenosis	80%	30%
Left-sided obstructive lesion	<5%	~30%
Heart block/bradycardia	Rare	25–70%

Table 27.3   Noncardiac Abnormalities in Right and Left Isomerisms

Right Isomerism	Left Isomerism
Asplenia in the majority of cases	Polysplenia in majority of cases
Intestinal malrotation virtually in all	Intestinal malrotation virtually in all
Partial thoracic stomach (hiatal hernia) in ~25%	Biliary atresia and/or hypoplastic or absent gallbladder in 20%
Heterogeneous anomalies encountered	Urinary anomalies in 17%
	Duodenal atresia 7%
	Extrahepatic portosystemic shunt, infrequently

- Increased risk of serious infections including meningitis and sepsis
□ Polysplenia syndromes with left isomerism:
  - Almost always (but not always) associated with congenital heart disease
  - More variable presentation related to the congenital heart disease; most frequently acyanotic heart disease
  - 25% show single-ventricle physiology
  - May present with congestive heart failure due to left-to-right shunt with or without left-sided obstructive lesion, atrioventricular valve regurgitation, or bradycardia
  - Bradycardia with atrioventricular dissociation is common; high mortality in fetal life due to heart block
  - Splenic dysfunction is common despite the presence of multiple spleens.

Chest Radiographic Findings

□ Best indicator of situs is the tracheobronchial anatomy, as the bronchial situs is a helpful marker of the atrial arrangement (**Fig. 27.2**).
  - Normal anatomy: the distance from the carina to the left upper lobe bronchus is 1.5 to 2 times the corresponding distance to the right upper lobe bronchus.
  - Right mainstem bronchus is referred to as eparterial, as it is located superior to the descending branch of the right pulmonary artery.
  - Left mainstem bronchus is referred to as hyparterial, as it is located inferior to the left pulmonary artery.
□ Less reliable but sometimes helpful in determining situs is identifying the position of the abdominal organs.
□ Left-sided stomach and right-sided larger lobe of the liver do not necessarily mean that there is situs solitus.

Left isomerism can show a similar abdominal visceral arrangement.
□ Right-sided stomach does not necessarily mean that there is situs inversus. The stomach can be right-sided in right and left isomerisms as well as in situs inversus.
□ Right isomerism
  - Findings regarding situs in right isomerism:
    – Bilateral symmetric eparterial right upper lobe bronchi
    – Bilateral horizontal fissures denoting symmetric trilobed lungs; the minor fissure when not seen is of no diagnostic value.
    – Both right and left pulmonary arteries positioned anterior to the upper lobe bronchi seen on the lateral image
    – Symmetric midline liver
    – Stomach on either side but tends to be close to the midline
    – Gastric fundus in the thorax
  - Findings regarding the cardiovascular status in right isomerism:
    – Any cardiac position
    – Normal or slightly large heart size
    – Decreased pulmonary vascularity due to pulmonary stenosis or atresia
    – Pulmonary venous hypertension when associated with obstructive type of total anomalous pulmonary venous connection
□ Left isomerism
  - Findings regarding situs in left isomerism:
    – Bilateral symmetric hyparterial upper lobe bronchi
    – Both right and left pulmonary arteries positioned posterior to the upper lobe bronchi seen on the lateral image

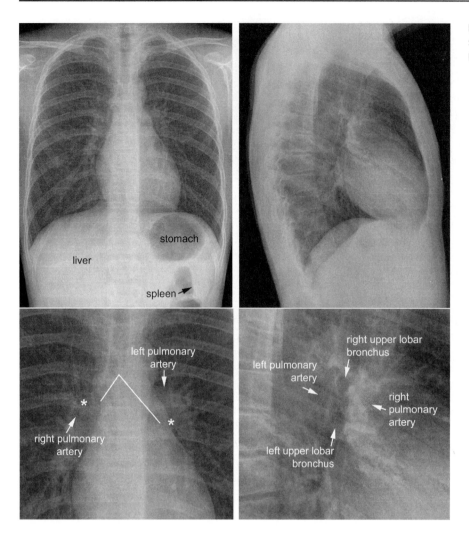

- Liver may be symmetric but typically less symmetric than in right isomerism. The larger lobe can be on either side.
- Splenic shadow can be identified along the greater curvature side of the stomach.
- Enlarged azygos venous arch at right or left tracheobronchial angle in cases with interruption of the inferior vena cava with azygos continuation. The inferior vena caval web filling the posterior cardiophrenic angle on the lateral view can be inconspicuous.

- Findings regarding the cardiovascular status in left isomerism:
  - Any cardiac position
  - Mild to moderate cardiomegaly
  - Increased vascularity with left-to-right shunt in the majority of cases
  - Decreased pulmonary vascularity when associated with pulmonary stenosis or atresia
  - May present with severe congestive heart failure due to a combination of a left-to-right shunt and left-sided obstructive lesions

- There is high concordance among abdominal, bronchopulmonary, and atrial situs, with a few exceptions.
- Position of the stomach is helpful in determining the situs but not a specific indicator.
  - Right-sided stomach only means that the situs is abnormal. The stomach can be right-sided in right and left isomerisms as well as in situs inversus.
- Bronchopulmonary arterial anatomy when seen is the most precise indicator of the situs.
- Cardiac malposition is defined as any combination of situs and cardiac position other than a combination of situs solitus and levocardia.
- Right isomerism is almost always associated with asplenia.
  - All cases with right isomerism have complex congenital heart disease, with single-ventricle physiology in over 70%.
  - Commonest combination of lesions consists of complete atrioventricular septal defects, transposition of the great arteries, and severe pulmonary obstruction.
  - Typical chest radiographic findings include symmetric liver with right- or left-sided stomach close to the midline, bilateral short eparterial bronchi, heart in any position with a normal size, prominent aorta, and diminished pulmonary vascularity.
  - Anomalies of pulmonary venous connection are common. Obstructive type of total anomalous pulmonary venous connection is associated with the worst outcome.
- Left isomerism is almost always associated with polysplenia.
  - Usually associated with less complex congenital heart disease
  - Single-ventricle physiology in only 25% and pulmonary obstruction in only 30%
  - Interruption of intrahepatic inferior vena cava with azygous or hemiazygous continuation is present in 80%.
  - Typical chest radiographic findings include bilateral hyparterial bronchi, stomach on either side, cardiomegaly, and increased vascularity. Dilated azygos venous arch is highly suggestive of left isomerism.
  - Extracardiac anomalies such as biliary atresia, and bradycardia with heart block are common.

Case 27.1

Situs solitus and dextrocardia in a newborn with absent right atrioventricular connection, transposition, and tubular hypoplasia of the aortic arch. Chest radiograph shows the stomach on the left. There is dextrocardia with the apex pointing to the right. Contrast-enhanced computed tomography (CT) image shows absent connection between the right atrium (RA) and the underlying main ventricular chamber of left ventricular morphology, inverted ventricular relationship with the rudimentary right ventricle (rv) to the left of the left ventricle (LV). LA, left atrium; RA, right atrium.

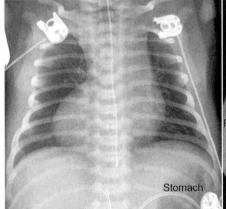
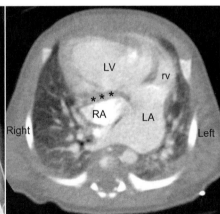

Case 27.2

Situs inversus and dextrocardia in a 12-year-old patient who underwent Rastelli operation followed by stent dilatation of the right ventricle–pulmonary artery conduit for complete transposition of the great arteries, ventricular septal defect, and pulmonary outflow tract obstruction. Chest radiograph shows situs inversus and dextrocardia. Airway anatomy correlates well with the anatomy of situs inversus seen at magnetic resonance (MR). There is mild cardiomegaly and the pulmonary vascularity is normal. AA, aortic arch; LMB and RMB, left and right main bronchi; LPA, descending branch of the left pulmonary artery; RPA, right pulmonary artery; black and white *asterisks*, right and left upper lobar bronchi.

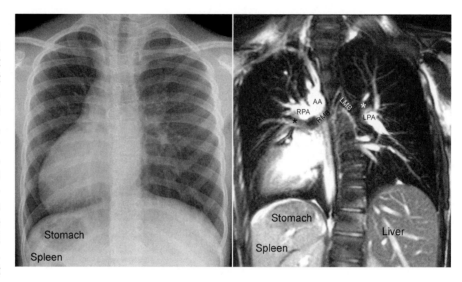

Case 27.3

Situs inversus and levocardia in an 8-year-old patient who underwent a left Blalock-Taussig shunt for congenitally corrected transposition of the great arteries, ventricular septal defect, and pulmonary atresia. Chest radiograph shows the stomach on the right and inverted branching pattern of the airway. Convex bulge of the right upper heart border is formed by the dilated ascending aorta (Ao), which is the mirror image of what is seen with the same disease in situs solitus.

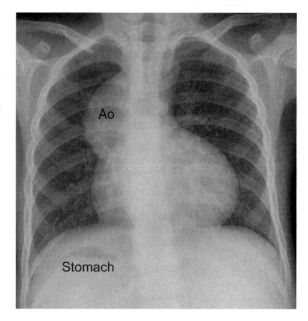

Case 27.4

Right atrial isomerism and levocardia in a newborn with complex congenial heart disease with pulmonary atresia, major aortopulmonary collateral arteries, and obstructed total anomalous pulmonary venous connection to the junction of the ductus venosus and inferior vena cava (IVC). Frontal radiograph of the chest and abdomen shows a horizontal symmetric liver and a right-sided stomach. The tip of an umbilical venous (UV) catheter is in the portal vein. Both lungs show increased interstitial markings due to pulmonary venous hypertension secondary to stenosis *(asterisk)* of the vertical vein as it connects to the inferior vena cava. Note the right isomeric pattern of the bronchial branching.

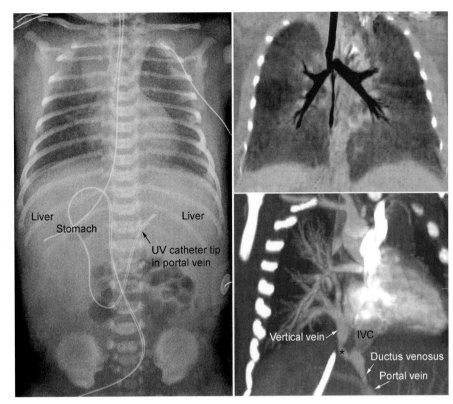

Case 27.5

Right isomerism and levocardia in a newborn with complex congenital heart disease, pulmonary atresia, and total anomalous pulmonary venous connection to the portal venous system. Chest radiographs show a symmetric transverse liver. The heart is normal in size, and both lungs show increased interstitial markings due to pulmonary venous hypertension. The upper lobar bronchi *(arrows)* are at a similar horizontal level on the lateral view.

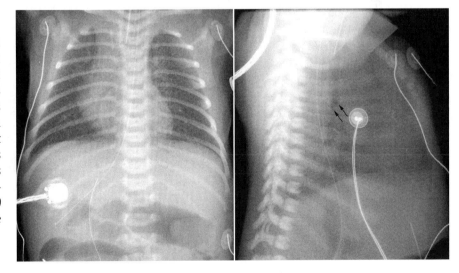

Case 27.6

Right atrial isomerism with complex congenital heart disease diagnosed unusually late at 6 years of age. Frontal chest radiograph shows the stomach on the right, suggesting an abnormal situs. The right main bronchus *(asterisk)* is above the descending branch of the right pulmonary artery (R) and therefore the relationship of the normal right lung. The bronchopulmonary anatomy of the left lung is not clearly shown. The presence of an eparterial bronchus on the same side of the stomach is a conclusive sign of right isomerism. Lateral chest radiograph shows the pulmonary arteries *(black arrows)* positioned anterior to the airway *(white arrows),* which is another sign of right isomerism. The patient had an absent left atrioventricular connection to the morphologic right ventricle, double-outlet right ventricle, and pulmonary stenosis. The heart is mildly enlarged and pulmonary vascularity is mildly reduced.

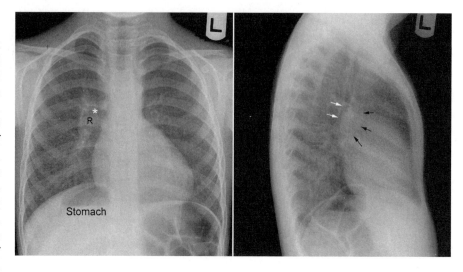

Case 27.7

Right atrial isomerism in a 7-month-old infant who underwent a right Blalock-Taussig shunt with clipping of the left ductus arteriosus for unbalanced right-dominant type of atrioventricular septal defect, transposition of the great arteries, and pulmonary atresia. Frontal chest radiograph shows the stomach medially located on the right and bilateral minor fissures. Lateral chest radiograph shows closely related end-on shadows of the upper lobar bronchi *(white arrows).* The pulmonary arterial shadows *(black arrows)* are seen mostly in front of and below the upper lobar bronchi. The patient also had obstructed total anomalous pulmonary venous connection, and both lungs show findings of pulmonary venous hypertension.

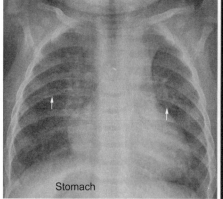
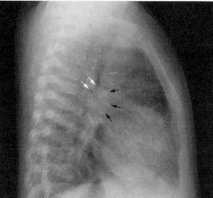

Case 27.8

Right isomerism with a part of the stomach in the thorax in a 4-month-old patient with the balanced form of complete atrioventricular septal defect, transposition of the great arteries, and pulmonary stenosis. Chest radiograph shows the gastric fundus located in the right lower thorax, which it is considered a manifestation of visceral heterotaxy. The right lower lobe shows collapse/consolidation.

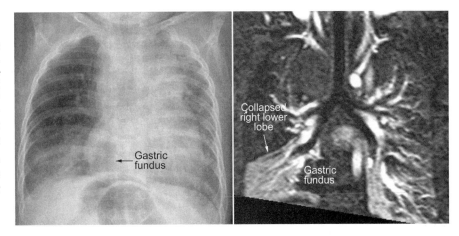

Case 27.9

Left isomerism and levocardia in a 9-month-old infant with a large ventricular septal defect, transposition of the great arteries, and pulmonary outflow tract obstruction. Frontal chest radiograph shows the stomach on the right and bilaterally long symmetric bronchi *(arrows)*. Lateral chest radiograph shows that the upper lobar bronchi *(white arrows)* are at the same horizontal level. The pulmonary arteries cast a shadow *(black arrows)* above and behind the upper lobar bronchi.

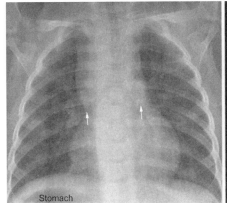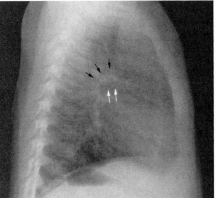

Case 27.10

Left isomerism with interrupted inferior vena cava in a 10-year-old patient with a secundum atrial septal defect. Frontal chest radiograph shows normal-looking visceral arrangement with levocardia. The bronchi, however, are symmetrically long, and a dilated azygos venous arch *(arrows)* is seen at the right tracheobronchial angle. On the lateral chest radiograph, the posterior cardiophrenic angle is unusually sharp *(arrow)* and empty due to the absence of the inferior vena cava web that normally fills this angle.

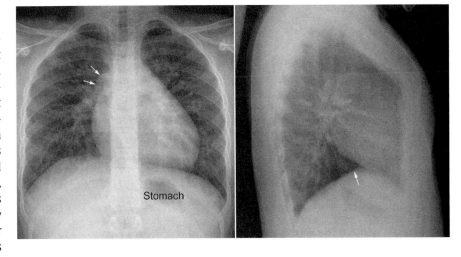

Case 27.11

Left isomerism with interrupted inferior vena cava in a 13-day-old neonate who had biliary atresia. Chest radiographs show the right-sided stomach located close to the midline and levocardia. On the lateral view, the posterior cardiophrenic angle *(arrow)* where normally the inferior vena cava web is seen is empty. The heart is moderately enlarged and pulmonary vascularity is markedly increased. The patient had a large perimembranous ventricular septal defect and a secundum atrial septal defect.

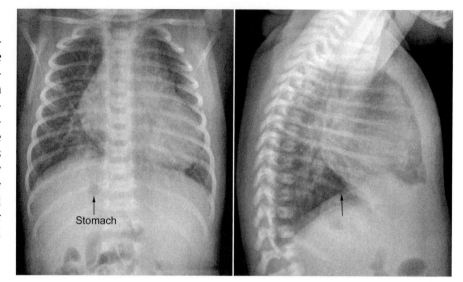

28 Rheumatic Fever and Acquired Valvular Heart Diseases

With Christian J. Kellenberger and Kevin S. Roman

Definition and Etiologic Consideration

- Rheumatic fever is a nonsuppurative diffuse inflammatory disease of connective tissue involving the heart, blood vessels, joints, central nervous system, and skin occurring as a delayed sequela postpharyngitis with rheumatogenic strains of group A β-hemolytic *Streptococcus*.
  - Jones criteria for diagnosis of acute rheumatic fever:
    - Major criteria: carditis, arthritis, chorea, erythema marginatum, subcutaneous nodules
    - Minor criteria: previous rheumatic fever, arthralgia, fever, elevated erythrocyte sedimentation rate, elevated white blood cell count, prolongation of PR interval, presence of C-reactive protein
  - Cardiac manifestations of acute rheumatic fever include pancarditis, pericarditis, and significant valvular inflammatory disease.
  - Approximately 25% of children with rheumatic fever develop chronic disease resulting in rheumatic heart disease due to thickening and scarring of the valves.
- Acquired valvular heart disease:
  - Rheumatic heart disease is the most common cause often associated with mitral valve disease. Mitral valve involvement occurs in approximately 75% and aortic valve involvement in 25% of all rheumatic heart disease.
  - Infective endocarditis is a less common cause of acquired valvular heart disease, which may affect congenitally deformed valves and less commonly a normal valve.
  - Traumatic injury
  - Conditions dilating the ascending aorta can result in aortic valve disease. Etiologies include the following:
    - Aortitis from a variety of conditions
    - Cystic medial necrosis often in association with Marfan syndrome, Loeys-Dietz syndrome, and idiopathic annuloaortic ectasia or associated with hypertension and dissecting aneurysm.
  - Conditions dilating a ventricle can result in valvar regurgitation.

Pathophysiology

- Rheumatic fever and rheumatic heart disease:
  - Postinfectious sequelae follow untreated pharyngitis with rheumatogenic strains of group A β-hemolytic *Streptococcus*. Susceptible host usually hypersensitized by repeated infections. Autoimmune response with antibodies, which cross-react with the organism and host tissues, causing tissue damage.
  - Carditis affects endocardium, myocardium, and pericardium, causing a pancarditis. Endocarditis involves mitral and aortic valves and rarely tricuspid or pulmonary valves.
  - Mitral regurgitation is the hallmark of acute rheumatic carditis in childhood.
  - Rheumatic endocarditis causes commissural fusion, thickened fibrous tissue, and calcification, leading to valvar stenosis and less commonly regurgitation.
  - Pulmonary arteriolar vasoconstriction develops to protect lung from congestion, which leads to pulmonary hypertension and right ventricular failure.
  - Aortic valve disease uncommon in childhood: scarred, thickened, and shortened leaflets, which are unable to coapt, resulting in aortic insufficiency.
  - Acquired aortic stenosis is a chronic sequela due to fibrosis, thickening, and fusion of commissures.
  - Very rare involvement of tricuspid and pulmonary valves
- Infective vegetations produce perforations or erosions, prevent valve coaptation, and destroy attachments of cusp tissue to the adjacent wall, leading to valvar regurgitation or a paravalvar leak.
- Traumatic laceration may involve a valve cusp or aortic wall, with dissection producing valvar regurgitation.
- Dilatation of ascending aorta or left ventricle leads to annular dilatation and separation of commissures, resulting in regurgitation.
- Pulmonary hypertension leads to dilatation of the pulmonary annulus, resulting in regurgitation.

Clinical Manifestations

- ☐ Diagnosis of acute rheumatic fever with one major and two minor Jones criteria
  - • Signs of carditis in acute rheumatic fever are cardiac enlargement, heart failure, pericardial effusion, and a new or changing murmur.
  - • Younger children more likely to present with moderate to severe carditis and develop rheumatic fever recurrences and chronic rheumatic heart disease
  - • Mitral regurgitation most common cardiac finding in children and adolescents; gradually develops mitral stenosis
  - • Aortic valve disease symptoms rare in childhood unless disease is severe
- ☐ Mitral and aortic disease may lead to left ventricular failure from volume overload or marked hypertrophy.
  - • Fatigue or syncope during exercise with fixed cardiac output
  - • Palpitation, exertional dyspnea, and angina with aortic insufficiency
- ☐ Pulmonary stenosis: symptomatic when severe with fatigue, dyspnea, syncope, and right ventricular failure
- ☐ Pulmonary insufficiency usually asymptomatic

Chest Radiographic Findings

- ☐ Cardiac involvement of rheumatic fever: cardiomegaly with signs of left atrial and left ventricular dilatation with findings of pulmonary venous hypertension; often associated with pericardial and pleural effusions
- ☐ Mitral vale disease produces a large left atrium with pulmonary venous hypertension and secondary pulmonary arterial hypertension.
- ☐ Mitral regurgitation produces a massively enlarged left atrium disproportionate to degree of left ventricular enlargement.
- ☐ Aortic regurgitation produces left ventricular enlargement disproportionate to degree of left atrial enlargement, prominent ascending aorta, and a tortuous descending aorta.
- ☐ Aortic insufficiency due to conditions dilating the ascending aorta may show severe aortic dilatation.
- ☐ Aortic stenosis results in poststenotic dilatation of the ascending aorta, mild cardiomegaly, with left ventricular hypertrophy, leading to ventricular failure and normal pulmonary vasculature or pulmonary venous hypertension.
- ☐ Pulmonary insufficiency due to pulmonary hypertension shows findings of pulmonary hypertension and right ventricular dilatation.

Pearls

- ☐ Cardiac involvement of acute rheumatic fever: pancarditis causing cardiomegaly with left atrial and left ventricular dilatation, pulmonary edema, pericardial effusion, and pleural effusions
- ☐ Chronic rheumatic fever is the most common cause of acquired valvular heart disease.

- ☐ Rheumatic heart disease most often leads to mitral valve stenosis.
- ☐ Other conditions most often lead to valve regurgitation.
- ☐ Conditions dilating the heart or great vessels lead to valve regurgitation.

Case 28.1

Rheumatic fever causing mitral, aortic, and tricuspid valve regurgitation and pericardial effusion in a 9-year-old child. Chest radiographs show markedly enlarged cardiac silhouette with effaced outline. Both lungs show findings of severe pulmonary venous hypertension with redistribution of vascularity and blurred vascular margins. The cardiac silhouette is rather smooth, which is consistent with an associated pericardial effusion.

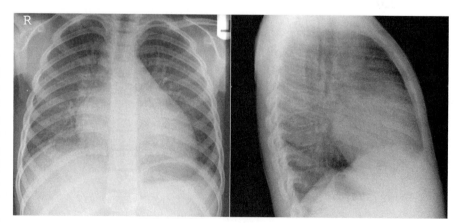

Case 28.2

Severe mitral regurgitation of rheumatic origin in a 7-year-old child. Chest radiographs show moderate cardiomegaly with predominant enlargement of the left atrium and left ventricle. The dilated left atrium forms a double contour on the right side *(arrow)* and widening of the carinal angle. The retrocardiac prespinal clear space is almost completely obliterated by left ventricular enlargement. Retrosternal space is also partially obliterated due to a lesser degree of right ventricular enlargement.

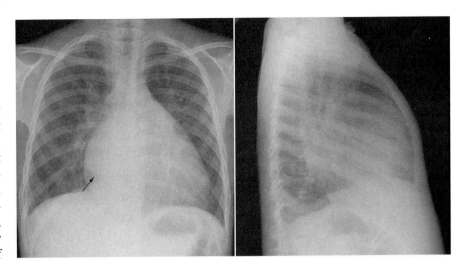

Case 28.3

Mitral regurgitation in an 11-year-old patient who has a history of rheumatic fever at 6 months of age. Chest radiographs show a classic triangular configuration with findings of left atrial and left ventricular enlargement. There is pulmonary vascular redistribution with dilatation of the upper lung zone vessels and collapse of the lower lung zone vessels. The interstitial markings are increased in both lungs.

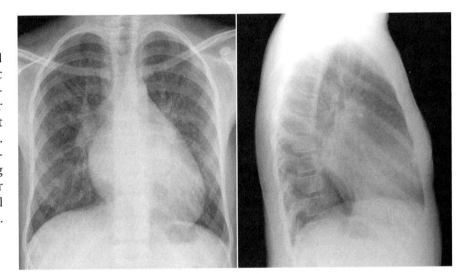

Case 28.4

Aortic and mitral regurgitation in a 14-year-old patient. Chest radiographs show signs of left atrial and ventricular enlargement. Although the dilated ascending aorta has not yet formed the right upper mediastinal border, the aortic knob and descending aorta are prominent.

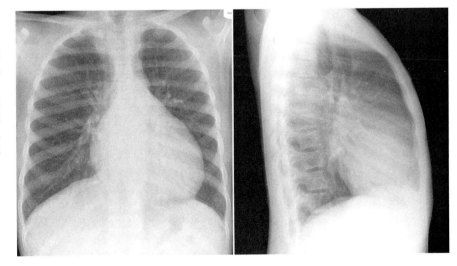

Case 28.5

Aortic regurgitation and mitral stenoinsufficiency in a 14-year-old patient. Chest radiograph shows moderately enlarged heart with signs of left ventricular dilatation. The ascending aorta is dilated forming a round contour of the right upper mediastinal border.

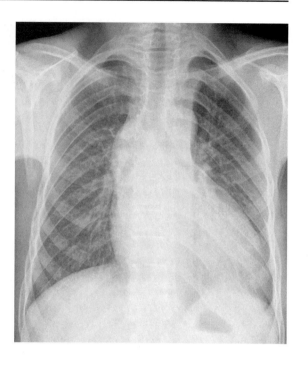

Case 28.6

Aortic regurgitation and mitral regurgitation in an 18-year-old patient with Marfan syndrome and severe skeletal deformity. The sternum shows severe bowing backward (*arrows*), leaving a small space for the heart as shown on magnetic resonance images. The heart is displaced into the left thorax. There is moderate cardiomegaly with dilatation of the left atrium (LA) and left ventricle (LV) due to aortic and mitral regurgitation. The aortic valve (AV) sinuses are markedly dilated. The right atrium (RA) and right ventricle (RV) are compressed. RVO, right ventricular outflow tract.

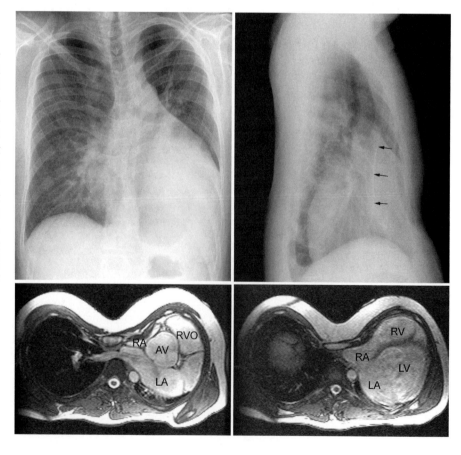

Case 28.7

Aortic regurgitation in Loeys-Dietz syndrome in a 16-month-old child. Frontal chest radiograph shows markedly dilated ascending aorta in the right upper mediastinum, prominent aortic knob, and tortuous descending aortic silhouette. There is cardiomegaly with left ventricular dilatation. Contrast-enhanced MR angiograms show characteristic features of Loeys-Dietz syndrome, including tortuosity and dilatation of the entire aorta , tortuous courses of the dilated aortic arch branches, and dilatation of the celiac axis (CA) and superior mesenteric artery (SMA). The vertebral arteries (VA) show a characteristic corkscrew appearance (right middle panel). A diastolic frame of the cine imaging in long-axis oblique view (right lower panel) shows a stream of aortic regurgitation (*arrows*) and a markedly dilated aortic root (Ao). There also was mitral valve regurgitation.

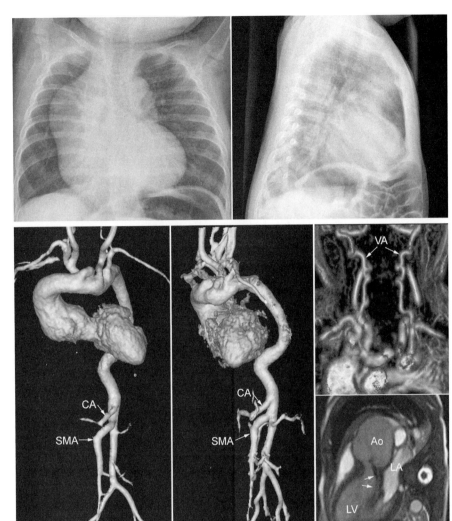

29 Cardiomyopathies and Related Conditions

With Kevin S. Roman

Definition and Classification

□ Traditionally, cardiomyopathies have been divided into primary and secondary forms. As the etiology of previously idiopathic disorders has been discovered, the distinction between primary and secondary forms has become increasingly tenuous. It has been proposed to define cardiomyopathy as a myocardial disorder in which the heart muscle is structurally and functionally abnormal, in the absence of known coronary artery disease, hypertension, valvular disease, and congenital heart disease sufficient to cause the observed myocardial abnormality.[1]

□ Classification (**Fig. 29.1**)[1]:
- Hypertrophic (HCM): presence of increased ventricular wall thickness or mass in the absence of loading conditions (hypertension, valve disease) sufficient to cause the observed abnormality
- Dilated (DCM): presence of left ventricular dilatation and left ventricular systolic dysfunction in the absence of abnormal loading conditions (hypertension, valve disease) or coronary artery disease sufficient to cause global systolic impairment
- Restrictive (RCM): restrictive ventricular physiology in the presence of normal or reduced diastolic volumes (of one or both ventricles), and normal or reduced systolic volumes

- Arrhythmogenic right ventricular cardiomyopathy (ARVC): presence of right ventricular dysfunction (global or regional), with or without left ventricular disease, in the presence of histologic evidence for the disease or electrocardiographic abnormalities in accordance with published criteria
- Unclassified:
  - Left ventricular noncompaction: presence of prominent left ventricular trabeculae and deep intertrabecular recesses
  - Takotsubo cardiomyopathy: presence of transient regional systolic dysfunction involving the left ventricular apex or midventricle in the absence of obstructive coronary disease on coronary angiography

□ Each class is then subclassified into familial and nonfamilial forms.

□ **Table 29.1**

Pathophysiology

□ Hypertrophic cardiomyopathy
- Rare form of cardiomyopathy in children
- May be obstructive or nonobstructive depending on the pattern of myocardial hypertrophy
- Myocardial hypertrophy develops in the absence of a hemodynamic afterload stress.
- Hypertrophy causes decreased ventricular compliance and elevates end-diastolic pressure, resulting in diastolic dysfunction.
- Ejection fraction and the rate of ejection are increased.

□ Dilated cardiomyopathy
- Both end-systolic and end-diastolic volumes are increased, with decreased stroke volume and ejection fraction.
- Mild to moderate atrioventricular valve regurgitation associated with ventricular dilation
- Myocarditis refers to inflammation of the myocardium and may be due to either infectious organisms, most commonly viral, or noninfectious inflammatory conditions, such as systemic lupus erythematous, polyarteritis nodosa, and Kawasaki disease.

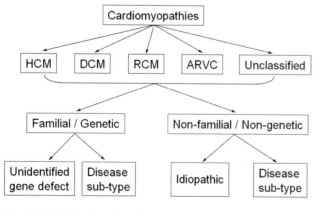

Fig. 29.1 Classification of cardiomyopathies.

Table 29.1 Examples of Different Diseases that Cause Cardiomyopathies

	Familial	Nonfamilial
HCM	Familial, unknown genetics	Obesity
	Sarcomeric protein mutations	Infants of diabetic mothers
	Glycogen storage diseases	Athletic training
	Lysosomal storage diseases	Amyloid (AL/prealbumin)
	Disorders of fatty acid metabolism	
	Carnitine deficiency	
	Phosphorylase B kinase deficiency	
	Mitochondrial cytopathies	
	Syndromic HCM	
	- Noonan's syndrome	
	- LEOPARD syndrome	
	- Friedreich's ataxia	
	- Beckwith-Wiedemann syndrome	
	- Swyer syndrome	
	Others	
	- Phospholamban promoter	
	- Familial amyloid	
DCM	Familial, unknown gene	Myocarditis: infective, toxic, immune
	Sarcomeric protein mutations	Kawasaki disease
	Z-band mutations	Eosinophilic (Churg-Strauss syndrome)
	Cytoskeletal gene mutations	Viral persistence
	Nuclear membrane mutations	Drugs
	Mildly dilated cardiomyopathy	Pregnancy
	Intercalated disc protein mutations	Endocrine
	Mitochondrial cytopathy	Nutritional: thiamine, carnitine, selenium, hypophosphatemia, hypocalcemia
		Alcohol
		Tachycardiomyopathy
RCM	Familial, unknown gene	Amyloid (AL/prealbumin)
	Sarcomeric protein mutations	Scleroderma
	Familial amyloidosis	Endomyocardial fibrosis
	Desminopathy	- Hypereosinophilic syndrome
	Pseudoxanthoma elasticum	- Idiopathic
	Hemochromatosis	- Chromosomal cause
	Anderson-Fabry disease	- Drugs (serotonin, etc.)
	Glycogen storage diseases	Carcinoid heart disease
		Metastatic cancers
		Radiation
		Drugs (anthracycline)
ARVC	Familial, unknown gene	Inflammation?
	Intercalated disk protein mutations	
	Cardiac ryanodine receptor mutations	
	Transforming growth factor-β3 (TGF-β3) mutations	
Unclassified	Left ventricular noncompaction	Takotsubo cardiomyopathy
	Barth syndrome	

Source: Data from Elliott P, Anderson B, Arbustini E, et al. Classification of the cardiomyopathies: a position statement from the European Society of Cardiology Working Group on myocardial and pericardial diseases. Eur Heart J 2008;29:270–276.

- Restrictive cardiomyopathy
  - Poor ventricular compliance with reduced diastolic filling
  - End-diastolic volume is usually normal or slightly reduced, and the ejection fraction is less than normal.
  - Loeffler's disease is due to an immunologic reaction to the eosinophil, resulting in infiltration of the myocardium, thrombi in the ventricular cavities, and characteristic scarring of the posterior mitral valve leaflet.
- Arrhythmogenic right ventricular cardiomyopathy
  - Desmosomal mutations causing detachment of myocytes and untimate; replacement of right ventricular myocardium with fibrous or adipose tissue causing arrhythmia of right ventricular origin
  - Right ventricular global or regional dysfunction

Clinical Manifestations

- Hypertrophic cardiomyopathy
  - Variable presentation with no correlation in the severity of symptoms between obstructive or nonobstructive types
  - Infants present with congestive heart failure, and disease may be fatal within the first year.
  - Older children are often less symptomatic and may be detected due to a cardiac murmur.
  - Infants of diabetic mothers show hypertrophy of the myocardium, which may be mild or moderate and usually resolves during the first 6 months.
- Dilated cardiomyopathy
  - Variable presentation with congestive heart failure
  - Newborns typically have a severe clinical course and may have a rapidly fatal illness, whereas older children usually have a less severe clinical course.
  - Often asymptomatic after initial phase of viral infection prior to cardiac manifestations
  - Preceding illness may be a mild respiratory or gastrointestinal infection.
  - Myocarditis may lead to ventricular dysrhythmias, atrioventricular block, and conduction abnormalities.
  - Mural thrombus may form in the dilated ventricle with associated risk of embolization.
- Restrictive cardiomyopathy
  - Restrictive cardiomyopathy presents with both left- and right-sided congestive heart failure.
- Left ventricular noncompaction
  - May cause left ventricular dysfunction and thrombus formation with cerebral stroke

Chest Radiographic Findings

- Findings depend on duration of disease and severity of hemodynamic disturbance as well as associated abnormalities
- No findings distinguish an etiologic cause of the cardiomyopathy.
- Overall size of the heart correlates well with the type of cardiomyopathy and degree of hemodynamic abnormality.
- Hypertrophic cardiomyopathy
  - Mild cardiomegaly due to ventricular hypertrophy and left atrial dilatation rarely severe
  - Mild pulmonary venous hypertension rarely progressing to pulmonary edema
- Dilated cardiomyopathy
  - Progressive enlargement of left ventricle, which is usually moderate to severe
  - Degree of left atrial enlargement and pulmonary venous hypertension correlates well with the degree of left ventricular failure.
  - Left atrial enlargement usually mild to moderate, with severe enlargement occurring when the papillary muscles become inadequate to maintain competence of the mitral valve.
  - Pulmonary venous hypertension progresses to interstitial and intraalveolar pulmonary edema.
  - Small pericardial effusions and small pleural effusions
  - Passive pulmonary hypertension may result, with mild right heart enlargement.
  - Heart size may be normal, with infants presenting with acute circulatory collapse or an older child with a dysrhythmia.
  - In young infants with clinical signs and radiographic features of dilated cardiomyopathy, anomalous origin of the left coronary artery from the pulmonary artery should be included in the differential diagnosis.
- Restrictive cardiomyopathy
  - Mild to moderate cardiomegaly due to dilatation of the atria, ventricular hypertrophy, and pericardial effusion
  - Moderate to severe pulmonary venous hypertension, which may progress to interstitial and intraalveolar pulmonary edema
  - Small to moderate pleural effusions

- Hypertrophic cardiomyopathy often appears normal.
- In dilated cardiomyopathy, left ventricular and atrial dilatation is associated with signs of pulmonary venous hypertension. In contrast to mitral valvular heart disease, the left ventricle may be disproportionately dilate.

- Dilated cardiomyopathy entails disproportionate enlargement of the heart without associated dilatation of the main pulmonary artery.
- Restrictive cardiomyopathy entails severe pulmonary venous hypertension and pulmonary edema with both right and left atrial enlargement.

Case 29.1

Hypertrophic cardiomyopathy in a 5-year-old patient. Chest radiograph shows mild cardiomegaly with a rounded configuration due to left ventricular hypertrophy and mild pulmonary venous hypertension.

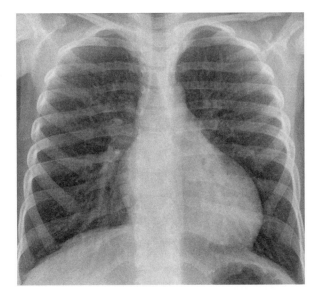

Case 29.2

Hypertrophic cardiomyopathy in a 7-month-old infant with Pompe's glycogen storage disease. Chest radiograph shows moderate cardiomegaly with a prominent left ventricular border due to left ventricular hypertrophy. Both lungs show findings of pulmonary venous hypertension.

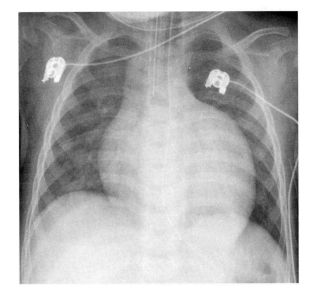

Case 29.3

Dilated cardiomyopathy of unknown etiology in a 2-year-old child. Chest radiographs show severe cardiomegaly with both left ventricular and left atrial enlargement and pulmonary venous hypertension. Left lower lung opacification is due to compressive atelectasis.

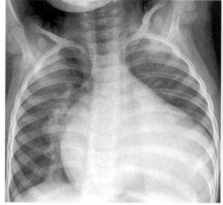
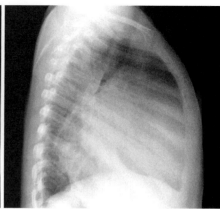

Case 29.4

Dilated cardiomyopathy in a 3-year-old child with mitochondrial encephalomyopathy, lactic acidosis, and stroke-like episodes (MELAS syndrome). Chest radiographs show moderate cardiomegaly with predominant left-side chamber enlargement and moderate right-side chamber enlargement. Both lungs show findings of pulmonary venous hypertension.

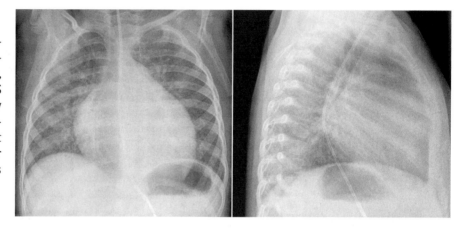

Case 29.5

Cardiomyopathy in a 4-month-old infant with an anomalous origin of the left coronary artery from the pulmonary artery. Chest radiographs show severe cardiomegaly with left ventricular and atrial enlargement associated with severe pulmonary venous hypertension, not distinguishable from the findings of dilated cardiomyopathy. This rare disease entity should be included in the differential diagnoses when a neonate shows features of severe left-sided heart failure. The left lower lobe is collapsed.

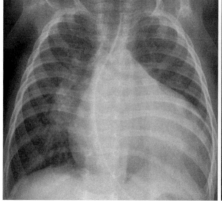
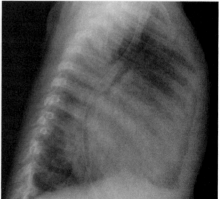

Case 29.6

Restrictive cardiomyopathy in a 5-year-old child. Chest radiograph shows mild cardiomegaly with dilatation of the atria associated with pulmonary venous hypertension and interstitial edema. Computed tomography (CT) image shows severe disproportionate dilatation of the right atrium (RA) and left atrium (LA) with a typical spade-configuration, findings of pulmonary venous hypertension and pleural effusions. The ventricles are neither dilated nor hypertrophied. LV, left ventricle; RV, right ventricle.

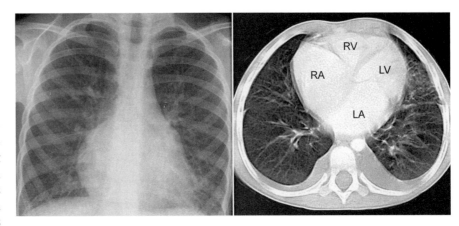

Case 29.7

Restrictive physiology in a 13-year-old patient with hypertrophic cardiomyopathy involving both ventricles. Chest radiograph shows moderate enlargement of the heart with disproportionate dilatation of the right atrium (RA) also shown in a magnetic resonance (MR) image and findings of pulmonary venous hypertension. Note severe myocardial hypertrophy of the left ventricle (LV) and lesser degree of hypertrophy involving the right ventricle (RV). The inferior vena cava (IVC) is dilated. LA, left atrium.

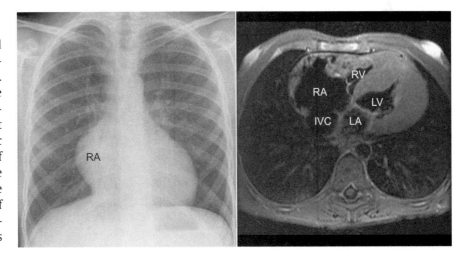

30 Kawasaki Disease

With Kevin S. Roman

Definition and Classification

- Also known as mucocutaneous lymph node syndrome
- Acute febrile illness associated with a generalized vasculitis in infants and young children
- Leading cause of acquired heart disease in children in developed world
- Disease course divided into three phases:
  - Acute stage: 1 to 2 weeks
    - Acute febrile period
    - Pancarditis with pericarditis, myocarditis, valvulitis, and coronary vasculitis
  - Subacute stage: 2 to 4 weeks
    - Begins with elevation of platelet count and ends with a return to nearly normal
    - Coronary artery aneurysms reach peak
  - Convalescent or chronic phase: months to possibly years
    - Abnormalities of coronary arteries most apparent
    - Expansion of giant aneurysms, smaller aneurysms tend to resolve, possible myocardial infarction

Pathophysiology

- Etiology unknown with an immunologic response likely triggered by an infectious agent based on clinical and epidemiologic features
- Epidemics in late winter and spring
- Genetic predisposition based on varying incidences among ethnic groups
- Vasculitis most severe in medium-sized and most importantly the coronary arteries
- Coronary artery aneurysms develop in 25% of untreated patients
- Immune system is highly activated with extensive production of cytokines.
- Generalized microvasculitis with inflammation in intima and adventitia, and smooth muscle necrosis in media
- Elastin and collagen fibers fragmented producing focal destructive lesions, leading to aneurysms
- Fibrosis and myointimal proliferation over time, leading to stenosis
- Stenosis most common in coronary arteries with giant aneurysms
- Luminal occlusion may occur by thrombosis or severe stenosis
- One half of coronary artery aneurysms resolve within 1 to 2 years, particularly the small and fusiform ones.

Clinical Manifestations

- No specific diagnostic assay
- Clinical features may not be present simultaneously.
- Hallmark clinical criteria are prolonged fever, generalized erythematous rash, conjunctival injection, cervical lymphadenitis, mucositis, and peripheral extremity changes.
- Peak frequency between 6 months and 5 years
- Goal of treatment: prevent coronary artery disease. Coronary artery aneurysms develop in less than 5 to 10% if treated with intravenous gamma globulin before the 10th day of illness.
- Carditis present to some degree in all cases; pericardium, myocardium, and endocardium can all be affected.
- Cardiovascular complications: once fever resolves, include myocardial dysfunction, rarely congestive heart failure, diffuse coronary artery ectasia and aneurysm formation, giant aneurysms, myocardial infarction, and rupture of coronary artery aneurysm with hemopericardium.
- Death usually from myocardial infarction secondary to thrombosis or rupture of large coronary aneurysm

Chest Radiographic Findings

- Acute stage important for baseline findings:
  - Main finding: pulmonary involvement due to pulmonary arteritis with increased vascular permeability and perivascular edematous changes, subclinical pneumonitis, and lower respiratory tract inflammation
  - Generalized interstitial lung changes with a diffuse reticulogranular pattern and peribronchial cuffing
  - Lung consolidation, atelectasis, and air trapping uncommon
- Pulmonary edema from congestive heart failure uncommon

- Heart size normal unless myocarditis causes cardiac enlargement or pericardial effusion present

- Rarely contour abnormalities by aneurysms
- Occasionally coronary aneurysms calcify as a late finding

Pearls

- Chest radiographs most often normal; about 15% will be abnormal
- Acute phase: pulmonary involvement with interstitial disease most common

- Chronic phase: coronary artery aneurysm calcifications are very characteristic

Case 30.1

Kawasaki disease in acute phase. Chest radiograph in a 4-month-old with an acute presentation of respiratory distress shows moderate cardiomegaly, which may be due to myocarditis with cardiac enlargement as well as a pericardial effusion. Lungs show generalized interstitial thickening, which would correlate with pulmonary edema secondary to congestive heart failure as well as lower respiratory tract inflammation and pneumonitis. A more localized focus of consolidation and atelectasis is seen within the left lower lobe associated with a left pleural effusion.

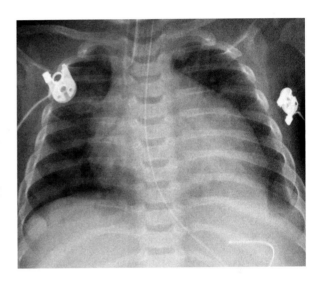

Case 30.2

Calcified aneurysm of the left coronary artery in a 13-year-old patient with a history of Kawasaki disease in early childhood. Chest radiographs show characteristic oval shell calcification (*arrows*) in the aneurysm of the left coronary artery. Heart size is normal and lungs are clear. Contrast-enhanced magnetic resonance (MR) angiogram shows aneurysms of both right and left coronary arteries (RCA and LCA, respectively). L, N, and R, left, non-, and right coronary sinuses; RVOT, right ventricular outflow tract.

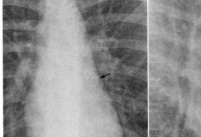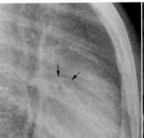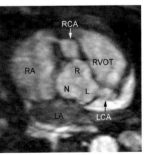

Case 30.3

Huge coronary artery aneurysm in a 1-year-old patient with Kawasaki disease. Chest radiograph shows moderate cardiomegaly and a focal contour bulge along the left upper heart border due to a giant coronary artery aneurysm.

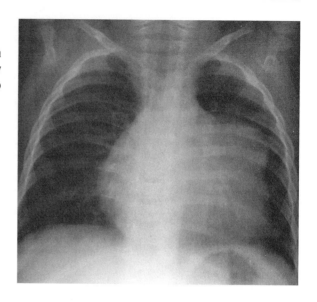

Case 30.4

Myocardial infarction as a late consequence of Kawasaki disease in early childhood in a 16-year-old patient. Chest radiograph shows moderate cardiomegaly with prominent elongated left ventricular margin and pulmonary edema and layered pleural effusion in the left thorax. Late gadolinium-enhancement images at MR show transmural infarct in the circumflex and right coronary arterial territories (arrows). LV, left ventricle; RV, right ventricle.

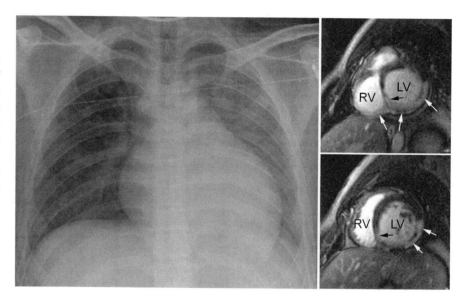

31 Pericardial Diseases

With Christian J. Kellenberger

□ Pericardial diseases include the following:
- Congenital pericardial defects
- Pericarditis and pericardial effusion
- Pneumopericardium
- Pericardial mass

■ Congenital Pericardial Defects

Classification

□ Total or partial defects
□ Left-sided defects more common when partial
□ Small percent associated with intracardiac anomalies

Clinical Manifestations

□ Complete defects almost always asymptomatic
□ Partial defects may present with intermittent chest pain, and rarely herniation of the left atrial appendage may become incarcerated, which is life threatening.

Chest Radiographic Findings

□ In complete absence of the pericardium, the heart is rotated leftward and is displaced away from the sternum and diaphragm.
□ Prominence of main pulmonary artery
□ Lung wedges between aorta and pulmonary artery
□ Lung interposed between heart and hemidiaphragm
□ Normal position of trachea and descending aorta
□ Partial defects: focal prominence of left atrial appendage along the left upper heart border

■ Pericardial Effusions and Pericarditis

Pathophysiology

□ Most common causes of pericardial effusions are infectious and iatrogenic.
□ Less common causes of pericardial effusions are neoplastic and connective tissue disorders.

□ Infectious pericarditis most commonly viral, less commonly bacterial, tuberculous, or fungal
□ Large pericardial effusion caused by bacterial pericarditis, malignancy, immune disorders, and sometimes never determined
□ Constrictive pericarditis with adherent, thickened, fibrotic pericardium restricting diastolic filling of all chambers
□ Pericardial effusion may complicate postoperative course with an unexplained enlargement of the cardiac silhouette size in a short interval.
□ Postpericardotomy syndrome is postulated to be an autoimmune response, perhaps triggered by a viral infection, 1 to 6 weeks following surgery in which the pericardial cavity has been entered with development of pericardial effusions.

Clinical Manifestations

□ Nonspecific fever and chest pain
□ Reduced cardiac output due to limited venous return to heart
□ Reduced ventricular filling causing fatigue, hypotension, tachycardia
□ Tamponade may occur when there is rapid development of effusion with severe compression of the heart.
□ Chest pain may be due to underperfused coronary arteries or compression of an epicardial coronary artery
□ Constrictive pericarditis presents similar to restrictive cardiomyopathy with elevated systemic venous pressures, resulting in ascites and hepatomegaly and pulmonary venous congestion with pulmonary edema
□ Postpericardotomy syndrome typically presents 2 to 4 weeks following surgery.

Chest Radiographic Findings

□ Insensitive unless effusion is large or rapidly expanding
□ Rapidly appearing cardiomegaly with a globular configuration and normal pulmonary vascularity
□ Fat pad sign on the lateral image due to separation of epicardial fat from retrosternal fat is unreliable.
□ Rarely pericardial calcification
□ Calcified pericardium not necessarily constricted
□ Pleural effusions

■ Pneumopericardium

- Most commonly due to air tracking from the pulmonary interstitium into the mediastinum
- A large amount can cause tamponade.

Chest Radiographic Findings

- Lucent halo of air encircling the heart extending between heart and diaphragm inferiorly and origin of great vessels superiorly
- Parietal and fibrous pericardium seen as a thin white strip between lung and pericardial air
- Distinguish from pneumomediastinum with air not extending above the great vessels

■ Pericardial Masses

- Pericardial cysts
- Pericardial teratoma most common tumor with mixed cystic and solid components

- Pericardial hemangioma
- Pericardial benign and malignant mesenchymal tumors and lymphoma are rare.

Clinical Manifestations

- Varies from an incidental finding to severe cardiorespiratory distress

Chest Radiographic Findings

- Pericardial cysts: well-defined mass most commonly at the right cardiophrenic angle
- Pericardial teratoma: massive enlargement of the cardiomediastinal silhouette due to a large pericardial effusion as well as a tumor mass
- Pericardial hemangioma: focal contour bulge most commonly along right heart border

Case 31.1

Partial eventration of pericardium in a 2-year-old child. Chest radiograph shows a focal contour bulge *(arrows)* along the left upper cardiac border due to protrusion of the left atrial appendage. Chest radiographic differential diagnosis includes partial pericardial defect, cardiac tumor, and left juxtaposition of the atrial appendages. T1-weighted magnetic resonance image shows marked dilatation of the left atrial appendage. There is a sharp indentation *(arrow)* at the junction of the left atrium and appendage (LAA). At operation, the pericardium overlying this region was not deficient but markedly thinned. Ao, ascending aorta; LA, left atrium; PA, pulmonary artery; RA, right atrium; RAA, right atrial appendage.

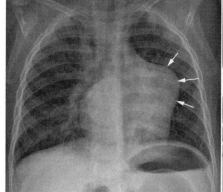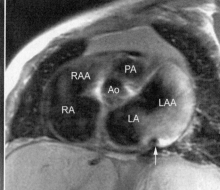

Case 31.2

Pericarditis in an 11-week-old infant. Chest radiographs show marked enlargement of cardiac silhouette, obscuring visualization of the lungs. Such a large pericardial effusion is more commonly seen with bacterial infections. Contrast-enhanced computed tomography (CT) images show the homogeneous low-density fluid surrounding the heart.

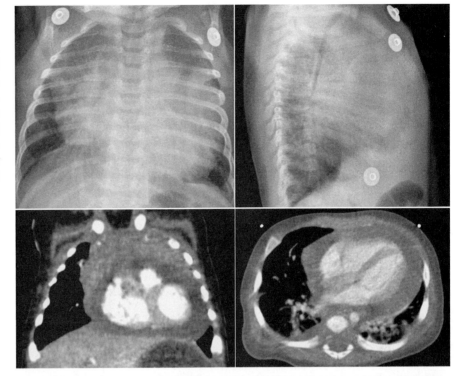

Case 31.3

Pericarditis in a 15-year-old patient. Chest radiographs show an enlarged cardiac silhouette with an unusually smooth margin, giving an appearance of a leather water bottle. The pulmonary vascularity is normal. Contrast-enhanced CT image obtained after pericardiocentesis shows complex fluid with pericardial thickening.

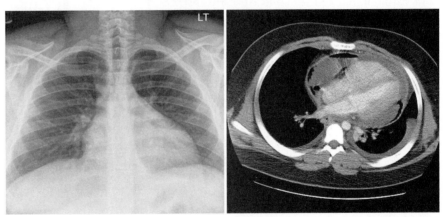

Case 31.4

Tuberculous pericarditis in an 18-year-old patient. Chest radiograph at 17 years of age showed superior mediastinal widening with a multilobulated contour. The patient was diagnosed as having pulmonary tuberculosis with mediastinal lymphadenopathy. The patient developed pericarditis despite antituberculosis medication. Chest radiograph at 18 years of age shows significant interval enlargement of the cardiac silhouette due to pericardial effusion and pleural effusion in the right thorax. The superior mediastinum is still wide. The pulmonary vascularity is normal.

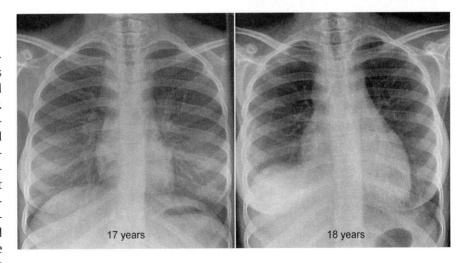

Case 31.5

Pneumopericardium in a newborn under ventilation. Chest radiographs show air encircling the heart, which does not extend above the origins of the great vessels. Both lungs show branching lucencies of interstitial emphysema through hazy parenchyma.

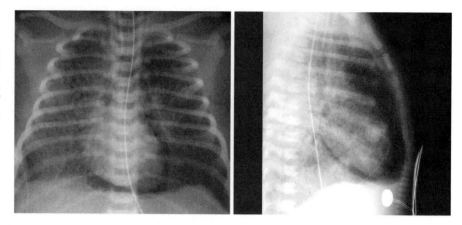

Case 31.6

Pericardial cyst in a 14-year-old patient. Chest radiographs show a well-defined mass (arrows) at the right cardiophrenic angle. Contrast-enhanced CT shows a cystic mass.

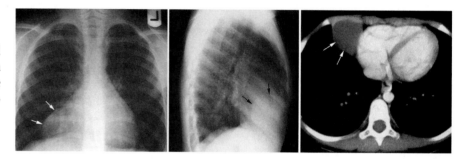

32 Cardiac Tumors

With Christian J. Kellenberger

General Consideration

□ Cardiac tumors are rare in the pediatric population.
□ The majority of cardiac tumors are benign.
□ Categorized by location:
   • Intracavitary
   • Intramural
   • Epicardial
   • Pericardial
   • Paracardiac
□ Categorized by histologic features and cellular differentiation:
   • Benign tumors
      – Muscle: rhabdomyomas
      – Fibrous tissue: fibromas
      – Fat: lipomas
      – Vascular tissue: hemangiomas
      – Other: myxomas
      – Nervous tissue: paragangliomas
      – Ectopic: teratomas
   • Malignant tumors
      – Mesenchymal: sarcomas
      – Lymphoid: lymphomas
      – Mesothelial: mesotheliomas

Pathophysiology

□ Rhabdomyomas
   • Most common pediatric cardiac tumor
   • Commonly associated with tuberous sclerosis complex, an autosomal dominant disorder with widespread tumors, called hamartomas, primarily affecting brain, heart, skin, kidneys
   • Most undergo partial or complete spontaneous regression
   • Usually multiple small discrete nodules; rarely a single lesion or rhabdomyomatosis with diffuse myocardial thickening
   • Cystic degeneration and calcification extremely uncommon
   • Conduction system involvement leads to various dysrhythmias.
   • Hemodynamic obstruction uncommon
□ Fibromas
   • Second most common pediatric cardiac tumor
   • Can be associated with Gorlin basal cell nevus syndrome

   • Spontaneous regression not often seen
   • Usually a large solitary mass
   • Intramural lesion most common locations interventricular septum and left ventricular free wall
   • Cystic degeneration and calcification may be present
   • Associated pericardial effusion not often present
   • Conduction system involvement leads to various dysrhythmias.
   • Hemodynamic compromise due to obstruction to inflow or outflow tracts
   • Coronary arteries may be compressed or incorporated into mass.
□ Lipomas
   • Large solitary infiltrating and insinuating mass
   • Epicardial lesion on the surface of an atrium or ventricle
   • Coronary arteries may be displaced, compressed, or incorporated into mass.
□ Hemangiomas
   • Association Kasabach-Merritt syndrome with multiple systemic hemangiomas
   • According to size of vascular channels, divided into capillary, cavernous, or venous types
   • Intracavitary, intramural, epicardial, or pericardial lesion, which can occur in any chamber
   • Calcifications often present
□ Myxomas
   • Rare in pediatric age
   • Associated with Carney complex, an autosomal dominant inherited disorder with multiple myxomas and other neoplasms, endocrine hyperfunction, and multiple lentigines
   • Solitary friable mass often pedunculated of variable size associated with surface thrombi and tendency to embolize
   • Intracavitary lesion: most common location left atrium attached to atrial septum
   • Classic triad of valvular obstruction, emboli, and constitutional symptoms
   • Small cysts may develop, and calcifications are more common in right atrial tumors.
   • Hemodynamic compromise due to mitral or tricuspid valvar obstruction
   • Fragmentation of the tumor may lead to systemic or pulmonary embolic event.

- Teratoma
  - Most present within the first year of life
  - Large mixed germ cell tumor mass with satellite nodules
  - Pericardial and rarely intramural lesion usually right-sided and typically connects to one of the great vessels through a pedicle
  - Multicystic, solid and fatty tissue, and calcifications
  - Hemodynamic compromise due to cardiac and great vessel compression as well as associated large pericardial effusions, which may cause tamponade
- Malignant tumors extremely rare with a poor prognosis; usually present with infiltrative disease and metastases
  - Sarcomas
    - Angiosarcoma most frequent usually within the right atrium arising from interatrial septum; spreads along epicardial surface, replacing right atrial wall
    - Large multilobular broad-base mass occupying most of affected cardiac chambers with pericardial and extracardiac invasion
    - Hemodynamic compromise with right-sided inflow obstruction or cardiac tamponade
    - Other types include rhabdomyosarcoma, fibrosarcoma, leiomyosarcoma, myxosarcoma, malignant fibrous histiocytoma, undifferentiated sarcoma, and liposarcoma
  - Primary cardiac lymphoma
    –Rare; typically non-Hodgkin type
    - Intracavitary, intramural, and pericardial originating from the heart or pericardium, involving more than one cardiac chamber in most cases
    - Contiguous invasion of surrounding myocardium, epicardium, pericardium, coronary arteries, and neighboring paracardiac structures
  - Metastases
    - Rare and may be secondary to hematogenous spread or from direct extension from abdominal masses through the inferior vena cava
    - Primary malignancies include leukemia or lymphoma, neuroblastoma, hepatoblastoma, Wilms' tumor, various sarcomas

Clinical Manifestations

- Majority of cardiac tumors are benign and do not metastasize or invade locally.

- Significant morbidity and mortality largely determined by the location and histology of the lesion.
- Often asymptomatic
- Intracavitary and intramural masses may cause either inflow or outflow tract obstruction, and presentation may be congestive heart failure, syncope, or superior vena cava syndrome.
- Intracavitary masses may cause hemolysis by mechanical damage to red cells.
- Intracavitary masses may damage valves, resulting in regurgitation.
- Intracavitary masses, which are friable, may lead to systemic or pulmonary embolism.
- Intramural masses can interfere with conduction pathways and produce dysrhythmias, which may present as palpitations, heart block, tachyarrhythmias, or sudden death.
- Intramural masses with extensive involvement of the myocardium may lead to myocardial dysfunction and congestive heart failure.
- Epicardial masses may obstruct coronary blood flow and present with chest pain.
- Pericardial masses are often asymptomatic until they compress cardiac chambers or produce large effusions, causing tamponade.

Chest Radiographic Findings

- Variable depending on the location and size of the tumor
- Small and intracavitary lesions frequently normal
- Extensive involvement of myocardium cardiomegaly with an abnormal cardiac contour
- Focal contour bulge with exophytic tumor masses
- Massively enlarged cardiomediastinal silhouette with epicardial and pericardial masses associated with pericardial effusions
- Specific chamber enlargement with obstructive masses and tumors causing valvar regurgitation
- Cardiac dilatation from ventricular failure
- Pulmonary venous hypertension when there is congestive heart failure due to obstruction or myocardial failure
- Rarely calcifications may be seen in tumor mass.

Pearls

- Small tumors do not show any radiographic changes.
- Fibromas most commonly cause a cardiac contour abnormality.

- Pericardial tumors almost always have significant pericardial effusions.

Case 32.1

Cardiac fibroma showing a cardiac contour change that would be unusual for chamber enlargement. Chest radiographs show enlarged cardiac silhouette with squared bulge of the left ventricular shoulder region. T1-weighted magnetic resonance (MR) images show a large mass with a homogeneous medium signal-intensity involving the left ventricular free wall.

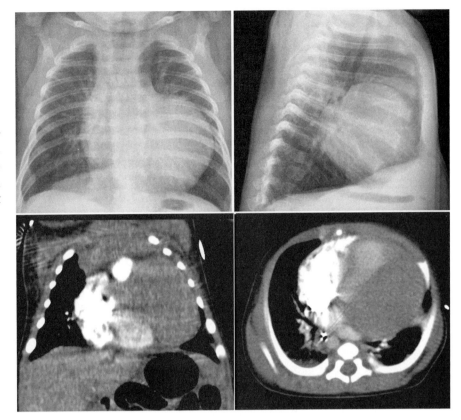

Case 32.2

Cardiac hemangioma in a 8-week-old neonate. Chest radiograph shows a large bulge of the right atrial border mimicking an enlarged right atrium (RA). MR images show that the bulge is due to a large mass. The mass was considered to arise from either the right atrial wall or the pericardial cavity. T1-weighted axial image and fat-saturated T1-weighted contrast-enhanced image reveal a mass with heterogeneous signal intensity showing dense contrast enhancement of the peripheral part. Biopsy of the tumor showed hemangioma with hemangioendothelioma component. The mass histology was more consistent with the mass arising from the right atrial wall. LA, left atrium; LV, left ventricle; RV, right ventricle.

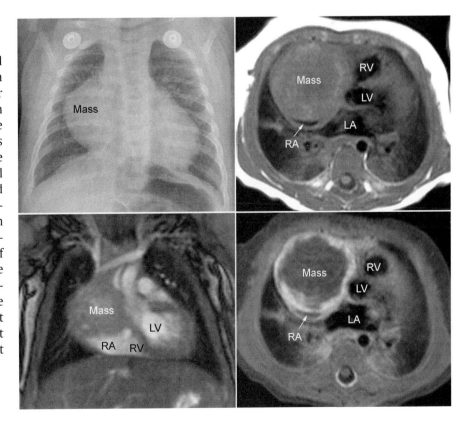

Case 32.3

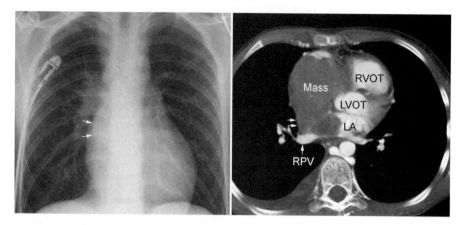

Primary cardiac lymphoma in a 15-year-old patient. Chest radiograph shows mild prominence of the right atrial contour and superior vena cava due to an intracavitary tumor mass as shown in the contrast-enhanced computed tomography (CT) image. The tumor mass forms a double contour (arrows) inside the right atrial border. The mass obliterates the right atrial cavity and protrudes into the left atrium. The orifice of a right pulmonary vein (RPV) is encroached on. LA, left atrium; LVOT and RVOT, right and left ventricular outflow tracts.

33 Pulmonary Thromboembolism

With Anne Geoffray

Pathophysiology

- Presence of an intraluminal clot within a pulmonary artery branch
- Pulmonary embolism is much rarer in children than in adults; the incidence is reported to be under 3% on autopsy series.
- Most often associated with indwelling intravenous catheter in children; less commonly with deep vein thrombosis.
- Predisposing factors to hypercoaguable state are nearly always present.
  - Central venous catheters
  - Recent vascular intervention
  - Recent surgery
  - Hyperalimentation, dehydration, septicemia, burns, asphyxia, trauma
  - Heart disease: intracardiac shunts, dilated cardiomyopathy
  - Renal diseases
  - Neoplasm: solid tumors, leukemias, lymphomas
  - Connective tissue diseases
  - Sickle cell disease
  - Disorders of coagulation: antithrombin III, protein C or protein S deficiency, antiphospholipid antibodies, coagulation-regulatory protein abnormalities
- Chronic pulmonary thromboembolism can lead to pulmonary arterial hypertension.

Clinical Manifestation

- Nonspecific or pleuritic chest pain, dyspnea, tachypnea, cough, rarely hemoptysis, cyanosis
- Symptoms often masked by intrinsic lung disease
- Often asymptomatic
- Pleural friction rub, tachycardia, accentuated pulmonic component of the second heart sound
- Plasma level of D-dimer, a fibrin degradation product (FDP), is elevated but can be normal.

Chest Radiographic Findings

- Most often normal when thromboembolism is not associated with pulmonary infarction
- Subtle perfusion abnormalities with generalized or localized oligemia: Westermark's sign
- Abrupt tapering of dilated pulmonary arterial branch: Palla's sign
- Nonspecific pulmonary consolidations often homogeneous and peripheral, abutting pleural surface in association with small effusions when thromboembolism is associated with pulmonary infarction: Hampton's hump
- Parenchymal opacity due to hemorrhagic edema may resolve rapidly.
- Pleural effusion is often bilateral.
- Elevation of ipsilateral diaphragm
- Radiographic Westermark sign and Hampton's hump are not sensitive but highly specific for diagnosis of pulmonary embolus.

Pearls

- Challenging diagnosis with no reliable symptoms; usually diagnosed when there is a high level of suspicious risk factors
- Chest radiographs are not sensitive, but certain findings are specific.
- Chest radiographs most often normal, unless thromboembolism is associated with parenchymal infarcts
- Consolidations due to parenchymal infarcts are often subpleural and associated with small effusions.
- Contrast-enhanced computed tomography (CT) is the diagnostic test of choice.

Case 33.1

Pulmonary thromboembolism in a 12-year-old patient with acute shortness of breath. Chest radiograph shows abrupt tapering *(arrow)* of the descending branch of the right pulmonary artery with obvious oligemia in the right lower lung (Westermark's sign). Contrast-enhanced CT image shows a long clot *(arrows)* extending into both branch pulmonary arteries. Large and small clots fill the descending branches of the right and left pulmonary arteries *(asterisks)*.

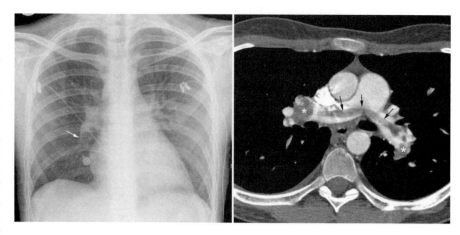

Case 33.2

Pulmonary thromboembolism in a 12-year-child injured in a motor vehicle accident. A large parenchymal subpleural consolidation is seen in the right upper lung associated with small pleural effusion. CT angiogram shows a clot *(asterisk)* in the right pulmonary artery (RPA) at the hilum, consolidation involving the posterior upper lobes, and bilateral pleural effusion.

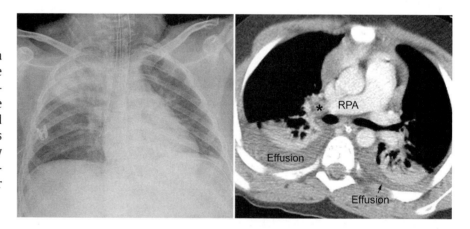

Case 33.3

Pulmonary thromboembolism in a 13-year-old patient with antiphospholipid syndrome and a thrombus in the right iliac vein. Two serial chest radiographs show deterioration with bilateral lower lung peripheral opacities and small effusions in keeping with parenchymal infarcts due to pulmonary emboli. Contrast-enhanced CT image shows emboli in the pulmonary arterial branches and parenchymal consolidation. Ultrasonogram of the right iliac vein shows a large clot *(arrows)*.

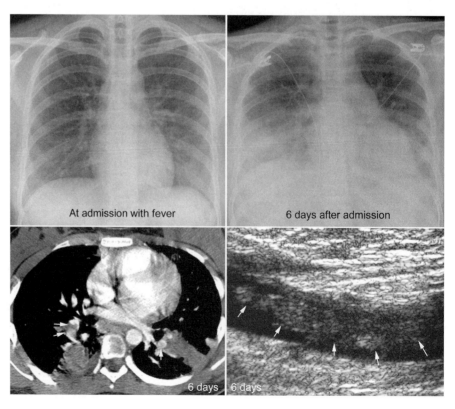

34 Pulmonary Hypertension

With Anne Geoffray

Definition and Classification

- Normal mean pulmonary arterial pressure ranges from 18 to 22 mm Hg. Pulmonary hypertension is defined as a mean pulmonary artery pressure greater than 25 mm Hg at rest and 30 mm Hg during exercise.
- Formerly classified as primary and secondary forms according to the absence or presence of underlying disease. New 2003 classification of the World Health Organization discarded the term *primary* and *secondary* (**Table 34.1**).

- Idiopathic and familial forms of pulmonary arterial hypertension
  - A mean pulmonary artery pressure greater than 25 mm Hg at rest and 30 mm Hg during exercise, with a normal pulmonary artery wedge pressure and the absence of identifiable causes or risk factors
  - One to two new cases per million each year
  - Pathophysiology of both idiopathic and familial pulmonary hypertension is poorly understood.

Table 34.1 World Health Organization Classification of Pulmonary Arterial Hypertension

1. Pulmonary arterial hypertension	1.1. Idiopathic
	1.2. Familial
	1.3. Associated with:
	1.3.1. Connective tissue disease
	1.3.2. Congenital systemic pulmonary shunts
	1.3.3. Portal hypertension
	1.3.4. Human immunodeficiency virus (HIV) infection
	1.3.5. Drugs and toxins
	1.3.6. Others (thyroid disorders, glycogen storage disease, Gaucher's disease, hereditary hemorrhagic telangiectasia, hemoglobinopathies, myeloproliferative disorders, splenectomy)
	1.4. Associated with significant venous or capillary involvement
	1.4.1. Pulmonary veno-occlusive disease
	1.4.2. Pulmonary capillary hemangiomatosis
	1.5. Persistent pulmonary hypertension of the newborn
2. Pulmonary hypertension associated with left-heart diseases	2.1. Left-sided atrial or ventricular heart disease
	2.2. Left-sided valvular heart disease
3. Pulmonary hypertension associated with lung respiratory diseases and/or hypoxemia	3.1. Chronic obstructive pulmonary disease
	3.2. Interstitial lung disease
	3.3. Sleep-disordered breathing
	3.4. Alveolar hypoventilation disorders
	3.5. Chronic exposure to high altitudes
	3.6. Developmental abnormalities
4. Pulmonary hypertension due to chronic thrombotic and/or embolic disease	4.1. Thromboembolic obstruction of proximal pulmonary arteries
	4.2. Thromboembolic obstruction of distal pulmonary arteries
	4.3. Nonthromboembolic pulmonary embolism (tumor, parasites, foreign material)
5. Miscellaneous	Sarcoidosis, histiocytosis X, lymphangiomatosis, compression of pulmonary vessels (adenopathy, tumor, fibrosing mediastinitis)

Source: Data from Simonneau G, Galie N, Rubin LJ, et al. Clinical classification of pulmonary hypertension. J Am Coll Cardiol 2004;43:Suppl:5S–12S.

- A hormonal, mechanical, or unidentified insult to the endothelium with an increased susceptibility to pulmonary vascular injury is considered to result in vascular scarring, endothelial dysfunction, and intimal and medial proliferation. As a result, the effective total cross-sectional area of the pulmonary vascular bed is reduced.
- Present with syncope, dyspnea on exertion, chest pain, and right heart failure
- Prognosis remains very poor, with a 5-year mortality rate of 35%.
- Vasodilator therapy with prostacyclin, sildenafil citrate and nitric oxide may be successful.
□ Pulmonary veno-occlusive disease
  - Pulmonary arterial hypertension secondary to intimal fibrosis and loss of luminal patency of the postcapillary pulmonary veins
  - One to two new cases per ten million each year
  - Very rare, but correct diagnosis is of paramount importance
  - Vasodilator therapy can be harmful and even fatal, whereas anticoagulation therapy can be helpful.
  - High index of suspicion at chest radiographic interpretation can lead to the right diagnosis. Computed tomography (CT) angiography is the diagnostic test of choice.
□ Pulmonary hypertension associated with systemic pulmonary shunts
  - Pulmonary arterial hypertension secondary to increased pulmonary blood flow
  - Normally, the pulmonary vascular bed has the capacity to recruit unused vasculature, accommodating an increase in blood flow. In the case of pulmonary hypertension, this capacity no longer exists, resulting in increased pulmonary pressure.
  - The vessels react with medial hypertrophy, intimal hyperplasia, and fibrosis, leading to occlusive changes and plexiform lesions.
  - Eventual right-to-left shunt causes cyanosis.

□ Persistent pulmonary hypertension of the newborn
  - Normally, the high prenatal pulmonary resistance decreases at birth, due to an increase in systemic vascular resistance after loss of the placenta, lung expansion, and alveolar oxygenation.
  - Persistent pulmonary hypertension of the newborn is the result of persistent elevated pulmonary vascular resistance after birth.
  - Results in right-to-left shunting through the fetal channels, including patent ductus arteriosus and patent foramen ovale
  - Three groups:
    - Associated with pulmonary parenchymal disease, such as hyaline membrane disease, meconium aspiration, or transient tachypnea of the newborn
    - No evidence of pulmonary parenchymal disease: known as persistent fetal circulation (PFC)
    - Associated with hypoplasia of the lungs, such as diaphragmatic hernia

Chest Radiographic Findings

□ Varies depending on the type
□ Pulmonary hypertension after the newborn period is characterized by dilated main and hilar pulmonary arteries, decreased peripheral vascularity, and right ventricular hypertrophy.
□ Pulmonary veno-occlusive disease is associated with diffuse interstitial thickening with interlobular septal lines, reflecting chronic capillary congestion with hemosiderin deposition, recruitment of venous channels, and lymphatic dilatation.
□ Pulmonary hypertension complicating systemic pulmonary shunts is characterized by diminishing heart size and peripheral vascular markings with dilatation of the central vessels.
□ Persistent pulmonary hypertension of the newborn has no specific radiographic findings, with the underlying lung pathology masking any hemodynamic changes.

Pearls

□ Characterize pattern to histologic subtype; critical in guiding treatment with vasodilators and anticoagulants
□ Pulmonary hypertension is characterized by dilatation of the central pulmonary vessels, diminished peripheral vascularity, and right ventricular hypertrophy.
□ Pulmonary hypertension due to veno-occlusive disease is characterized by increased interstitial markings with other findings of pulmonary hypertension.

Case 34.1

Idiopathic pulmonary hypertension in a 15-year-old patient. Frontal chest radiograph shows a markedly dilated main pulmonary arterial segment *(arrow)*, rather small peripheral vessels, and moderate cardiomegaly. Lateral radiograph shows dilated central pulmonary arteries forming a mass *(arrows)* in the hilar region, from which small vessels arise. The retrosternal clear space is obliterated by the hypertrophied right ventricular outflow tract and dilated main pulmonary artery. The lungs are clear. CT angiograms show enlarged central pulmonary arteries with tapered tortuous peripheral branches and no interstitial thickening.

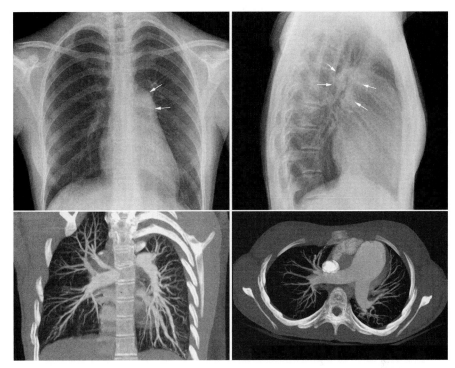

Case 34.2

Pulmonary veno-occlusive disease in a 15-year-old patient. Chest radiograph shows dilatation of the central pulmonary arteries with mild cardiomegaly and a diffuse pattern of interstitial thickening with subpleural septal lines. The diffuse pattern of lung disease due to chronic venous congestion with recruitment of collaterals and lymphatic dilatation is well shown on the CT image.

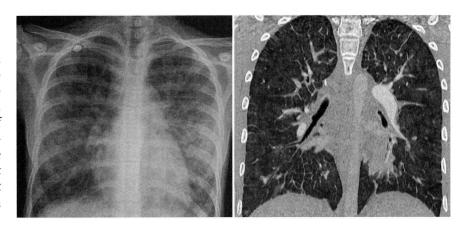

Case 34.3

Pulmonary veno-occlusive disease in a 15-year-old patient before *(left panel)* and after *(right panel)* administration of a vasodilator. There is obvious worsening of pulmonary edema after vasodilator therapy.

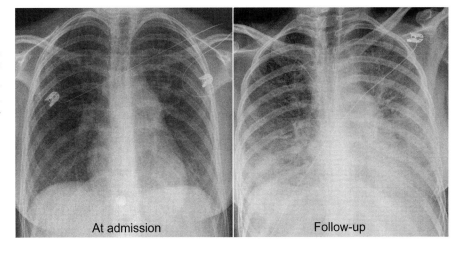

At admission   Follow-up

Case 34.4

Pulmonary hypertension in a 4-year-old child with a large ventricular septal defect. Chest radiographs show markedly dilated central pulmonary arteries. Normal heart size with prominent pulmonary vascularity is highly suggestive of pulmonary hypertension. On the lateral view, the retrocardiac clear space is obliterated by the hypertrophied right ventricular outflow tract and dilated main pulmonary artery. The pulmonary vascular resistance was increased at catheterization and responded to oxygen administration.

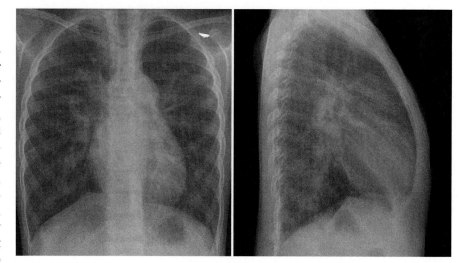

Index

Note: Page numbers followed by *f* and *t* indicate figures and tables, respectively.